Lanchester Library

LANCHESTER LIBRARY

WITHDRAWN

3 8001 00518 4944

ZU8

19

KT-197-856

Contraception and Contraceptive Use

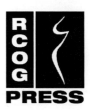

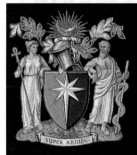

Since 1973 the Royal College of Obstetricians and Gynaecologists has regularly convened Study Groups to address important growth areas within obstetrics and gynaecology. An international group of eminent scientists and clinicians from various disciplines is invited to present the results of recent research and to take part in in-depth discussions. The resulting volume, containing the papers presented and also edited transcripts of the discussions, is published within a few months of the meeting and provides a summary of the subject that is both authoritative and up-to-date.

SOME PREVIOUS STUDY GROUP PUBLICATIONS AVAILABLE

Infertility
Edited by AA Templeton and JO Drife

Intrapartum Fetal Surveillance
Edited by JAD Spencer and RHT Ward

Early Fetal Growth and Development
Edited by RHT Ward, SK Smith and D Donnai

Ethics in Obstetrics and Gynaecology
Edited by S Bewley and RHT Ward

The Biology of Gynaecological Cancer
Edited by R Leake, M Gore and RHT Ward

Multiple Pregnancy
Edited by RHT Ward and M Whittle

The Prevention of Pelvic Infection
Edited by AA Templeton

Screening for Down Syndrome in the First Trimester
Edited by JG Grudzinskas and RHT Ward

Problems in Early Pregnancy: Advances in Diagnosis and Management
Edited by JG Grudzinskas and PMS O'Brien

Gene Identification, Manipulation and Treatment
Edited by SK Smith, EJ Thomas and PMS O'Brien

Evidence-based Fertility Treatment
Edited by AA Templeton, ID Cooke and PMS O'Brien

Fetal Programming: Influences on Development and Disease in Later Life
Edited by PMS O'Brien, T Wheeler and DJP Barker

Hormones and Cancer
Edited by PMS O'Brien and AB MacLean

The Placenta: Basic Science and Clinical Practice
Edited by JCP Kingdom, ERM Jauniaux and PMS O'Brien

Disorders of the Menstrual Cycle
Edited by PMS O'Brien, IT Cameron and AB MacLean

Infection and Pregnancy
Edited by AB MacLean, L Regan and D Carrington

Pain in Obstetrics and Gynaecology
Edited by AB MacLean, RW Stones and S Thornton

Incontinence in Women
Edited by AB MacLean and L Cardozo

Maternal Morbidity and Mortality
Edited by AB MacLean and J Neilson

Lower Genital Tract Neoplasia
Edited by Allan B MacLean, Albert Singer and Hilary Critchley

Pre-eclampsia
Edited by Hilary Critchley, Allan MacLean, Lucilla Poston and James Walker

Preterm Birth
Edited by Hilary Critchley, Phillip Bennett and Steven Thornton

Menopause and Hormone Replacement
Edited by Hilary Critchley, Ailsa Gebbie and Valerie Beral

Implantation and Early Development
Edited by Hilary Critchley, Iain Cameron and Stephen Smith

Contraception and Contraceptive Use

Edited by

Anna Glasier, Kaye Wellings
and Hilary Critchley

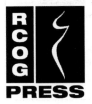

Contraception and Contraceptive Use

The Royal College of Obstetricians and Gynaecologists gratefully acknowledges the support of Organon Laboratories, Pfizer Ltd and Schering Health Care Ltd for both the 49th Study Group on Fertility Control and the subsequent Study Group follow up meeting 'Contraception and Contraceptive Use'.

Published by the **RCOG Press** at the Royal College of Obstetricians and Gynaecologists, 27 Sussex Place, Regent's Park, London NW1 4RG

www.rcog.org.uk

Registered Charity No. 213280

First published 2005

© 2005 Royal College of Obstetricians and Gynaecologists

ISBN 1 904752 15 2

No part of this publication may be reproduced, stored or transmitted in any form or by any means, without the prior written permission of the publisher or, in the case of reprographic reproduction, in accordance with the terms of licences issued by the Copyright Licensing Agency in the UK [www.cla.co.uk]. Enquiries concerning reproduction outside the terms stated here should be sent to the publisher at the UK address printed on this page.

The use of registered names, trademarks, etc. in this publication does not imply, even in the absence of a specific statement, that such names are exempt from the relevant laws and regulations and therefore for general use.

While every effort has been made to ensure the accuracy of the information contained within this publication, the publisher can give no guarantee for information about drug dosage and application thereof contained in this book. In every individual case the respective user must check current indications and accuracy by consulting other pharmaceutical literature and following the guidelines laid down by the manufacturers of specific products and the relevant authorities in the country in which they are practising.

The right of Hilary Critchley, Anna Glasier and Kaye Wellings to be identified as Editors of this work has been asserted by them in accordance with the Copyright, Designs and Patents Act, 1988.

DECLARATION OF INTEREST

All contributors to the Study Group were invited to make a specific Declaration of Interest in relation to the subject of the Study Group. This was undertaken and all contributors complied with this request. David Baird is an occasional consultant to Organon, Schering, Wyeth, Johnson & Johnson, TAP Pharmaceuticals, Toni Belfield is Director of Information, fpa, a leading charity addressing contraception and sexual health; Hilary Critchley has been an invited speaker for Leiras and Schering on the subject of Mirena and has received laboratory study support from Leiras, Schering, Jenapharm and TAP Pharmaceuticals; Anna Glasier is a member of an advisory group to Pfizer giving information about a new formulation of Depo Provera; Anna Graham is a member of the Publications Committee of Brook Advisory Centres; Stephen Killick holds research grants and acts as a consultant to the pharmaceutical industry, in particular, Schering, Wyeth and Organon; Diana Mansour has received honoraria, research support and travelling financial support from a number of pharmaceutical companies; Carolyn Westhoff is a consultant to Barr Laboratories, Pfizer-Pharmacia and Organon, she has received grant support from Berlex Laboratories, Besins International, Organon, Pfizer-Pharmacia, Ortho-McNeil, and Wyeth-Ayerst and is on the speaker's bureau for Organon and Danco Laboratories.

RCOG Editor: Jane Moody
Index: Cath Topliff, SfEP accredited indexer
Design: Karl Harrington, FiSH Books, Enfield, Middx.
Printed by Henry Ling Ltd, The Dorset Press, Dorchester, DT1 1HD, UK

Coventry University

Contents

Participants vii

Preface xi

SECTION 1 THE CURRENT SITUATION

1   **Agenda setting: from population control to reproductive health**
Kaye Wellings (with Ian Diamond) 3

2   **The converse of contraception: fertility trends in England and Wales**
Steve Smallwood 5

3   **Trends in sexual behaviour**
Kaye Wellings 12

4   **Unintended pregnancy**
Geraldine Barrett 19

5   **Women's need for abortion in Britain**
Ellie J Lee 33

6   **Overview of contraceptive methods: a provider's perspective**
Diana Mansour 44

7   **Contraception: users' perspectives and determinants of choice**
Toni Belfield 78

8   **Patterns of contraceptive use: cross-sectional surveys**
Stephen R Killick 88

9   **Longitudinal studies of birth control and pregnancy outcome among women in an urban Swedish population**
Ian Milsom 98

10   **Contraceptive adherence and continuation rates**
Carolyn Westhoff 108

11   **Highly effective contraception and sexually transmitted infections in the Western European context**
Charles S Morrison, Abigail Norris Turner, Kathryn Curtis, Patricia Bright and Paul D Blumenthal   119

12   **Hormonal contraception update on safety: breast and cervical cancer**
Philip C Hannaford   136

13   **Hormonal contraception and cardiovascular safety**
Kathryn M Curtis and Polly A Marchbanks   148

14   **Contraception for young people**
Anna Graham   169

15   **Contraception for older women**
Ailsa E Gebbie   184

SECTION 2 MAKING THINGS BETTER

16   **Potential new targets for female contraception**
David T Baird   197

17   **Improving male contraceptive methods**
Fred CW Wu   208

18   **Strategies to reduce unintended pregnancy among young people**
Catherine Dennison and Cathy Hamlyn   217

19   **Fertility control: improving prescribing**
Gillian Penney   225

20   **Improving services: increasing options and encouraging use**
Anna Glasier   236

21   **Improving sexual health education**
Judith M Stephenson   249

SECTION 3 CONSENSUS VIEWS

22   **Consensus views arising from the 49th Study Group**   261

Index   269

Participants

David T Baird
Emeritus Professor, Contraceptive Development Network, UCE Centre for Reproductive Biology, University of Edinburgh, 51 Little France Crescent, Old Dalkeith Road, Edinburgh EH16 4SA, UK

Geraldine Barrett
Lecturer, School of Health Sciences and Social Care, Brunel University, Osterley Campus, Borough Road, Middlesex TW7 5DU, UK

Toni Belfield
Director of Information, fpa, 2–12 Pentonville Road, London N1 9FP, UK

Kathryn M Curtis
Epidemiologist, Women's Health and Fertility Branch, Division of Reproductive Health, Centers for Disease Control and Prevention, MS K-34, 4770 Buford Highway NE, Atlanta, GA 30341, USA

Hilary OD Critchley
Professor of Reproductive Medicine and Consultant Gynaecologist, Centre for Reproductive Biology, University of Edinburgh, The Queen's Medical Research Institute, 47 Little France Crescent, Edinburgh EH16 4TJ, UK.

Catherine Dennison
Research Manager, Children and Young People's Public Health, Department of Health, Skipton House, 80 London Road, London SE1 6LH, UK

Ian Diamond
Chief Executive, Economic and Social Research Council, Polaris House, North Star Avenue, Swindon, Wiltshire SN2 1UE, UK

Ailsa E Gebbie
Consultant Gynaecologist, Family Planning Centre, 18 Dean Terrace, Edinburgh EH4 1NL, UK

Anna Glasier
Director of Family Planning and Well Woman Services and Honorary Professor, University of Edinburgh and University of London, Lothian Primary Care NHS Trust, 18 Dean Terrace, EH4 1NL, UK

Anna Graham
Clinical Lecturer and GP Principal, Academic Unit of Primary Health Care, University of Bristol, 1 Woodland Road, Clifton, Bristol BS8 1AU, UK

Cathy Hamlyn
Acting Head, National Programme Delivery, Department of Health, Skipton House, 80 London Rd, London SE1 6LH, UK

Philip C Hannaford
NHS Grampian Professor of Primary Care, University of Aberdeen, Foresterhill Health Centre, Westburn Road, Aberdeen AB25 2AY, UK

Stephen R Killick
Professor of Reproductive Medicine and Surgery, University of Hull, Women's and Children's Hospital, Anlaby road, Hull HU3 2JZ, UK

Ellie Lee
Lecturer in Social Policy, University of Kent at Canterbury, Canterbury, Kent CT2 7NS, UK

Diana Mansour
Deputy Medical Director, Head of Service, Consultant in Community Gynaecology and Reproductive Health Care, Newcastle Primary Care Trust, Graingerville Clinic, Newcastle General Hospital, Westgate Road, Newcastle upon Tyne NE4 6BE, UK

Ian Milsom
Professor and Consultant Gynecologist, Department of Obstetrics and Gynecology, Sahlgrenska University Hospital, Östra, SE-416 85 Göteborg, Sweden

Charles S Morrison
Senior Epidemiologist, Family Health International, PO Box 13950, Research Triangle Park, NC 27709, USA

Gillian Penney
Senior Lecturer and Programme Director, Scottish Programme for Clinical Effectiveness in Reproductive Health, University of Aberdeen, Aberdeen Maternity Hospital, Cornhill Road, Aberdeen AB25 2ZD, UK

Steve Smallwood
Head of Family Demography Unit, Office for National Statistics, B6/3, I Drummond Gate, London SW1V 2QQ, UK

Judith M Stephenson
Senior Lecturer in Epidemiology, Centre for Sexual Health and HIV Research, Royal Free and University College Medical School, 3rd Floor, Mortimer Market Centre, off Capper Street, London WC1E 6AU, UK

Kaye Wellings
Professor of Sexual and Reproductive Health, London School of Hygiene and Tropical Medicine, Keppel Street, London WC1E 7HT, UK

Carolyn Westhoff
Professor, Obstetric and Gynecological Epidemiology, College of Physicians and Surgeons, Columbia University, 630 168th Street, New York, NY 10032, USA

Fred CW Wu
Department of Endocrinology, University of Manchester, Manchester Royal Infirmary, Oxford Road, Manchester M13 9WL, UK

Discussants

Alison Bigrigg
Director, Faculty of Family Planning and Reproductive Health Care Sandyford Initiative, Sandyford Place, Glasgow G7 7NB, UK

Additional contributors

Paul D Blumenthal
Associate Professor, Department of Obstetrics and Gynecology, Johns Hopkins University, U940 Easterne Avenue, Baltimore, Maryland 21226, USA

Patricia L Bright
International Research Coordinator, Johns Hopkins University, School of Medicine, 600 North Wolfe Street, Carnegie Rm 443, Baltimore, Maryland 21287, USA

Ann Furedi
Chief Executive, British Pregnancy Advisory Service, Austy Manor, Wooton Wawen, West Midlands B95 6BX, UK

Polly A Marchbanks
Epidemiologist, Team Leader, Fertility Epidemiology Studies, Women's Health and Fertility Branch, Division of Reproductive Health, Centers for Disease Control and Prevention, MS K-34, 4770 Buford Highway NE, Atlanta, GA 30341, USA

Abigail Norris Turner
Doctoral student, Department of Epidemiology, School of Public Health, University of North Carolina at Chapel Hill, McGavran-Greenberg Hall, Pittsboro St, CB#7435, Chapel Hill, North Carolina 27599-7435, USA

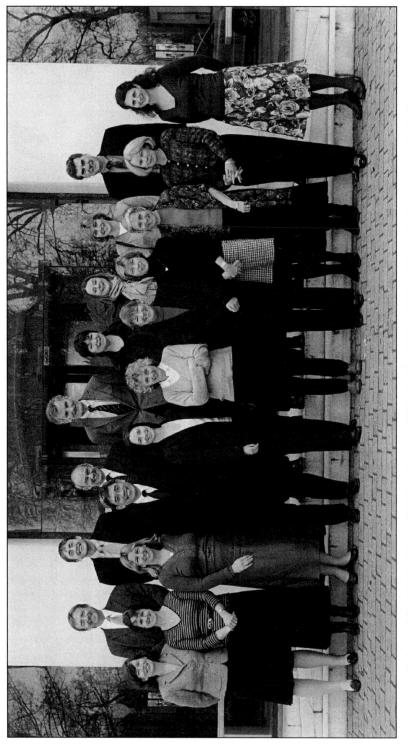

Back row: (*left to right*): Ian Milsom, Phil Hannaford, Steve Killick, David Baird, Kaye Wellings, Ellie Lee, Judith Stephenson, Charlie Morrison
Front row: (*left to right*): Kate Curtis, Diana Mansour, Alison Bigrigg, Fred Wu, Geraldine Barrett, Anna Glasier, Gillian Penney, Ailsa Gebbie, Carolyn Westhoff,
Toni Belfield, Anna Graham

Preface

It is a fundamental desire of men and women to wish to regulate their own fertility. Birth control has been practiced since classical times. The need for fertility control to stem population growth is a more recent phenomenon and a great deal has been achieved in this respect in the past half century. As a result, there are those who question the continued need for a focus on family planning programmes. However, as the landmark 1994 Cairo conference made clear, population control is not only about controlling the size of the population but also about ensuring that individual men and women are able to decide when and whether to have children, how many to have and how to ensure their health and wellbeing.

We have seen a marked shift in the last decade of the 20th century from goals driven by demography towards those focusing on reproductive health and an improvement in the lives of parents and their children. There is, however, no room for complacency. Changes and improvements to health systems and services are still needed even in developed countries. Contraception in the UK is now widespread and available to all, whatever their means or marital status, a range of methods is available from general practitioners and community family planning clinics and condoms and emergency contraception are available without the need to see a health provider. But there is still work to be done to realise the ideals of the birth control pioneers of the first half of the 20th century. Despite easy access to contraception, abortion rates in the UK are among the highest in Europe and most unintended pregnancies occur among couples using no contraception or using a method inconsistently. Elsewhere in the developed world, unintended pregnancy is common. The challenge remains one of meeting the needs of individuals in their search for reliable, effective contraceptive methods that are easy to use, and to access.

The programme for the 49th RCOG Study Group was designed to explore the big picture of contraceptive use and to discuss the demographic, social and behavioural issues that affect it.

The 'Consensus Views' expressed in this volume are not formal recommendations but the conclusions of independent experts. Each of the chapters within this book has provided the authors with an opportunity to share personal views in greater depth and to provide a more comprehensive and evidence-based description of their specialist topic. It is intended that this publication will provide a source of expertise for all those with an interest in improving fertility control, whether involved in research, clinical practice, education or policy making.

Anna Glasier
Kaye Wellings
Hilary Critchley

SECTION 1
THE CURRENT SITUATION

Chapter 1
Agenda setting: from population control to reproductive health

Kaye Wellings (with Ian Diamond)

Introduction

The desire on the part of men and women to regulate their fertility has a long history. Evidence of the use of birth control is available from classical times. In Crete, homosexuality was, according to Aristotle, officially supported as a population control tactic and concern for limitation of number of offspring is known to have been motivated by concern for the division of the estate in Roman times (McLaren).[1] Low population growth in the Middle Ages is partly attributable to low expectation of life but, even then, the contribution of the practice of birth control, using methods such as withdrawal and abstinence, was not inconsiderable (Potts and Campbell).

The rationale for fertility control to curb population growth is more recent. The impetus for population control had begun in the 1800s, following the famous declaration of Thomas Malthus in 1798 that, while population was increasing geometrically, the Earth's food supply could at best be increased only arithmetically. At the start of the 19th century, the Western world was in 'demographic transition'; the ratio of births to deaths was growing larger each year. Between 1650 and 1850 the world's population is believed to have more than doubled. This was attributed largely to a marked decline in the death rate.[2] In the absence of modern sanitation and medicine, annual death rates of 38 or more per thousand had been characteristic but by the 19th century the death rate in certain European countries and North America had fallen to 30 per thousand and below.

The use and development of modern methods of contraception can be attributed at least in part to the momentum of this demographic explosion.[3] By the turn of the 20th century, many other birth control methods were known and used, although they tended to be practised more widely among the middle classes. Birth control was not taught in medical schools until 1928 and awareness of the needs of poorer people to limit the size of their families was not high among the medical profession. Malthusian arguments were then joined by the likes of Margaret Sanger and Marie Stopes, who tried to bring acceptance of birth control to all sectors of society and to find new and effective methods of contraception.[4]

By the 1930s, the most popular methods of contraception in the UK were still withdrawal, condoms and rhythm but pessaries had also started to be used.[5] Further developments came in the 1950s and 1960s with the introduction of oral contraception.

Alongside the development of increasingly effective methods of contraception came the introduction of national family planning programmes aimed at reducing population growth. These were supported by international agencies and by national governments. Comtemporaneously with the introduction of family planning programmes there has been a reduction in childbearing in many parts of the world. However, it is a matter of much serious debate whether these programmes have had a direct effect on attitudes to childbearing or whether by making contraception available to all couples they have had a largely indirect effect. With the reduction in childbearing some international donor funding ids diminishing. Do we still need family planning programmes?

Today, the assumption is made by many that population is no longer a vitally important world policy area, on the grounds that fertility rates are declining everywhere; contraception is widely available and used and growth rates are in decline. The parallel assumption has also gained currency, that there is no longer a need for government-sponsored population programmes, on the grounds that family planning and reproductive health can be provided by private means (with some public support); that service delivery is simply a matter of getting the market right; that education, rather than contraception, is likely to impact most dramatically on unplanned pregnancy and that population and 'development' are not linked.

Yet antagonists point out that fertility rates are not falling everywhere; that contraceptive use is not increasing everywhere; and that service delivery – despite improvements – is still patchy. More profoundly, there are those who point out that population change is not simply about births (and deaths) but about the health and wellbeing of men and women and their children.[6]

By the early 1990s, there became broad agreement that women were rarely able to exercise their right to reproductive and sexual choices.[7] The International Conference on Population and Development (ICPD) held in Cairo in 1994 recognised explicitly the close link between global population dynamics and the life events of individuals. In so doing, the conference called for a shift in the focus of programmes from demographic objectives towards those relating to reproductive health and improvements in women's situation.

The Cairo Conference moved explicitly towards reproductive health and mandated the integration of family planning and modern contraception with other interventions aimed at creating a state of reproductive wellbeing. Improving women's reproductive health and social status became a central issue.[8] Reproductive health was seen as encompassing the ability to enjoy satisfying sexual relations without fear of infection, pregnancy, coercion or violence; the ability to regulate fertility without unpleasant or dangerous adverse effects and in a manner and to a degree of one's own choosing; and the ability to bear and raise healthy children. Fertility regulation is thus seen as a preventive health measure and also a way of achieving gender equality. Significantly, Cairo was the first World Population Conference at which women contributed to the agenda on a large scale.[9]

The situation in the UK

Use of contraception in the UK is now widespread (see Chapter 20). It has been available to all women, regardless of marital status, since the early 1970s and to all, regardless of ability to pay, since it became available free of charge on the National Health Service in 1972. Yet trends suggest that there is a long way to go with respect to achieving optimal reproductive health for all. As many of the contributions to this volume point out, we are not yet reaching all parts of our populations. Many of the problems remaining are the most intractable and the mediating effect of fertility control in the relationship between health and poverty continues to challenge us with the need to focus on hard to reach and disadvantaged groups.

References

1. McLaren A. *A History of Contraception from Antiquity to the Present Day*. Oxford: Blackwell Publishing; 1990. p. 50.
2. Ehrlich P, Ehrlich A. The population explosion: why isn't everyone as scared as we are? Amic J 1990;12(1):22–9.
3. Benagiano G, Testa G, Cocuzzi L. [The meaning of fertility control in an integrated world.] *Minerva Ginecol* 2004;56(3):271–81 [Italian].
4. McLaren A. *A History of Contraception from Antiquity to the Present Day*. Oxford: Blackwell Publishing; 1990. p. 208.
5. McLaren A. *A History of Contraception from Antiquity to the Present Day*. Oxford: Blackwell Publishing; 1990. p. 235.
6. Caldwell JC, Phillips JF, Barkat-e-Khuda. The future of family planning programs. *Stud Fam Plann* 2002;33(1):1–10.
7. Shallat L. Rights of life. Sexuality and reproduction. *Womens Health J* 1993;3:31–7.
8. Humble M. Women's perspectives on reproductive health and rights. Overview. *Plan Parent Chall* 1995;(2):26–31.
9. Coleman E, Reardon C. Out of Cairo: forging a new population policy. *Ford Found Rep* 1994;25(3):33–5.

Chapter 2

The converse of contraception: fertility trends in England and Wales

Steve Smallwood

Introduction

The use of contraception is primarily predicated by the desire of men and women to control their level and timing of fertility. The last half of the 20th century saw major changes in both aspects of childbearing across the world. In areas with developed-world mortality, replacement fertility is at an average of 2.1 children per woman. In most countries in the developed world, fertility has fallen to around or below (in some cases well below) replacement level. Fertility is also falling across the developing world. For example, China has had levels of developed-world fertility for more than two decades. Wilson and Pison[1] have estimated that half the world's population now lives in countries or regions with fertility at or below an average of 2.1 children per woman. However, in those countries in which mortality is still high, replacement level would be well above 2.1 and fertility rates may be below their replacement level.[2] It is, therefore, likely that more than half the world's population live in areas of below replacement fertility. Together with falls in the level of fertility many developed countries have seen a trend towards later childbearing in the last few decades.

Measures of fertility

Total fertility rate

Data for England and Wales illustrate trends towards both a falling level of fertility and delays in fertility. Figure 2.1 shows births for each year from 1940 to 2003. A brief baby boom after World War II was followed by a more sustained baby boom in the mid-1960s. Numbers of births then fell dramatically in the 1970s, a decline which coincided with increased availability and use of contraception generally, and that of the birth control pill in particular.[3] A rise in the number of births was seen around 1990, although the second measure in Figure 2.1, the total fertility rate, illustrates that this rise was largely the result of the increase in the number of women of childbearing age. The total fertility rate controls for the age distribution of the female population and gives a better indication of the changing level of fertility in the population. Prior to the 1980s, the total fertility rate broadly followed the trend in births. Since then,

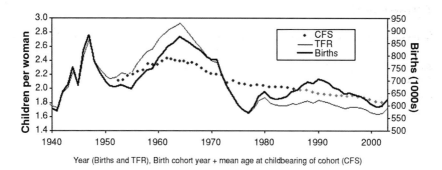

Figure 2.1. Births, total fertility rate (TFR) and completed family size (CFS), England and Wales, 1940–2003 and cohorts born 1924–1973 (source: Office for National Statistics)

the overall trend in the total fertility rate has been a drift downwards. Underlying the drift downwards has been a fall in fertility at younger ages and an increase in fertility at older ages, as seen in Figure 2.2, which shows the total fertility rate split between the contributions of women under 30 years of age and those of 30 years and over.

Completed family size

The third measure of fertility shown in Figure 2.1 is completed family size. Whereas the total fertility rate measures fertility in a specific year, completed family size measures fertility for a group of women born in a particular year. Measures such as

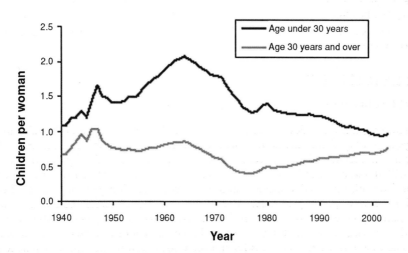

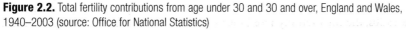

Figure 2.2. Total fertility contributions from age under 30 and 30 and over, England and Wales, 1940–2003 (source: Office for National Statistics)

completed family size are referred to as cohort measures. Although measured in a different time dimension, by plotting the cohorts at the mean age of their child-bearing we can see that cohorts that were at the peak of their childbearing in the 1960s had a lower completed family size than the fertility level indicated by the total fertility rate. Conversely, cohorts at their peak childbearing ages in the 1980s and 1990s had, or are likely to have, higher fertility than indicated by the total fertility rate. These differences are the results of changes in timing of childbearing. For example, the current level of the total fertility rate is likely to be depressed (in comparison with completed family size) as women are foregoing childbearing at younger ages but may go on to have children at older ages.

Other measures of fertility

A key determinant of overall childbearing timing is the timing of a woman's first birth. Figure 2.3 shows the mean age at first birth for cohorts of women in England and Wales. Women born in the 1940s commenced their childbearing early but women since then have, on average, started their childbearing successively later. Projections of fertility assume that this trend will continue. The same pattern of later childbearing can be seen across Europe, although the exact timing of the upturn in mean age at first birth varies.[4]

In addition to changes in timing of childbearing, there has been a rise in the prevalence of childlessness. For cohorts just completing their childbearing (born around 1960) one in five women is likely to be childless. The proportion of childless women in a cohort is projected to increase slightly to around 23% for cohorts currently commencing their childbearing.[5] This compares with only around 10% of women born in the mid-1940s who remained childless.

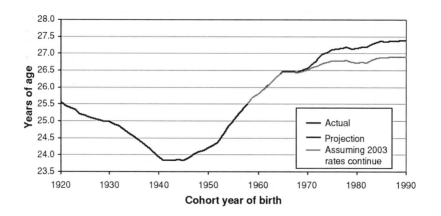

Figure 2.3. Standardised mean age at first birth, England and Wales, cohorts born 1920–1990

Fertility trends

Thus, different measures of fertility can give different messages about fertility trends. Live births are an important measure, as they will determine population size and therefore also resource requirements. The number of births is related to the number of women of childbearing age, and the total fertility rate provides a measure controlling for the number and age distribution of that population. However, this measure can be affected by the timing of births; cohort measures provide a truer measure of the ultimate level of fertility for women.

As will be seen in Chapter 3, not only has the mean age of first intercourse fallen but the range has also narrowed. It is therefore clear that women are spending an ever-longer period of time during which they are potentially sexually active but not having children.

Examining the proportion of conceptions that end in abortion provides further evidence for the change in timing of childbearing, as well as perhaps the increased use of abortion resulting from increased exposure of risk to conception possibly coupled with lack of contraception or contraceptive failure.

Abortion

For each age group under 30 years, there has been a steady rise in the percentage of conceptions ended by abortion, although there is some evidence for the latest year available that the rising trend has ceased. This long-term rise may be the result of greater prevalence of sexual activity, lack of contraception, simply a reflection that abortion is a more acceptable option for unplanned pregnancy, or combinations of all of these possibilities. The trend has been reasonably stable for the 30–34 years age group but at older ages the proportion of conceptions ending in abortion has fallen. Recourse to abortion for the older age groups in the 1970s and 1980s is likely to have

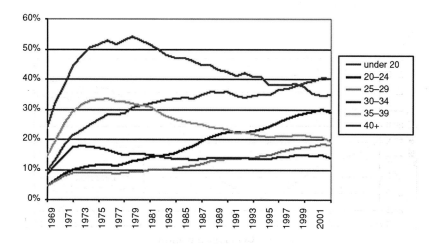

Figure 2.4. Abortion as a percentage of conception rates, England and Wales, 1969–2002

been an option used to limit larger families. As family sizes have dropped there will be fewer women to take up this option. Conversely, there are now more women who want to have first or second children at these later ages.[6]

Timing of childbearing

Further information about the changing timing of childbearing comes from survey data. For the last 25 years, the General Household Survey has included a module that asks all women of childbearing age about their family-building intentions. The survey asks three main questions: whether the woman thinks she will have any more children; how many children the woman thinks she will have in total; and, where the woman expressed an intention for a further birth, at what age she thought she would be at her next birth.

In the General Household Survey, like many such surveys in this and other countries, the resulting completed family size is around two children but, in general, such surveys do not provide accurate predictions of actual completed family size when compared with fertility outcomes at the macro level.[7] However, it is clear from the question about the timing of childbearing that women have expressed the thought that they would have children later. One of the reasons for this delay is the increase in female education and employment. There is evidence for cohorts that have recently completed their childbearing (born 1954–58) that women with higher educational attainment commenced their childbearing on average 5 years later than those with lower levels of education.[8]

Figure 2.5 shows the proportions of women intending a birth within 3 years and within 3–5 years, for women aged 21–23 years by educational status. Although the beginning of the 1990s saw a fall for the higher educated women, there has subsequently been a slight rise in the proportions of more highly educated women saying

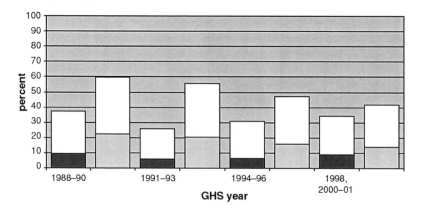

Figure 2.5. Percentage of women aged 21–23 years with different educational levels who intend to have a child within the next 3 years and 3–5 years, England and Wales, 1988–2001 (General Household Surveys)

that they would have a birth within 5 years. This rise may reflect the greater heterogeneity of this group as the numbers entering higher education have increased. For women without higher education the proportion saying that they will have a birth in the next 5 years has fallen from 60% to 40% and is now approaching the level of the more highly educated women. Thus, the birth timing intentions of women with lower levels of education appears to be becoming more like their more highly educated peers.

Conclusions

These changes in fertility trends are only one aspect of larger changes in society. Changes in relationships, such as decreasing prevalence of marriage, increase in divorce and prevalence of cohabitation, have changed the environment in which becoming a parent and childrearing occurs. Economic changes, including increased female labour force participation, and other social changes such as the moving towards individualisation will have also had an effect on decisions about childbearing. All of these contexts will also affect decision making about use of contraception both for prevention of conception or to control timing of conception.

References

1. Wilson C, Pison G. More than half of the global population lives where fertility is below replacement level. *Population & Societies* 2004; (405):1–4.
2. Espendshade T, Guzman J, Westoff C. The surprising global variation in replacement fertility. *Popul Res Policy Rev* 2003;22:575–83.
3. Murphy M. The contraceptive pill and women's employment as factors in fertility change in Britain 1963–1980: a challenge to the conventional view. *Popul Stud* 1993;47:221–43.
4. Population Statistics. Theme 3: Population and Social Conditions. Eurostat. 2004 [www.eustatistics.gov.uk/Download. asp?KS-NK-04-002-__-N-EN_tcm90-17102.pdf].
5. Smallwood S. Fertility assumptions for the 2002-based national population projections. *Popul Trends* 2003;114:8–18.
6. Smallwood S. New estimates of trends in births by birth order in England and Wales. *Popul Trends* 2002;108:32–48.
7. Smallwood S, Jefferies J. Family building intentions in England and Wales: trends outcomes and interpretations. *Popul Trends* 2002;112:15–28.
8. Rendall R, Smallwood S. Higher qualifications, first birth timing and further childbearing in England and Wales. *Popul Trends* 2002;111:18–26.

Chapter 3
Trends in sexual behaviour

Kaye Wellings

Introduction

In this chapter, we examine changes that have occurred in sexual behaviour in recent decades, the influences on the trends and their implications for sexual health status and for intervention. Patterns of sexual behaviour are key determinants of fertility patterns and the transmission dynamics of sexually transmitted infection and, hence, diversity in human behaviour is a major focus of academic interest and research.[1-3]

In 1990, the first National Survey of Sexual Attitudes and Lifestyles (Natsal 1990) was carried out in Britain in response to the urgent need for estimates of sexual practices in the context of prediction and prevention of further transmission of HIV/AIDS. In the event, the results were not only useful in modelling the extent of the HIV epidemic in Britain and guiding public health strategies but were also widely used in a range of policy areas, including sex education, contraception services and fertility control. In 1999–2001, a further survey (Natsal 2000) was carried out, using similar questions to Natsal 1990 but with some methodological improvements to provide new estimates of sexual behaviour patterns and assess changes in reported behaviour over time.[4] This time, questions were added specifically to allow the data to be used in the widest possible context.

In the case of repeat cross-sectional surveys of a population of a wide age range, there are two possibilities in terms of examining secular trends in sexual behaviour. For events that occur only once in a lifetime (such as first intercourse) or at certain defined ages (for, example teenage pregnancy) we can compare estimates in successive age cohorts of the sample, (the oldest of which, in Natsal, were born between 1931 and 1936). For behaviours which continue through life, such as the accumulation of partners and experience of sexual activities, where the influence of historical time cannot easily be distinguished from life-stage related change, the comparison is made between surveys; that is, comparing reports made in 2000 with those made in 1990.

What are the changes?

A number of important changes in sexual behaviour occurred in the second half of the 20th century. Description of these trends is organised by three main themes:

1. An increase in the prevalence in risk behaviours.

2. An increase in the interval between first sexual activity and age at first child-bearing and an increase in the proportion of older people who are again 'on the sexual market'.

3. A convergence in the patterns of sexual behaviours of men and women over time.

There is clearly overlap between these themes but their organisation helps to identify key changes which have occurred over the last half century.

Increase in risk behaviours

The first, and the most dramatic, increase in risk behaviours is the progressive decline in the age at which first intercourse occurs. Median age at first intercourse decreased from 21 years for women, and 20 years for men born in the early 1930s and sexually active in the 1950s, to 16 years for both sexes born in the early 1980s becoming sexually active in the late 1990s. The most precipitous decline occurred during the 1950s, when median age for women dropped by 2 years. This was followed by a decline of a further year during the 1960s, and a more gradual decline thereafter. Median age thus fell by 5 years for women, from 21 years for those born in the early 1930s and having first sex in the early 1950s, to 16 years for those born in mid-1980s becoming sexually active at around the turn of the century. The 1990s, however, saw the first signs in half a century of a stabilisation of age at first heterosexual intercourse among women, although a longer time series would be needed before this could be confirmed.

In parallel with this trend, the proportion of young people who are sexually active before the age of 16 years has increased over the period. At the end of the 20th century, 25% of young women had intercourse before the age of sexual consent, compared with fewer than 1% of those becoming sexually active in the 1950s. With respect to the circumstances of first intercourse, the event is much less likely to occur within a long-term relationship than was the case hitherto. First sexual intercourse now predates marriage for the vast majority (fewer than 1% of women, and no men, in the youngest cohort of Natsal 1990 were married before having sexual intercourse). Thirty-nine percent of women and 14% of men born in the early 1930s married before having sexual intercourse and a further 14% of women and 6% of men were engaged to be married before doing so. Not surprisingly, given the earlier onset of sexual activity, recent decades have seen higher rates of partner change. A comparison of reports from Natsal 1990 and 2000 shows higher rates of new partner acquisition among men and women aged under 25 years and single.

Compared with 1990, estimates for the prevalence for all risk behaviours were higher in 2000. Both men and women were more likely to report having had more than five lifetime partners and less likely to report having only one, and the difference was particularly striking for women. A wide range of behaviours associated with increased risk of HIV/AIDS transmission had all increased by 2000 compared with 1990, including concurrency of partnerships, numbers of heterosexual partners, homosexual partnerships, heterosexual anal sex and payment for sex.

At the same time, there is evidence for the increasing adoption of risk reduction practices. First sexual experience is increasingly less likely to lead to conception. For only a small minority of young people (11% in Natsal 2000) was first intercourse unprotected against infection and conception. The data show a striking increase in condom use at first intercourse, sustained during the 1990s despite predictions that the weaker impact of AIDS-linked safer sex messages might have brought about complacency. Further, 25% of young women are now already using oral contraception at their first experience of sexual intercourse.

Between the two surveys, we also saw an increase in consistent condom use suggesting that sexual health promotional messages had an effect. The increase was not, however, sufficient to offset the increased risk contingent on numbers of partners. Combining data on condom use and numbers of partners as an indicator of 'unsafe sex', the data showed that, overall, the proportion of the population who reported two or more partners in the past year and who did not use condoms consistently had increased between the surveys. The proportion of the population who reported two or more sexual partners in the past year and inconsistent condom use in the past month (an indicator of safe sex) had increased significantly in men and women between the surveys: a continuation of the increase in condom use and the decrease in the proportion using no contraceptive method at first intercourse and an increase in the importance of school in the sexual education of the young, particularly men, in recent birth cohorts.

Intervals between life events

The duration of time between onset of sexual activity and childbearing also has important implications for sexual health. Plotting median ages for first sexual intercourse and first live-in relationship, and between first live-in relationship and first birth, shows the recent increase in the time period between the three events with successive cohorts. Comparing the cohort born in the late 1950s with that born in the early 1930s, the interval between median age at first intercourse and first cohabitation increased from 4 to 7 years for men and from 1 to 3 years for women; the interval between age at first cohabitation and birth of first child has increased from 4 to 5 years for men and from 3 to 4 years for women and the interval between first intercourse and first birth has increased from 8 to 12 years for men and from 4 to 7 years for women.

For both men and women, the time period between first sexual intercourse and first birth has increased markedly in recent decades.[5] While median age at first intercourse has fallen, age at first birth has risen. The increase in age at first birth is more marked for the upper quartile. More than 25% of women in the more recent cohorts delayed motherhood until their 30s and the same proportion of men delayed fatherhood until after the age of 35 years.

The data also show a trend towards greater uniformity in terms of sexual debut. The interquartile range for age at first intercourse has decreased over time: for men born between 1931 and 1936 it was 5 years and for women of this age it was 4 years, compared with 2 years for men and women born in the mid-1980s. By contrast, the data show greater diversity in terms of birth of the first child. The social clock seems to be exerting a more powerful effect on age at onset of sexual activity and a weaker effect on age of onset of cohabitation and reproductive activity. As might be expected, (since their fertility is more time-limited) the age range within which women have their first child is narrower than for men but even so, comparing them with older cohorts it has increased fairly markedly among those who became parents in the late 1970s and early 1980s.

One consequence of the increasing interval between life events and, in particular, the extension of the time period between onset of sexual activity and settling with a partner in a committed relationship is that there is clearly greater opportunity to accumulate larger numbers of sexual partners. As expected, there is a relationship between the length of the interval between life events and number of lifetime sexual partners. Men with ten or more lifetime partners have a median interval between first sexual intercourse and first child of 9 years, compared with only 4 years for men who, at the time of interview, had been monogamous. The median interval between first sex and first child for women with ten or more partners is 7 years, compared with 3 years for monogamous women. The time period during which partners are most likely to be accumulated is between first sexual intercourse and first live-in relationship and the longer this period is, the larger the number of sexual partners.

Gender convergence in behaviour

The changes in sexual behaviour described above have been more marked among women than men. Although there are continuing differences in reporting between men and women in a number of areas of sexual behaviour – number of lifetime partners, for example – there has been some convergence in many of the behaviours of men and women over recent times. Comparing successive birth cohorts in Natsal 1990 and 2000, for the cohort born in the early 1930s median age at first intercourse was a year earlier for men than for women (20 compared with 21 years), while for cohorts born after the 1970s the age was the same for both, that is 17 years decreasing later to 16 years.[6]

Despite the convergence in the behaviour of men and women with respect to the age at which first intercourse occurs, there remain gender differences in the experience of the event. The proportion of those who are sexually competent according to the criteria adopted here, (that is, the experience was consensual, free from regret, autonomous and protected from infection and unplanned pregnancy) has increased with time among men but not women. Women are twice as likely as men to regret their first experience of intercourse and three times as likely to report being the less willing partner. These findings are confirmed by others.

Are the changes real?

Are these real changes in behaviour or are they the result of changes in methodology, or changes in respondents' willingness to report disapproved behaviours, or both? It has been said that patterns of behaviour change less through time than does the manner in which it is reported. Certainly, as attitudes become more lenient, people are increasingly willing to report behaviours that they might once have believed or feared were socially prohibited.

There are strong grounds for believing that there have been real changes in behaviour. The increase in prevalence in risk behaviours is also consistent with evidence from external sources. The period between 1990 and 1999 saw increases in new diagnoses in UK genitourinary medicine clinics of acute sexually transmitted infections in men and women of 56% and 20%, respectively.[7] Substantial increases in unprotected anal intercourse have also been recorded in social venue surveys of homosexual men in London.[8]

There was also little evidence of a methodological effect. Prior to carrying out Natsal 2000, an experiment conducted to explore whether computer-assisted self-interviews and computer-assisted personal interviews (CASI and CAPI) and pencil and paper interviews did not produce different estimates for sensitive behaviours. There were no significant differences in measurements of key variables. We were also able to look at the internal consistency of the data by comparing the reports of time specific behaviours in the age cohorts eligible for both surveys (that is, those born between 1956 and 1974, aged 16 to 34 years in Natsal 1990 and 26 to 44 years in Natsal 2000) with those of representatives of the same age cohort, aged 16 to 34 years in Natsal 1990 born between 1956 and 1974. Where there were differences, they were in the direction of increased reporting of sensitive behaviours but they were not of a sufficient magnitude to explain much of the difference in reporting seen between the surveys.[9]

What are the factors which have contributed to these changes?

The factors contributing to changes in behaviour are predominantly social. Although early menarche is independently associated with early age at first intercourse, the decrease in age at first menstruation accounts for little of the decline in age at first intercourse. There has undoubtedly been a relaxation in social attitudes towards sexual behaviour and, particularly, towards the sexual behaviour of the young. Attitudes towards homosexual behaviour, nonexclusive sexual relationships and sex outside of marriage have all softened over recent decades. In part, this is attributable to an increasing secularisation. Absolute morality, as dictated by religious scriptures, has gradually been replaced by a situational ethic, in which people are encouraged to consider the implications of their behaviour on its merits.

The trends towards greater gender equality in sexual matters also reflect fluctuations in the economy, increasing female participation in the workforce and the influence of the women's movement. The need for women to work during the Second World War helped to change attitudes towards women's independence, which did not revert subsequently.

Changes in the timing of sexual and reproductive events occur in response to a number of factors. Advances in contraception have freed sexual expression from its reproductive consequences. Progress in obstetric medicine has enabled more choice to be exercised over the timing of birth and ensured that later birth is safer. Years spent in formal education and levels of educational attainment also influence life event schedules and the historical trend has been towards an increase in both. Later age at marriage and childbearing has to an extent been contingent on the increasing length of time spent in education and training.

The increase in sexual activity of the young, and of women, is often also attributed to the so-called 'sexual revolution' of the 1960s. Although it is often said that the availability of reliable contraception was a prime determinant in this, the evidence is more complex. As we have seen, the sharpest drop in age at first intercourse occurred in the 1950s. It was to be another decade before the advent of the oral contraception in Britain in 1961, and more than two decades before the pill was generally available to single women in 1972, when family planning clinics were mandated to supply oral contraception to all women, regardless of marital status. It was not available to women of all financial means, regardless of ability to pay, until 1975, when contraception was made available under the NHS.

The 1960s were certainly a decade of legislative reform around sexual matters. 1967 saw the decriminalisation of both abortion and homosexuality, followed in 1969 by reform of the divorce laws. Yet the shift in attitudes which was to lead to these liberalising legislation had begun at least a decade earlier.[10] The Wolfenden report, for example, which made the recommendation that consensual sex between two men should not be unlawful, was published in 1957. It is almost certainly as true to say that the softening of attitudes towards sexual matters provided the impetus to the liberalising reforms of the 1960s, as it is to say that the reforms triggered a less censorious Britain.

What are the implications for sexual health?

We have seen marked changes, in little more than a generation, in the onset of sexual activity, in the prevalence of risk behaviours, in the timing and spacing of life events and in the behaviour of women relative to men. A corollary of changes in sexual behaviour is self-evidently a change in sexual health status.

The increase in risk behaviours clearly has implications for the prevalence of sexually transmitted diseases. Since the period before settling down with one partner is longer than was previously the case and the number of sexual partners is larger, the chances of infection are greater. Changes in the timing and phasing of first sexual intercourse, first live-in partnership and first birth life events have important implications for the timing of sex education and for the provision of services for contraception and abortion. The extension of the period between first intercourse and first birth has consequences for contraceptive usage. A large proportion of men and women today are likely to be requiring a reliable method of contraception for between one and two decades before the birth of their first child and for a period of the same magnitude after completing their family. An increase in the length of time during which young people are sexually active and at risk of unplanned pregnancy will also have implications for the demand for abortion. Further, 25% of women today have their first child in their 30s and will be medically designated as 'elderly primigravidae'.

We hear a great deal about the current crisis in sexual health in this country and it is often assumed that the situation in England is worse than in other countries. Yet the trends described above are not unique to Britain but are broadly consistent with those which have occurred in other resource-rich countries in the comparable time period. The fall in age at first intercourse has been documented in other European countries, as have the increases in the prevalence of risk behaviours. A comparison of data from contemporaneous surveys in the UK and France[11] and between those from the UK and the USA[12] showed few differences in trends. Comparative evidence does, however, suggest that young people in Britain are sexually active at an earlier age than they are in other countries and less likely to use contraception on their first occasion of sexual intercourse.[13]

Rates of sexually transmitted infections have been increasing but current incidence still does not compare with the high rates seen earlier in the 20th century. Teenage pregnancy rates are worse than in the rest of Europe but the comparative situation has not deteriorated in the 1990s and 2000s. A little over one in 20 women give birth to a child while under the age of 18 years and the proportion has changed little over the latter half of the 20th century.

Much of the commentary on changes in the sexual health of the young tends to conflate risks of sexually transmitted infection and early pregnancy, constructing a generic sexual health risk. Yet the risk factors for sexually transmitted infections and teenage pregnancy, for example, are different. This is an important distinction. Preventive efforts need, perhaps to heed, not so much variability through time, as between different social groups in the population.

References

1.   Laumann EO, Gagnon JH, Michael RT, Michaels S. *The Social Organization of Sexuality: Sexual practices in the United States*. Chicago and London: University of Chicago Press; 1994.

2.   Turner CF, Danella RD, Rogers SM. Sexual behavior in the United States, 1930–1990: trends and methodological problems. *Sex Transm Dis* 1995;22:173–90.

3.   ACSF investigators. AIDS and sexual behaviour in France. *Nature* 1992;360:407–9.

4.   Johnson AM, Mercer CH, Erens B, Copas AJ, McManus S, Wellings K, *et al*. Sexual behaviour in Britain: partnerships, practices and HIV risk behaviours. Lancet 2001;358:1835–42.

5.   Manning WD. Cohabitation, marriage and entry into motherhood. *J Marriage Fam* 1995;57:191–200.

6.   Wellings K, Nanchahal K, Macdowall W, McManus S, Erens B, Mercer CH, *et al*. Sexual behaviour in Britain: early heterosexual experience. *Lancet* 2001;358:1843–50.

7.   Public Health Laboratory Service, England, Wales and N. Ireland DHSS and PS Northern Ireland and the Scottish ISD D 5 Collaborative Group ISD SCIEH and MSSVD. *Trends in Sexually Transmitted Infections in the United Kingdom 1990–1999*. London: PHLS; 2000.

8.   Dodds JP, Nardone A, Mercey DE, Johnson AM. Increase in high risk sexual behaviour among homosexual men, London 1996-8: cross sectional questionnaire study. BMJ 2000;320:1510–11.

9.   Copas AJ, Wellings K, Erens B, Mercer CH, McManus S, Fenton KA, *et al*. The accuracy of reported sensitive sexual behaviour in Britain: exploring the extent of change 1990–2000. *Sex Transm Infect* 2002;78:26–30.

10.   Petigny A. Illegitimacy, post war psychology and the reperiodization of the sexual revolution. *J Social History* 2004;38:63–80.

11.   Bajos N, Wadsworth J, Dudcot B, Johnson AM, Le Pont F, Wellings K, *et al*. Sexual behaviour in HIV epidemiology: comparative analysis in France and Britain. *AIDS* 1995;9:735–43.

12.   Michael RT, Wadsworth J, Feinleib J, Johnson AM, Laumann E, Wellings K. Private sexual behaviour, public opinion, and public health policy related to sexually transmitted diseases: A US–British comparison. *Am J Public Health* 1998;88:749–54.

13.   Currie C, Roberts C, Magan A. *Young People's Health in Context. Health Behaviour in School-aged Children: International Report from the 2001/2002 Survey*. Health Policy for Children and Adolescents, No. 4. Copenhagen: WHO Regional Office for Europe; 2004.

Chapter 4
Unintended pregnancy

Geraldine Barrett

Introduction

The concept of an unintended or unplanned pregnancy is relatively recent. Although methods of contraception have been known about since ancient times,[1] their use did not become common in most developed nations until the first part of the 20th century, leading to the fall in birth rates which characterises the 'demographic transition'.[2] The widespread use of highly effective artificial methods of contraception was a feature only of the latter part of the 20th century.[3] Contraception allows women and couples to choose if and when they begin a pregnancy and with this choice emerges the concept of an intended or planned pregnancy.

The desirability of planned pregnancies has been an accepted tenet of family planning and maternal and child health policy in Britain and elsewhere in the world for many years.[4-8] The assumption of such policy is that there are a number of costs to the individual and society from unintended pregnancies. Unintended pregnancies that result in abortion carry a financial cost to the healthcare system or the woman herself, as well as a potential personal and emotional cost and physical risk (albeit small, with legal abortion) to the woman. In Britain, there are about 190 000 abortions every year, comprising over one-fifth of all conceptions[9-11] and in the USA it has been estimated that approximately half of all unintended pregnancies end in abortion.[7] Further, women who have unplanned pregnancies which continue to term have fewer opportunities to benefit from preconceptual and early antenatal care (such as taking folic acid and giving up smoking) and there has been some evidence (albeit equivocal) linking unplanned pregnancies to poor infant outcomes.[7,12-16] More generally, unintended pregnancy has been taken as an indicator of the state of reproductive health[5,8,17,18] and in Britain this has most recently been restated in the English Strategy for HIV and Sexual Health[19] and the draft Scottish Sexual Health Strategy.[20]

The prominence of policy aims to reduce the number of unintended pregnancies has meant that there have been many attempts at measurement, varying from studies in which the concept is assumed to be self-evident to those in which more sophisticated measurement strategies have been used. In recent years, however, the concept of unintended pregnancy has undergone a re-evaluation and critical attention has been paid to its measurement. In this chapter I outline the ways in which national estimates of unintended pregnancy have been produced in the UK and USA and describe the latest developments relating to the measurement of pregnancy planning, including the development of a new British measure. I conclude by discussing the insights and implications that measurement of unintended pregnancy has for our approaches to fertility control.

National estimates of unintended pregnancy in Britain

The first national estimates of unintended pregnancy in Britain were by Ann Cartwright at the end of the 1960s. In a nationwide survey of new mothers (all of whom were married) she asked a question about reactions to pregnancy (Table 4.1). Pregnancies about which the mother was "sorry it happened at all" or "rather it happened a bit later" were classified as unintended.[21] Cartwright also included a question on contraceptive use around the time of conception and found that for each 'reaction to pregnancy' response category there were contraceptive users and non-users. In subsequent surveys, Cartwright added a further summative question (Table 4.1) on which estimates of unintended pregnancy were based.[22,23] The last estimates using Cartwright's questions were by Ann Fleissig in 1991, based on 1989 data, where 31% of live births were classified as unintended.[24] It was clear, however, that during the 1980s Ann Cartwright became more circumspect about the ability of her questions to elicit pregnancy intention status. In each survey, she had found evidence

Table 4.1. Ann Cartwright's questions

Study	Years	Survey information	Question
Cartwright[21]	1967–68	Included: 1495 women with a legitimate live birth Pregnancy status questions asked about most recent birth (5–7 months ago) and any previous legitimate births	'Apart from what you feel now – looking back to the time when you found you were pregnant – at the time, would you rather it happened a bit later or earlier or were you pleased when you were pregnant then or sorry it happened at all?' Pleased = planned Rather earlier = planned Rather later = mistimed (unplanned) Sorry ... at all = unwanted (unplanned)
Cartwright[22,23] Fleissig[24]	1973, 1984, 1989	Included: 1973: 1437 married women 1984: 1508 women (married and single) 1989: 1483 women (married and single) Pregnancy status question: 1973: legitimate live births 1984: all live births 1989: all live births	1) When you first found out you were pregnant, how did you feel about it then? Would you rather it had happened a bit later or were you pleased you were pregnant then, or sorry it had happened at all? 2) Around the time you became pregnant, were you or your husband or partner generally using a method of birth control? 3) So would you say you intended to become pregnant that time or not? Answer to question 3 defines unintended/unplanned (* question 1 in 1973 still included the 'rather it happened a bit earlier' category)

that there was no neat fit between 'reactions to pregnancy', contraceptive use and intention status, and concluded in 1988 "that 'intentions' seem somewhat indefinite for some couples".[23]

In the period of the 1970s and 1980s, Ann Cartwright's questions were the most influential by virtue of the fact that they were used most frequently but Margaret Bone and Karen Dunnell also made important contributions (Table 4.2),[25–27] the latter's work forming Britain's submission to the World Fertility Survey.[28] Karen Dunnell was also the first to ask unmarried women about the intention status of their pregnancies. Her questions are interesting in that they acknowledge that there might be pregnancies which were intended by the woman but not overtly planned by the couple or that a woman might not have any particular intentions. Unfortunately, in neither Dunnell's, Bone's nor Cartwright's studies is any description given of how the questions were developed or why particular categories were used and there is no evidence of qualitative or other empirical work being carried out to inform question development. To criticise, however, is not to diminish the importance of their contributions. The focus of their surveys was primarily on contraceptive use and family formation and the questions on pregnancy intention status were small parts of these surveys. At the time of the surveys, there were still high rates of birth within marriage and the majority of

Table 4.2. Bone's and Dunnell's questions

Study	Years	Survey information	Question
Bone[25,26]	1970, 1975	Included: 1970: 2520 married women aged 16–40 years and 974 single women aged 16–35 years 1975: 3898 ever married women aged 16–55 years and 749 single women aged 16–40 years Pregnancy status questions only asked of all legitimate births and current pregnancies	Long series of questions for each birth. From these questions, pregnancy status was defined on the following criteria: Planned: pregnancies where couples stopped contraception in order to have a child Unplanned: pregnancies that occurred before couples started using contraception Unplanned and accidental: pregnancies that occurred when couple 'took a chance' and pregnancies that occurred while the couple were using contraception Bone also uses Cartwright's (1970) question but calls this 'reactions to pregnancy'. Bone uses the 'sorry it happened at all' category to define 'unwanted' pregnancies
Dunnell[27]	1976	Included: 6589 women (married and single) aged 16–49 years Pregnancy status questions asked of all pregnancies (including live and stillbirths, miscarriages, abortions and current pregnancies)	'When you became pregnant that time would you say you were trying to get pregnant or not trying to get pregnant?' If not: 'Would you say then it was a complete accident, a kind of accident on purpose, or did you just not mind if you got pregnant?'

sexual activity took place within marriage. This made questioning more straight-forward as women tended to be in similar situations. Also, widespread free contraception only became available during the 1970s, the broad assumption being that unintended pregnancies occurred because of deficiencies in family planning services. The expectation that unintended pregnancies would decrease as women were given the tools with which to plan their pregnancies was reasonable. It is only with current knowledge that we can see that these expectations have not been met and it is now apparent that intentions, planning and decision making around pregnancy (and therefore measurement of pregnancy intention status) is likely to be more complicated.

In the 1990s, there were a number of calls for new methodological work on the measurement of pregnancy planning[4,29–31] and in 1998 we began a study to develop a new British measure[32,33] (discussed more fully below). Unfortunately, a recent national survey of women with live births, the Millennium Cohort Survey,[34] failed to capitalise on the new work on pregnancy planning or even to use Cartwright's older questions. Instead, when fieldwork was carried out with over 18 000 mothers in 2001/02, a single question was used, incorporating the term 'planned' (Were you planning to get pregnant or was it a surprise?), which is likely to be of limited validity.[32,35,36] As such, the survey represents a missed opportunity to provide new national prevalence estimates of unplanned pregnancy.

National estimates of unintended pregnancy in the USA

The USA has, by far, the most extensive history of attempts to measure pregnancy status and the experience there usefully augments that in Britain. National attempts to measure the intention status of pregnancies began in the 1950s with the Growth of American Families Survey, followed by the National Fertility Surveys and then, subsequently, the federally sponsored National Survey of Family Growth (NSFG).[7,37,38] There have been six rounds of the NSFG since the early 1970s and it is now the main source of estimates of unintended pregnancy for the USA. In the NSFG, pregnancy intention status is assessed by a series of questions on intentions and wantedness (Table 4.3). From these questions, women are allocated to specific categories of intended, mistimed, and unwanted:

● intended: intended at conception, i.e. wanted at that time or sooner (irrespective of contraceptive use)
● mistimed: conceptions that were wanted by the woman at some time but which occurred sooner than they were wanted (irrespective of contraceptive use)
● unwanted conceptions that occurred when the woman did not want to have any (more) pregnancies at all (irrespective of contraceptive use)

Mistimed and unwanted pregnancies are then classified as unintended pregnancies.[7] On this classification, the proportion of live births that resulted from an unintended pregnancy has, since 1973, ranged from 31% to 38%.[39–41]

The NSFG questions have been influential. For instance, most other US surveys that attempt to measure pregnancy intention status either include the NSFG questions or use questions based on the concepts of mistimed and unwanted.[13,16,42,43] In the World Fertility Survey in the 1970s and 1980s, the pregnancy intention status questions included in the core module (which was used in most countries) were also closely related to the NSFG questions.[28,44] The World Fertility Survey questions have continued to be used in the Demographic and Health Surveys which have been run since

Table 4.3. US National Survey of Family Growth

Study	Years	Survey information	Question
National Survey of Family Growth	Cycle I: 1973 Cycle II: 1976 Cycle III: 1982 Cycle IV: 1988 Cycle V: 1995 Cycle VI: 2002	Included: women of ages 15–44years: Ever-married women for cycles I and II, all women after that Women were asked about births up to 5 years before survey (interviews)	1) Was the reason you (were not/had stopped) using any method of contraception because you, yourself, wanted to become pregnant? (yes/no) 2) At the time you became pregnant, did you, yourself actually want to have a(nother) baby at some time? (yes/no/ don't know) 3) It is sometimes difficult to recall these things but, just before that pregnancy began, would you say you probably wanted a(nother) baby at *some* time or probably not? 4) Did you become pregnant sooner than you wanted, later than you wanted, or at about the right time? (Sooner/ later/right time/didn't care) Additional questions added in 1995: 5) (for unwanted pregnancies) So when you became pregnant, you thought you did not want to have any children *at any time in your life*, is that correct? 6) (for mistimed pregnancies) How much sooner than you wanted did you become pregnant? (Answers recorded in months or years) Additional questions added in 2002: 7) (for intended pregnancies) Right before (the/this/that) pregnancy, did you want to have a(nother) baby with that partner? Definitely yes/probably yes/probably no/definitely no 8) (for mistimed or unwanted pregnancies) Right before (the/this/that) pregnancy, did you think you might ever want to have a(nother) baby with that partner? Definitely yes/probably yes/probably no

1984 by ORC Macro, funded by the US Agency for International Development.[45-47] The Demographic and Health Surveys are now the main source of data for the international family planning movement.

Despite the well-established nature of the NSFG (and related) questions, there has been a growing awareness of their limitations, resulting in a number of commentaries and methodological studies in the last few years by the NSFG survey organisers and others.[17,35,48-58] Concern about the NSFG questions began after the 1988 survey, when a large proportion of teenage women seemed to be indicating that their pregnancies were unwanted (i.e. they had never wanted children). Further investigation showed that this was due to a lack of understanding of the questions.[48,49] Further questions of clarification were added to the 1995 and 2002 surveys to try to improve validity of the question module (Table 4.3). The NSFG survey organisers and others have also examined questions on related topics, such as ambivalence about pregnancy and happiness with becoming pregnant, in order to explore their relationship with the NSFG intendedness categories.[17,53,55] Unsurprisingly, no neat fit between concepts was found. Trussell *et al.*,[17] for instance, described (in a manner reminiscent of Ann Cartwright) some of the inconsistencies: 'Women with contraceptive failures classified as intended pregnancies almost never reported being unhappy or very unhappy with that pregnancy, and 90% said they were happy or very happy. These results are consistent with one another, but it is still not clear why these women were practicing contraception. On the other hand, although a majority (59%) of women with contraceptive failures classified as unintended pregnancies reported being unhappy or very unhappy, 25% said they were happy or very happy.

One of the problems with the NSFG questions has been that they were developed for use with married women (in an era of no legal abortion and higher marital stability), when concern was greatest about excess fertility at the end of family building. The difficulties of knowing lifetime reproductive preferences have been exacerbated over time with the move to more fluid patterns of relationship and family formation. As the NSFG intendedness concepts are so well established in the USA, it has been difficult for US researchers to move away from them, despite the evidence about their limitations. Even those who have carried out innovative work have related their new ideas to the NSFG concepts.[54,57] So far only one North American team has suggested a different form of measurement.[56]

Development of a British measure of unplanned pregnancy

When we began the study to develop a new British measure of pregnancy planning and intention, it was clear that it was not only the measurement of unintended pregnancy that needed to be reconsidered but also the concept itself. Also, to make good the deficiencies of previous questions and to capitalise on advances in research methodology, lay understandings of unintended pregnancy needed to be taken into account. Pregnancies ending in abortion needed to be included and psychometric techniques of measure development needed to be employed. We therefore developed a study design which incorporated all these elements.[32,33] The main aim of the study was to develop a measure of unplanned pregnancy which is valid, reliable and appropriate in the context of contemporary demographic trends and social mores and can be used to establish population estimates of unplanned pregnancy. We used a two-stage study design: firstly, qualitative methods in order to delineate the construct of pregnancy planning and intention; and, secondly, quantitative and psychometric methods to establish the means of measurement. Data collection took place across

CONTEXT

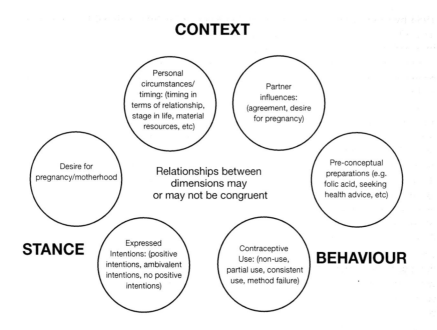

Figure 4.1. Conceptual model of pregnancy planning and unplanned pregnancy

eight health service providers (comprising 14 clinics, including antenatal, abortion and one general practitioner) across London, Edinburgh, Hertfordshire, Salisbury, and Southampton.

The study began with qualitative in-depth interviews with 47 women to explore their accounts of the circumstances in which they became pregnant and to find out if and how they used terms such as 'planned', 'unplanned', 'unintended', 'unwanted'. We found that women tended not to use the terms spontaneously and, when offered them, did not interpret or define the terms in any consistent way.[36] There was great variety in women's accounts of the circumstances of their pregnancies. A conceptual model was built to represent this, based on the key elements of the interviews, through which an understanding of women's experiences could be gained. The conceptual model has six dimensions: expressed intentions, desire for pregnancy and motherhood, contraceptive use, preconceptual preparations, personal circumstances and timing, and partner influences. These, in turn, fall into three domains: stances, behaviour and context (Figure 4.1). In keeping with the complexity of women's accounts, each dimension of the model represents a number of positions (positive, ambivalent, negative) and a feature of the model is that it does not assume, or require, congruence between the dimensions of the domains.

Twenty women who continued their pregnancies to term were re-interviewed after the births of their babies so that we could examine the stability of their accounts over time. Stability relating to the dimensions of the conceptual model was high. The conceptual model was then used to inform the item development at the quantitative stage of the project and the items were pre-tested with 26 women using qualitative/

cognitive techniques to check understanding. A field test with 390 women was carried out and psychometric techniques were used for item analysis and selection. The resulting set of items was then tested in a second field test with 651 women. Psychometric evaluation demonstrated the measure's high internal consistency (Cronbach's alpha greater than 0.90), high stability (test–retest coefficient greater than 0.90), and excellent face, content and construct validity.

A self-completion measure of pregnancy planning and intention is now ready for use with British women (Appendix 4.1). Compared with previous questions used to assess pregnancy planning, the measure has a number of advantages:

- it makes no assumptions about the nature of women's relationships
- it does not rely on women having fully formed childbearing plans
- it does not assume a particular form of family building
- it is suitable for use with any pregnancy regardless of outcome (i.e. continued pregnancy, miscarriage, abortion).

Also, because of its conceptual basis, the measure does not presume that women have clearly defined intentions and behaviour in accordance with their intentions. The measure is short (only six items) and field testing demonstrated that it was highly acceptable (i.e. easy to understand, inoffensive and quick to complete), attributes which make the measure suitable for use in large-scale surveys and other research studies.

The range of positions that women have in relation to pregnancy planning are represented by the measure's range of scores, from 0 to 12 (a higher score indicating a greater degree of intention/planning). These scores provide more sophisticated information about pregnancy planning than has been previously available with the dichotomous categories of planned and unplanned. For instance, it can be seen in

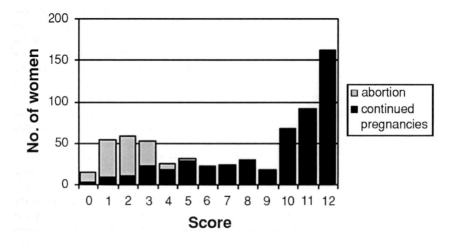

Figure 4.2. Scores according to outcome of pregnancy

Figure 4.2 that approximately 25% of the women in the study fell into the middle 'ambivalent' part of the scale. Of the women whose pregnancies ended in abortion, 9% had a score of 4 or higher (indicating that they had a degree of ambivalence or positive intention prior to their pregnancy) and of the women who continued their pregnancies to term, 36% had scores lower than 10 (indicating less than high levels of planning/intention).

How can a new measure of unintended pregnancy benefit fertility control in the UK?

A new measure of pregnancy planning/intention can provide us with a more accurate understanding of the circumstances surrounding women's conceptions and therefore help us to make better informed and more sophisticated judgements about strategies for preventing unintended pregnancies. Currently, rates of abortion and teenage pregnancy tend to be used as proxy measures of unintended pregnancy. Data from the development study showed that some abortions were preceded by ambivalent or positive intentions and that a number of teenage pregnancies were intended. These proxy measures are therefore insufficiently sensitive and specific to provide true estimates of unintended pregnancy. The pregnancies of women who are ambivalent (or indeed positive) about conception are unlikely to be prevented by improvements to contraceptive services and we should not consider such pregnancies to be failures of the family planning system. A better understanding of the risk factors for unintended pregnancy at different stages in the reproductive life course would enable us to target contraceptive services more effectively. We may also be able to learn which groups of women might benefit from interventions other than those related to contraceptive advice and provision. Further, by looking at the long-term outcomes of unintended pregnancies that continue to term, we may be able to tell if there are indeed negative consequences for these children and their mothers.

At the macro level, information produced by the measure could be used to help evaluate the impact of policy. For instance, a current aim of the Strategy for Sexual Health and HIV is to reduce rates of unintended pregnancy.[19] At the same time, the Strategy is supporting a programme of work to increase the accessibility of abortion services. While there is no conflict between these two objectives, it is possible that, without comprehensive data on unintended pregnancy (i.e. without monitoring women whose unintended pregnancies continue to term), an increase in the abortion rate (caused by the increased accessibility of abortion services) could be interpreted as a failure to reduce unintended pregnancies when, in fact, all that has happened is that fewer unintended pregnancies are being continued to term. Monitoring the levels of unintended pregnancy among women whose pregnancies result in birth would provide a more complete understanding of abortion rates. In the same vein, such monitoring would also aid our understanding of teenage conceptions, relevant to the Teenage Pregnancy Strategy.[59]

At the individual level, the measure may also be suitable for use in clinical consultations. Clinicians often have reason to ask pregnant women about the planning status of their pregnancies, for instance in antenatal clinics and abortion services and in some services the answers are recorded systematically for all women. Where this happens, there may be value in substituting the measure (which women can fill in prior to consultation, in the waiting room if necessary), thus providing a ready summary of the planning status of a woman's pregnancy for the consulting clinician. The recorded scores would also provide useful intelligence at the service level. An evaluation of the use of the measure in clinical practice would, however, need to be carried out first in order to check that the measure:

- remains valid when answers are not anonymous but are shared with clinic staff
- provides information above and beyond that which clinicians ordinarily collect in the consultation.

Indications from the validation study suggest that women are mainly worried about information about them being known outside a service, rather than shared within it, which augurs well for possible clinical use.

Finally, further methodological work on unplanned pregnancy, building on developments so far, is desirable. Clinicians involved in fertility control are primarily concerned with preventing unplanned pregnancies among the nonpregnant women that they see, yet the measure of unplanned pregnancy that has been recently developed relates to pregnancies that have already occurred (that is, the pregnancies of currently pregnant or recently pregnant, women). The logical next step from this work, therefore, is to develop a measure that identifies women at risk of an unplanned pregnancy, designed specifically for use in clinical practice

Conclusion

The history of the measurement of unintended pregnancy has consistently shown over many years that, for a proportion of women, pregnancy intentions, feelings about pregnancy and contraceptive behaviour are not consistent, yet it has only been recently that measurement of the construct of unintended pregnancy has been reassessed in light of this. The new British measure, with its conceptual basis, represents a clear break with the forms of measurement found in the previous (and some current) British surveys and the current US and Demographic and Health Surveys. As such, the measure avoids the assumption that members of modern (post-demographic transition) societies are universally rational and instrumental in terms of their fertility decisions and control: an assumption that some have seen as characterising research on fertility and fertility change in the 20th century.[2,60] Instead, the measure permits representation of a range of positions (for example, actions congruent with intentions, actions inconsistent with intentions, ambivalence in fertility intentions and actions), thereby providing a more complex and realistic portrayal of human fertility behaviour than existing questions. We need to use the data that the measure can produce to increase our understanding of which women experience unintended pregnancies and why.

References

1. McLaren A. *A History of Contraception: From Antiquity to the Present Day*. London: Blackwell; 1990.
2. Szreter S. *Fertility, Class and Gender in Britain, 1860–1940*. Cambridge: Cambridge University Press; 1996.
3. Weeks J. *Sex, Politics and Society: the Regulation of Sexuality since 1800*. London: Longman; 1989.
4. Royal College of Obstetricians and Gynaecologists. *Report of the RCOG Working Party on Unplanned Pregnancy*. RCOG: London; 1991.
5. Department of Health. *The Health of the Nation*. London: HMSO; 1992.
6. UNICEF. *The Progress of Nations: the nations of the world ranked according to their achievements in health, nutrition, education, family planning, and progress for women*. New York: UNICEF; 1993.
7. Brown SS, Eisenberg L, editors. *The Best Intentions: Unintended Pregnancy and the Well-Being of Children and Families*. Washington: National Academy Press; 1995.

8.   Lee PR, Stewart FH. Failing to prevent unintended pregnancy is costly. *Am J Public Health* 1995;85:479–80.

9.   Office for National Statistics. *Birth Statistics: Review of the Registrar General on births and patterns of family building in England and Wales, 2002.* Series FM1 no. 31. London: Stationery Office; 2004.

10. Government Statistical Service, Department of Health. *Abortion Statistics, England and Wales: 2002 Statistical Bulletin 2003/23.* London: Stationery Office; 2003, revised 2004.

11. Information and Statistics Division of NHS in Scotland. Abortion data. May 2004 [www.isdscotland.org].

12. Fergusson DM, Horwood LJ. Childhood disadvantage and the planning of pregnancy. *Soc Sci Med* 1983;17:1223–7.

13. Baydar N. Consequences for children of their birth planning status. *Fam Plan Perspect* 1995;27:228–34, 245.

14. Montgomery MR, Lloyd CB, Hewett PC, Heuveline P. *The Consequences of Imperfect Fertility Control on Children's Survival, Health, and Schooling.* Analytical Report 7. Calverton, MD: Macro International Inc; 1997.

15. Sable MR, Spencer JC, Stockbauer JW, Schramm WF, Howell V, Herman AA. Pregnancy wantedness and adverse pregnancy outcomes: differences by race and medicaid status. *Fam Plan Perspect* 1997;29:76–81.

16. Joyce TJ, Kaestner R, Korenman S. The effect of pregnancy intention on child development. *Demography* 2000;37:83–94.

17. Trussell J, Vaughan B, Stanford J. Are all contraceptive failures unintended pregnancies? Evidence from the 1995 National Survey of Family Growth. *Fam Plan Perspect* 1999;31:246–7, 260.

18. Cates W, Spieler J. Contraception, unintended pregnancies, and sexually transmitted infections: still no simple solutions. *Sex Transm Dis* 2001;28:552–4.

19. Department of Health. *The National Strategy for Sexual Health and HIV.* London: DH; 2001.

20. Scottish Executive. *Enhancing Sexual Wellbeing in Scotland: A Sexual Health and Relationships Strategy: Proposal to the Scottish Executive.* Edinburgh: Scottish Executive Health Department; 2003.

21. Cartwright A. *Parents and Family Planning Services.* London: Routledge Kegan Paul; 1970.

22. Cartwright A. *How Many Children?* London: Routledge and Kegan Paul; 1976.

23. Cartwright A. Unintended pregnancies that lead to babies. *Soc Sci Med* 1988;27:249–54.

24. Fleissig A. Unintended pregnancies and the use of contraception: changes from 1984 to 1989. *BMJ* 1991;302:147.

25. Bone M. *Family Planning Services in England and Wales.* London: HMSO; 1973.

26. Bone M. *The Family Planning Services: changes and effects.* London: Department of Health and Social Security; 1978.

27. Dunnell K. *Family Formation 1976.* London: HMSO; 1979.

28. United Nations. *Fertility Behaviour in the Context of Development: Evidence from the World Fertility Survey.* Population Studies, no. 100. New York: United Nations; 1987.

29. Faculty of Public Health Medicine. *UK Levels of Health.* London: FPHM; 1991.

30. Wellings K. *Report of the HEA's Expert Working Group on Teenage Motherhood and Lone Parenthood.* London: Health Education Authority; 1997.

31. Newman M, Bardsley M, Morgan D, Jacobson B. *Contraception and Abortion Services in London.* London: The Health of Londoners Project; 1997.

32. Barrett G. Developing a measure of unplanned pregnancy. PhD thesis. University of London; 2002.

33. Barrett G, Smith SC, Wellings K. Conceptualisation, development and evaluation of a measure of unplanned pregnancy. *J Epidemiol Community Health* 2004;58:426–33.

34. Dex S, Joshi H, editors. *Millennium Cohort Survey First Survey: A User's Guide to Initial Findings.* London: Institute of Education, University of London; 2004.

35. Fischer RC, Stanford JB, Jameson P, DeWitt MJ. Exploring the concepts of intended, planned, and wanted pregnancy. *J Fam Pract* 1999;48:117–22.

36. Barrett G, Wellings K. What is a "planned" pregnancy? Empirical data from a British study. *Soc Sci Med* 2002;55:545–57.

37. Freedman R, Whelpton PK, Campbell AA. *Family Planning Sterility and Population Growth.* New York, NY: McGraw Hill; 1959.

38. Ryder NB, Westoff CF. *Reproduction in the United States, 1965.* New Jersey: Princeton University Press; 1971.

39. Williams LB. Determinants of unintended childbearing among ever-married women in the United States: 1973-1988. *Fam Plan Perspect* 1991;23:212–15.

40. Henshaw SK. Unintended pregnancy in the United States. *Fam Plan Perspect* 1998;30:24–9, 46.

41. Abma JC, Martinez GM, Mosher WD, Dawson BS. Teenagers in the United States: Sexual activity, contraceptive use, and childbearing, 2002. National Center for Health Statistics. *Vital Health Stat* 2004;23(24).

42. Kost K, Landry DJ, Darroch JE. Predicting maternal behaviors during pregnancy: does intention status matter? *Fam Plan Perspect* 1998;30:79–88.
43. Dietz PM, Adams MM, Spitz AM, Morris L, Johnson CH, PRAMS Working Group. Live births resulting from unintended pregnancies: is there variation among States? *Fam Plan Perspect* 1999;31:132–6.
44. Cleland J, Scott C. *The World Fertility Survey: an Assessment*. Oxford: Oxford University Press; 1987.
45. Westoff CF. *Reproductive Preferences: A Comparative View*. DHS Comparative Studies, no. 3. Columbia, MD: Institute for Resource Development; 1991.
46. Macro International. *Model 'A' Questionnaire, with commentary for high contraceptive prevalence countries*. Demographic and health Surveys, phase 3, number 1. Calverton, MD: Macro International Inc; 1995.
47. Macro International. *Model 'B' Questionnaire, with commentary for low contraceptive prevalence countries*. Demographic and health Surveys, phase 3, number 2. Calverton, MD: Macro International Inc; 1995.
48. London K, Peterson L, Piccinino L. The National Survey of Family Growth: principal source of statistics on unintended pregnancy: supplement to chapter two. In: Brown SS, Eisenberg L, editors. *The Best Intentions: Unintended Pregnancy and the Well-Being of Children and Families*. Washington DC: National Academy Press; 1995.
49. Kaufmann RB, Morris L, Spitz AM. Comparison of two question sequences for assessing pregnancy intentions. *Am J Epidemiol* 1997;145:810–16.
50. Moos MK, Petersen R, Meadows K, Melvin CL, Spitz AM. Pregnant women's perspectives on intendedness of pregnancy. *Womens Health Issues* 1997;7:385–92.
51. Luker K. Contraceptive failure and unintended pregnancy: a reminder that human behavior frequently refuses to conform to models created by researchers. *Fam Plan Perspect* 1999;31:248–9.
52. Zabin LS. Contraceptive failure and unintended pregnancy: ambivalent feelings about parenthood may lead to inconsistent contraceptive use - and pregnancy. *Fam Plan Perspect* 1999;31:250–1.
53. Piccinino L, Peterson LS. Ambivalent attitudes and unintended pregnancy. In: Severy LJ, Miller W, editors. *Advances in Population: Psychosocial Perspectives, Volume 3*. Philadelphia, PA: Jessica Kingsley Publishers; 1999.
54. Stanford JB, Hobbs R, Jameson P, DwWitt J, Fischer RC. Defining dimensions of pregnancy intendedness. *Matern Child Health J* 2000;4:183–9.
55. Sable MR, Libbus MK. Pregnancy intention and pregnancy happiness: are they different? *Matern Child Health J* 2000;4:191–6.
56. Morin P, Payette H, Moos MK, St-Cyr-Tribble D, Niyonsenga T, De Wals P. Measuring the intensity of pregnancy planning effort. *Paediatr Perinat Epidemiol* 2003;17:97–105.
57. Speizer IS, Santelli JS, Afable-Munsuz A, Kendall C. Measuring factors underlying intendedness of women's first and later pregnancies. *Perspect Sex Reprod Health* 2004;36:198–205.
58. Kendall C, Afable-Munsuz A, Speizer I, Avery A, Schmidt N, Santelli J. Understanding pregnancy in a population of inner-city women in New Orleans: results of qualitative research. *Soc Sci Med* 2005;60:297–311.
59. Social Exclusion Unit. *Teenage Pregnancy*. London: HMSO; 1999.
60. Fisher K. Uncertain aims and tacit negotiation: birth control practices in Britain, 1925-50. *Popul Dev Rev* 2000;26:295–31.

Appendix 4.1

The London self-completion measure of unplanned pregnancy

CIRCUMSTANCES OF PREGNANCY

Below are some questions that ask about your circumstances and feelings around the time you became pregnant. Please think of your current (or most recent) pregnancy when answering the questions below.

Scoring: 1) In the month that I became pregnant...
   (Please tick the statement which <u>most</u> applies to you):

2   ☐ I/we were not using contraception

1   ☐ I/we were using contraception, but not on every occasion

1   ☐ I/we always used contraception, but knew that the method had failed (i.e. broke, moved, came off, came out, not worked etc) at least once

0   ☐ I/we always used contraception

2) In terms of becoming a mother *(first time or again)*, I feel that my pregnancy happened at the...
   (Please tick the statement which <u>most</u> applies to you):

2   ☐ right time

1   ☐ OK, but not quite right time

0   ☐ wrong time

3) Just <u>before</u> I became pregnant...
   (Please tick the statement which <u>most</u> applies to you):

2   ☐ I intended to get pregnant

1   ☐ my intentions kept changing

0   ☐ I did not intend to get pregnant

4) Just <u>before</u> I became pregnant...

(Please tick the statement which <u>most</u> applies to you):

2   ☐ I wanted to have a baby

1   ☐ I had mixed feelings about having a baby

0   ☐ I did not want to have a baby

In the next question, we ask about your partner: this might be (or have been) your husband, a partner you live with, a boyfriend, or someone you've had sex with once or twice.

5) <u>Before</u> I became pregnant...

(Please tick the statement which <u>most</u> applies to you):

2   ☐ My partner and I had agreed that we would like me to be pregnant

1   ☐ My partner and I had discussed having children together, but hadn't agreed for me to get pregnant

0   ☐ We never discussed having children together

6) <u>Before</u> you became pregnant, did you do anything to improve your health <u>in preparation for pregnancy</u>?

(Please tick <u>all</u> that apply)

       ☐ Took folic acid

       ☐ Stopped or cut down smoking

2 = 2 or   ☐ Stopped or cut down drinking alcohol
more actions
1 = 1 action   ☐ Ate more healthily

       ☐ Sought medical/health advice

       ☐ Took some other action, please describe _____

or

0   ☐ I did not do any of the above **before** my pregnancy   ☐

Chapter 5
Women's need for abortion in Britain

Ellie Lee

Introduction

Abortion is a commonplace experience for British women and it has become increasingly so. The trend has been towards a rising abortion rate, particularly for women in their early 20s (Tables 5.1 and 5.2), while important recent innovations in policy and practice suggest growing acceptance of women's need for abortion.[1-5]

The absence of any decline in demand for abortion remains a source of controversy. Media coverage of the release of abortion statistics is guaranteed and its tone mostly is to bemoan the fact that abortion rates continue to increase. The question often asked is: why, when contraception is accessible and the promotion of its use forms a significant part of sexual health policy, do women still experience unwanted pregnancy and seek abortion? How could this be the case for a greater proportion of women than previously?

More controversial still is a particular aspect of the demand for abortion – that for abortion procedures later in pregnancy. In 2004, disquiet about 'late abortion' arose, when it became the subject of intense and extensive media debate. "I still support it",

Table 5.1. Abortions, all women, England and Wales (source: National Statistics 2004)

Year	Number (1000s)	Percentage aborted	Age-standardised rate/1000 residents
1976	129.7	–	10.2
1981	162.5	–	11.9
1986	172.3	–	13.0
1991	179.5	19.4	15.0
1996	177.5	20.8	16.0
1997	179.7	21.3	16.3
1998	187.4	22.3	17.2
1999	183.2	22.6	16.8
2000	185.4	22.7	17.0
2001	186.3	23.3	17.1
2002	185.4	22.5	17.0
2003	190.7	–	17.5

Coventry University

Table 5.2. Abortion rates per 1000 residents by age, England and Wales (source: National Statistics 2004)

Year	Age (years)						
	Under 16	**16–19**	**20–24**	**25–29**	**30–34**	**35–44**	**45 and over**
1976	3.4	24.0	23.6	19.3	14.6	14.7	0.5
1981	3.5	31.4	34.3	21.9	18.7	17.6	0.6
1986	3.9	33.8	45.3	28.7	18.0	17.5	0.4
1991	3.2	31.1	52.7	38.6	23.4	17.9	0.4
1996	3.6	28.8	46.4	39.3	28.2	21.1	0.4
1997	3.4	29.9	45.0	40.2	28.9	22.3	0.5
1998	3.8	33.2	45.8	40.4	30.4	23.8	0.5
1999	3.6	32.8	45.0	38.5	29.1	24.1	0.5
2000	3.7	33.2	47.1	37.9	28.7	24.4	0.5
2001	3.7	33.4	48.3	36.5	28.8	25.2	0.5
2002	3.7	33.0	48.4	35.8	28.5	26.0	0.5
2003	3.7	33.4	48.3	36.5	28.8	25.2	0.5

commented *Sunday Times* journalist Jasper Gerard, of the British abortion law. "But as my wife prepares to give birth, just thinking of an abortion makes me shudder".[6] Many journalists appeared similarly to express almost total incomprehension, verging on revulsion, when commenting on abortion performed in the second trimester of pregnancy, especially late in the second trimester.

This chapter responds to such disquiet about abortion by explaining why women seek abortion. Since 'late' abortion has emerged as a particular issue of debate, I begin by briefly discussing the reasons for this aspect of demand for abortion in Britain. I then consider women's need for abortion more generally, assessing the relationship between contraceptive use and abortion. Finally, I consider trends in fertility, and explanations for them, on the grounds that these trends may help to contextualise current demand for abortion in Britain.

'Late' abortion

Almost 90% of abortions occur in the first 12 weeks of pregnancy.[7] Given that most women will not even realise they are pregnant until they have missed at least one period, this suggests that women generally act very quickly indeed to resolve unwanted pregnancies. Regardless of the impression that might be given by the controversy about it, demand for 'late abortion' remains quite low and relatively stable.

From 1985 to 2002, the percentage of all abortions that were performed after 20 weeks remained fairly static. The proportion carried out between 13 and 19 weeks changed little: from 10% (16 709) in 1985 to 12% (19 328) in 2002. The proportion carried out at 20+ weeks is less than 2% of the total number of terminations. In 1985, there were 141 101 abortions, of which 2116 were performed at 20+ weeks. In 2002, the figures were 175 932 and 2874, respectively.[7] Yet however small the rates, the question must still be asked, why do these abortions take place at this gestational stage?

Some of the incidence of late abortion can be accounted for by delays confronting women who have requested abortion at a much earlier gestational stage.[8] Research evidence suggests that women's need for late abortion is not, primarily at least, a function of whether women have speedy access to early abortion services.[9] Diagnosis of fetal abnormality, which occurs during (and sometimes late during) the second trimester, accounts for some of the demand, although more than 60% of the approximately 2000 terminations for fetal abnormality that occur annually take place before the end of the 19th week of pregnancy.[10]

Two other main categories of reasons for late abortions can be identified. The first comprises women who fail to recognise their pregnancy earlier because of irregular, infrequent periods, failed contraception (particularly with methods that can cause amenorrhoea or irregular bleeding) and denial of pregnancy (sometimes associated with occasional episodes of bleeding that are interpreted as menstruation). The second category is made up of women who know that they are pregnant but delay seeking abortion because of indecision, apprehension (difficulty in confiding in parents or partner), failure of anticipated emotional or economic support (from family, partner, and employer) and unanticipated change in socio-economic circumstances.[8]

In all these cases, women may not request abortion until their pregnancy is relatively advanced, sometimes well into the second trimester, as the following extracts from a study of women requesting 'late' abortion[11] indicate.

Age 17 years; abortion at 20 weeks
"Cause I started on the pill about the end of August … I'd never been on the pill before, you're never quite sure about it and I didn't know what to expect anyway … When I'd been to the GP I'd worked out I was two months pregnant … then I went in to have the internal examination [at consultation] … he was like, 'well actually … you're more like four and a half months pregnant' … and I hadn't known, 'cause I hadn't been having my periods normally."

Age 17 years; pregnancy confirmed at 8 weeks, abortion at 19 weeks
"I told my partner … he seemed all right with it as well. But then I started getting mixed feelings about whether or not I should keep it and I started coming up with all the reasons in my head … it's happened to my mum before and my mum's got seven kids, so … I just thought 'I can't bring a child into the world the way things are at the moment, 'cause I ain't working, I'm still at home, I've got no support or nothing' … it's from there it started to change."[11]

Women who terminate pregnancies late are not, as some media coverage has implied, a 'different breed' to those who do so earlier on. The most distinctive feature of such women is that they tend to be of younger age. In 2002, 3.1% of abortions to women aged under 16 years and 2.2% of abortions to women aged 16–19 years were performed at 20+ weeks (2.3% of all abortions to all women aged under 20 years) compared with 1.4% for those aged 30–39 years.[7] As discussed above, their route into late abortion is characterised by experiences that mean they do not request abortion until relatively late in gestation, for reasons largely beyond their control. They may, for example, experience unforeseen difficulties in their personal relationships. Like many women who have abortions, some find contraceptive availability and use has not allowed them to prevent unwanted pregnancy, and it is to this experience more generally that we now turn.

Contraceptive use and abortion

Some analyses of the relationship between contraception and abortion suppose that the abortion rate will be highly sensitive to levels of contraceptive use and efficacy and that, over time, a situation will emerge whereby contraception will largely enable women to manage their fertility.[12-16] Demand for abortion will fall to zero, it is argued, 'only in the "perfect contraceptive population", in which women are protected by absolutely effective contraceptive use at all times, expect for the relative short periods when they want to conceive'. Since this population does not exist, there is always a 'residual demand for abortion', the extent of which is contingent on levels of contraceptive use and choice of methods.[16]

Contraceptive use has thus been viewed as tending to lead to a reduced demand for abortion, although that demand will never fall to zero. A parallel increase in both the abortion rate and contraceptive use appears to confound such expectations and has therefore been the subject of specific investigation. The conclusion has been drawn that a rise in abortion and in use of contraception may exist, where contraceptive use alone is insufficient to meet a growing need for fertility regulation, when fertility is falling rapidly.[16] An increased use of abortion and of contraception at the start of the shift from high to low fertility[12] is a phenomenon presented as an aspect of 'fertility transition'. High demand for abortion for this reason has been seen as especially relevant for the developing world. Countries in which this aspect of 'fertility transition' has been clearly identified include Cuba, between 1967 and 1985,[16] and South Korea, from 1963 to 1979,[16] yet a similar pattern is also identifiable at particular points in time in Denmark, the Netherlands and the USA. In these instances, a rise in the incidence of abortion was then followed by decline (in the early 1970s in the Netherlands, the mid-1970s in Denmark and early 1980s in the USA).[12]

Discussion of trends for Britain does not feature specifically in most commentaries about the relationship between contraception and abortion. Given that contraception is easily available, the general hypothesis outlined above may imply that the abortion rate should be low. Yet, while it might be predicated on the basis of statistical models that contraceptive availability should reduce demand for abortion in Britain, evidence points to a rather different picture of 'real life'.

British women's accounts of their reasons for seeking abortion indicate that they cannot manage their fertility solely by means of contraceptive use. A survey of more than 2000 women requesting abortion at clinics run by the British Pregnancy Advisory Service, Britain's largest specialist abortion provider, found that almost 60% of women claimed to have been using contraception at the time they became pregnant and nearly 20% said they were on the pill.[17] Other studies have shown similar results.[18]

The number of women who claim they experienced a split or slipped condom or that they had missed only one or two pills is undoubtedly inflated. Unprotected sex resulting in unplanned pregnancy is a source of stigma[19] and some women requesting abortion may falsely claim to have used contraception, believing that they will be treated more sympathetically if the pregnancy is 'not their fault'.[20] Even so, it is clear that contraceptives let couples down. All methods of contraception have a recognised failure rate.[21,22] Even older couples sometimes fail to use contraception effectively and efficiently, despite greater experience of contraceptive use.[20] Pregnancies that occur because the condom split or because the couple failed to get it out of the packet are thus both aspects of the experience of the tens of thousands of women who seek abortion each year, who are primarily not inexperienced teenagers.

This suggests that many British women seek abortion despite having tried to use, or having used, contraception but have become pregnant regardless. It is necessary to take full account of the realities of sexual interactions and use of contraception in order to understand women's need for abortion. Unplanned pregnancy is a 'fact of life' for British women, regardless of contraceptive availability[17] and this must form the starting point for any discussion of the demand for abortion. Yet such factors do not fully account for increases in the abortion rate in Britain.

Outcomes associated with contraception, for example the effects of the 'pill panic' of the mid-1990s, have been discussed as explanations for the increase in women resorting to abortion in the 1990s.[23] The demand for abortion has, however, either remained stable or has increased since the 'pill panic', suggesting the need for further explanation. The concept of a 'second demographic transition' (a social trend characterised by postponement of first births and low total fertility, together with the rise of cohabitation, the postponement of marriage, the decrease in marriage rates and rise in divorce, and an increase in nonmarital births) may help in this regard.[24]

The 'second demographic transition'

Changes to birth rates, as set out in Table 5.3, constitute a noteworthy development of the past 40 years,[25] with those of the 1990s being the subject of a great deal of both scholarly and more popular discussion.[26-28] Figures for 2003 show the highest number of births since 1999 (621 469 births), giving an annual increase of 4.3%.[29] It is too early to know whether this constitutes a longer-term trend. It does not diminish the age-specific pattern, which is of a decline in fertility among women in their 20s and an increase, although less sizeable, in the birth rate to those aged 35 years and over.

The decline in fertility among women in their early 20s is a long-term trend, evident since the mid-1960s. For women in their late 20s, a trend to declining fertility is more recent, dating from the late 1980s. In general, fertility rates for older women have increased over the same period of time. The age group in which women are most likely to give birth is still 25–29 years but, since 1992, those aged 30–34 years have been more likely to give birth than those aged 20–24 years. As a result, age of first birth has risen considerably.[30] The mean age of mothers at first birth in 1971 was 24.0 years, in 1984 it was 27.0 years and in 1999 it was 29.4 years. The trend is towards not only delayed motherhood but also to childlessness.[31] There has been an increase in the proportion of women remaining childless in each age cohort born since 1950. Proportions of women who would have no children at 40 years stood at 9% in 1986 but had risen to 19% in 1998. Projections from the Office for National Statistics suggest that about 23% of women born after 1972 will be childless when they reach 45 years of age.[30]

For an increasing proportion of women, therefore, motherhood is either marginal throughout their lives or for a longer period than before. How can we understand these fertility patterns? What explanations have been offered for them and what effect do they have on the demand for abortion?

Childlessness

As noted above, childlessness has become a specific subject of discussion, particularly the extent to which childlessness may be understood as 'voluntary'.[24,25,32] Childlessness resulting from an active choice based on negative views towards having children has been found to exist at lower levels than might be expected across Europe.[32] Fewer than

Table 5.3. Live births (*n*, 1000s)/age-specific fertility rates (source: National Statistics 2004)[47]

Year	Age of mother at birth (years)						
	All	**< 20**	**20–24**	**25–29**	**30–34**	**35–39**	**40+**
1961	811.3/89.2	59.8/37.3	249.8/172.6	248.5/176.9	152.3/103.1	77.5/48.1	23.3/15.0
1966	849.8/90.5	86.7/47.7	285.8/176.0	253.7/174.0	136.4/97.3	67.0/45.3	20.1/12.5
1971	783.2/83.5	82.6/50.6	285.7/152.9	247.2/153.2	109.6/77.1	45.2/32.8	12.7/8.7
1976	584.3/60.4	57.9/32.2	182.2/109.3	220.7/118.7	90.8/57.2	26.1/18.6	6.5/4.8
1981	634.5/61.3	56.6/28.1	194.5/105.3	215.8/129.1	126.6/68.6	34.2/21.7	6.9/4.9
1986	661.0/60.6	57.4/30.1	192.1/92.7	229.0/123.8	129.5/78.0	45.5/24.6	7.6/4.8
1991	699.2/63.6	52.4/33.0	173.4/89.3	248.7/119.4	161.3/86.7	53.6/32.1	9.8/5.3
1992	689.7/63.6	47.9/31.7	163.3/86.2	244.8/117.5	166.8/87.3	56.7/33.4	10.2/5.8
1993	673.5/62.7	45.1/30.9	152.0/82.6	236.0/114.4	171.1/87.3	58.8/43.1	10.5/6.2
1994	664.7/62.0	42.0/28.9	140.2/79.1	229.1/112.4	179.6/89.3	63.1/35.8	10.7/6.4
1995	648.1/60.5	41.9/28.5	130.7/76.4	217.4/108.7	181.2/88.2	65.5/36.4	11.3/6.8
1996	649.5/60.6	44.7/29.7	125.7/77.0	211.1/106.8	186.4/89.7	69.5/37.5	12.1/7.2
1997	643.1/60.0	46.4/30.3	118.6/75.9	202.8/104.5	187.5/89.9	74.9/39.3	12.9/7.6
1998	635.9/59.3	48.3/31.3	113.5/74.8	193.1/101.5	188.5/90.7	78.9/40.4	13.6/7.9
1999	621.9/57.9	48.4/31.3	110.7/73.1	181.9/98.4	185.3/89.7	81.3/40.6	14.3/8.1
2000	604.4/56.0	45.8/29.5	107.7/70.2	170.7/94.5	180.1/88.1	85.0/41.4	15.1/8.4
2001	594.6/54.8	44.2/28.1	108.8/69.2	159.9/91.9	178.9/88.2	86.5/41.6	16.3/8.8
2002	596.1/54.8	43.5/27.1	110.9/69.2	153.4/91.6	180.5/89.9	90.5/43.2	17.3/9.1

10% of women are childless by choice in all countries except Belgium and Austria; in Britain the proportion is only 7–8% at 42 years. Men and women who are uncertain whether to have children comprise a larger group: in Britain, 12% of women and 21% of men at 42 years and 33% of women and almost 50% of men at 30 years.[32]

The relatively large size of the group of those who are uncertain about whether to have children has led to the conclusion that ambivalence about childbearing and delay in making decisions about whether and when to have children plays a more dominant role than a definite decision to be 'childfree'.[24,33,34]

Childbearing is now very susceptible to situational factors (such as changes in the incidence of marriage) and to the social, economic and policy environment.[32] In other words, delaying having and not having children are largely neither the result of circumstances entirely beyond individual control, such as the effects of war, nor for the most part the result of voluntarism. Rather, current fertility patterns can be best understood in relation to how individuals interact with range of factors, some of which are discussed below, that impact on experiences and perceptions of parenthood.

Employment

One aspect of the social and economic environment discussed in many studies of fertility is the increase in the percentage of women in employment. This has increased from 58.3% in 1984 to 68.9% in 2000. In 1981, women formed 3% of the total occupied population and, by 1998, over 46%.[30] Women's participation in the labour force is often on a part-time basis and in certain sectors of the economy. However, the numbers of women who expect to continue working through their adult lives has increased considerably.

The effect of this development on fertility is a source of debate. On the one hand, it is argued that there is an identifiable relationship between employment patterns and fertility patterns.[35] While some argue that increased female participation in the labour force is almost inevitably linked with deferred childbearing, others see a more complex relationship between the changed position of women in regard to the labour force and their postponement or rejection of parenthood. The British Social Attitudes Survey, for example, suggests that, 'it is less than clear that fertility decisions and family life are taking second place to employment in the minds of the majority of women'. At the same time, a significant proportion of women (25%) who do not have dependant children work part-time.[24]

Qualitative research suggests that childless women are not mostly 'driven by ambition'.[24] The evidence challenges the notion that large numbers of women are manifestly placing their commitment to their paid work above having children. As Hakim notes,[32] the fact that a high proportion of professional women remains childless may be the result of a drive to succeed at work. However, these women constitute a 'tiny fraction' of those without children, since it is still the case that very few women reach the top of their chosen profession. Childlessness, rather, is mostly accounted for by those in 'middle and lower-grade occupations' who are by no means necessarily career-oriented nor strongly rejecting of the prospect of eventually having children.

This is not to argue that changes to employment patterns are not important in explaining why fertility has declined but it suggests that the relationship between fertility and employment is not straightforward. According to McAllister and Clarke,[24] fertility outcomes may be better understood as a result of the interaction of employment with other trends, notably those relating to formation of partnerships.

Marriage

Marriage patterns also impact on fertility. Marriage now happens in general later in life and less frequently. The average age of marriage for women rose from 23.8 years in 1985 to 27.7 years in 1998.[30] The proportion of all unmarried women aged 18–49 years who were cohabiting in Britain more than doubled between 1979 and 1998–99, from 11% to 29%. Additionally, the proportion of people living in couples of any kind, married or cohabiting, is falling. The proportion of people living 'solo' has been identified as growing,[36] as has 'living together apart', whereby partners choose to live in separate households.[37]

These trends are significant for fertility in that nonmarital relationships are more likely to be childless. Cohabitation has not simply replaced marriage in this regard.[25,30] Qualitative research suggests that people who are married tend to have different expectations. In particular, women who are single are three to four times more likely to say they will remain childless than married women.[24]

Ambivalence characterises choices relating to marriage just as it does those relating to having children.[39,40] With both possible life events it can be argued that a fairly widespread perception has emerged in which the difficulty looms large of reaching a point of certainty about what is the best life choice and whether or not to take on the responsibilities associated with certain choices.

Childcare

Finally, public policies impacting upon parenthood are also important in shaping fertility trends, primarily those affecting provision of childcare.[38] Social policies about 'family-friendly working' and childcare are likely to make little difference to the 'childfree' but may have a significant effect for the numerically larger group that is uncertain about childbearing.[32] Fertility outcomes are likely to be affected to some degree at least by policies relating to the availability of childcare, working arrangements and maternity leave.

Policy may also influence fertility through its reflection and amplification of themes associated with the problem of 'parenting'. The nature of parent–child interactions has been placed increasingly under the spotlight and policy has been shaped with this in mind.[41] Increasing credence has been given to the notion that the experience of the 'early years' is decisive for a person's future development and, as a result, emphasis on the 'early years' now strongly influences the agenda for childcare policy.[42] This, in turn, has given added impetus to the idea that it is far better for pregnancies to be planned and wanted, thus impacting on reproductive health policy.

No research specifically addresses the extent to which ideas about 'parenting' influence decisions about having children. However, a focus on parenting may have heightened concerns about being 'good enough parents', increasing a sense of uncertainty about when is the 'right time' to take on what might now seem to be a considerable challenge.

Abortion and the 'second demographic transition'

The trends discussed above form the backcloth against which the demand for abortion can be viewed. Research has not specifically and systematically examined the relationship between these trends and fertility regulation in general, including abortion. However, certain conclusions can be drawn. The increase in prevalence of abortion has contributed to but does not fully account for the trends in fertility.

There is a statistical relationship between abortion rates for young women, particularly those in their early 20s, and towards increased female participation in education and employment. Qualitative research suggests that those in these age groups who terminate pregnancies perceive finishing education and establishing themselves at work as the most significant aspects of their immediate futures.[43] Moreover, abortion

Table 5.4. Conceptions by marital status and outcome, England and Wales (source: National Statistics 2004)[48]

	1987	1991	1995	1998
Conceptions inside marriage leading to maternities (%)	56	52	49	44
Conceptions inside marriage leading to legal abortions (%)	5	4	4	4
Conceptions outside marriage leading to maternities inside marriage (%)	5	4	3	3
Conceptions outside marriage leading to maternities outside marriage (%)	20	25	28	30
Conceptions outside marriage leading to legal abortions (%)	14	15	16	18
All conceptions (%)	850 000	854 000	790 000	797 000

rates among cohabitees are more similar to those among single women, which are far higher than among married women. In 1998, for example, overall, 22% of all conceptions led to abortion. Nine percent of conceptions within marriage were terminated compared with 35% of those of unmarried women (Table 5.4).

It could also be argued that abortion may now be viewed as an option by women in a way that was not the case in the past.

Parenthood is an experience that is increasingly viewed as a choice. There is consequently a widespread sense that children should be planned, wanted and born only 'when the time is right'. It could be that women are now more comfortable with the idea of requesting abortion than they might have been even a decade ago and pregnancies may therefore be terminated which may previously have been tolerated. Unplanned pregnancies that in other social contexts may have been accepted and continued may now be rejected and terminated. In this case, a relatively high and sometimes increasing abortion rate is best understood as the outcome of abortion being perceived by women as an option to an extent that has not previously been the case.

Conclusions

In public debate in Britain, explanations for an increasing abortion rate has tended to represent the demand for abortion as in substantial part related to problems of contraception, yet women throughout the world use abortion to regulate their fertility, albeit unintentionally. As Kulczycki *et al.* point out, while abortion alone is an inefficient means of fertility control, 'no society can meet the desire of all women (or couples) for fertility spacing or limitation without resort to abortion'.[12] It is, therefore, unrealistic to imagine that there will ever be anything other than a considerable demand for abortion, regardless of how accessible and effective contraception becomes.

This does not mean that problems of contraception are unimportant, but it does imply that explanations for the increasing demand for abortion which focus exclusively on inadequacies of contraceptive methods in services are at best only partial.[23,44-46] There is not enough research that considers in detail British women's contemporary experiences in making decisions about whether to terminate pregnancy, and on perceptions of motherhood. The recent coincidence of a stable or increasing abortion rate with a range of other trends relating to fertility suggests, at least, that a relatively high abortion rate is not a sign of the failure of sex education and family planning programmes. Rather, it is an understandable and acceptable outcome of the current socio-cultural context.

The current context is one in which women have fewer children than before and later in life; where cohabitation and solo living are more commonplace; where a very high primacy is placed on pregnancies being planned and wanted; where women expect, and are expected to, take on responsibilities other than motherhood through their 20s; and where 'parenting' has come to be viewed as a skill that is demanding and needs to be acquired rather than something that 'comes naturally'. It is unsurprising, given all of this, that abortion rates fail to decline. Abortion has come to be perceived as a choice that can be considered when unplanned pregnancies occur, in a way that has not been the case previously.

Turning lastly to the problem of late abortion, numerically, late abortion forms a relatively insignificant part of the demand for abortion. However, in the light of recent public debate that has largely represented late abortion as a particular problem, the issue needs to be accorded careful consideration. At least two points can be made. First, there is no surge in the demand for late abortion. Second, the existing demand will not, for the most part, be reduced by improvements to the early abortion service, since it is mostly a product of factors that lead women to request abortion late. It is to these two factors that attention must be paid, in order to diminish still further the problem of late abortion.

References

1. Department of Health. *The National Strategy for Sexual Health and HIV*. London: Department of Health; 2001.
2. Royal College of Obstetricians and Gynaecologists. *The Care of Women Requesting Induced Abortion.* Evidence-based Clinical Guideline No. 7. London: RCOG Press; 2000.
3. British Pregnancy Advisory Service. *Abortion Review*. Wooton Wawen: bpas; Winter 2003.
4. All-Party Parliamentary Pro-Choice and Sexual Health Group. *NHS Abortion Services, A Report of Primary Care Trusts Carried out by Voice for Choice*. London: All-Party Parliamentary Pro-Choice & Sexual Health Group; 2004.
5. Furedi, A. Wrong but the right thing to do: British public opinion and abortion. In: Lee E, editor. *Abortion Law and Politics Today*. Basingstoke: Macmillan; 1998.
6. Gerard, J. A blurring of the abortion battle lines. *The Sunday Times*, 18 April 2004.
7. Clements, S. Abortion at 20 or more weeks: trends and statistics. In: *Late Abortion: A Review of the Evidence. A Briefing Compiled by Prochoice Forum*. London: Prochoice Forum; 2004. p. 7–10 [www.prochoiceforum.org.uk].
8. Lee E. Debating late abortion: time to tell the truth. *J Fam Plann Reprod Health Care* 2005;31:7–9.
9. George A, Randall S. Late presentation for abortion. *Br J Fam Plann* 1996;22:12–15.
10. Statham H, Dimavicius J, Gillott J. Termination of pregnancy after prenatal diagnosis of fetal abnormality. In: *Late Abortion: A Review of the Evidence. A Briefing Compiled by Prochoice Forum*. London: Prochoice Forum; 2004. p. 22–4 [www.prochoiceforum.org.uk].
11. Lee, E. Why women have late abortions. In: *Late Abortion: A Review of the Evidence. A Briefing Compiled by Prochoice Forum*. London: Prochoice Forum; 2004 p. 13–14 [www.prochoiceforum.org.uk].
12. Kulczycki A, Potts M, Rosenfeld A. Abortion and fertility regulation. *Lancet* 1996;347:1663–8.
13. Alan Guttmacher Institute. The Role of Contraception in Reducing Abortion. Issues in Brief. New York: Alan Guttmacher Institute; 1998 [www.agi-usa.org/pubs/ib19.html].
14. Henshaw SK, Singh S, Haas T. Recent trends in abortion rates worldwide. *Int Fam Plan Perspect* 1999;25:44–8.
15. Bongaarts J, Westoff C. The potential role of contraception in reducing abortion. *Stud Fam Plann* 2000;31:193–202.
16. Marston C, Cleland J. Relationships between contraception and abortion: a review of the evidence. *Int Fam Plan Perspect* 2003;29:6–13.
17. Furedi, A. The causes of unplanned pregnancy. Information Resources Library. Contraception. Prochoice Forum. 1997 [http://www.prochoiceforum.org. uk/ri1.asp]
18. MORI Consumer Survey of 1258 women aged 16 to 49, throughout the UK. Conducted in March 1993 on behalf of Roussel Laboratories [unpublished].
19. Freely, M. Hidden reasons for having kids. *Sunday Times Magazine*, 15 February 2004.
20. Furedi, A. *Unplanned Pregnancy, Your Choices*. Oxford: OUP; 1996.
21. Vessey M. Efficacy of different contraceptive methods. *Lancet* 1982;i(8276):841–3.
22. Wheble. Contraception: failure in practice. *Br J Fam Plann* 1987;13:40–5.
23. Hall, C. Abortion rate rises 8.3pc. *The Daily Telegraph*, 23 July 1997.
24. McAllister F, Clarke L. *Choosing Childlessness*. London: Family Policy Studies Centre; 1998.
25. Kiernan, KE. Who Remains Childless? *J Biosoc Sci* 1987;21:387–9.
26. Family Policy Studies Centre. *Families in Britain*. London: FPSC; 1998.
27. Hewlett, SA. *Baby Hunger*. London: Atlantic Books; 2002.
28. Taylor L, Taylor, M. *What Are Children For?* London: Short Books; 2003.
29. National Statistics. Live births, largest annual rise since 1979. 2004 [www.statistics.gov.uk/cci/nugget.asp?id=951].
30. Halsey AH. A hundred years of social change. In: Matheson J, Summerfield C, editors. *Social Trends 30*. London: The Stationery Office; 2000.
31. Kiernan, KE. Who Remains Childless? *J Biosoc Sci* 1987;21:387–9.

32. Hakim C. Childlessness in Europe. Summary of Research Results for the Economic and Social Research Council (ESRC) project funded by research grant RES-000-23-0074, running December 2002–July 2003 [unpublished].
33. Veevers JE. *Childless by Choice*. Toronto: Butterworths; 1980.
34. Letherby, G. Childless and bereft? Stereotypes and realities in relation to 'voluntary' and 'involuntary' childlessness and womanhood. *Sociol Inq* 2002;72:7–20.
35. Jensen, TK, Anderson, AN, Skakkbaek NE. Is human fertility declining? In: Daya S, Harrison RF, Kempers RD, editors. *Advances in Fertility and Reproductive Medicine. Proceedings of the 18th World Congress on Fertility and Sterility held in Montreal, Canada 23–28 May 2004*. International Congress Series 1266. Amsterdam: Elsevier; 2004. p. 32–44.
36. Centre for Research on Families and Relationships. Solo living across the adult lifecourse [www.crfr.ac.uk/Research/sololiving.htm].
37. Drew E. Re-conceptualising families. In: Drew E, Emerek R, Mahon E, editors. *Women, Work and the Family in Europe*. London and New York: Routledge; 1998.
38. McDonald P. Gender equity, social institutions and the future of fertility. *J Popul Res* 2000;17:1–16.
39. Lewis J. *The End of Marriage?* Cheltenham: Edward Elgar; 2001.
40. Bristow J. *Maybe I Do: Marriage and Commitment in Singleton Society*. London: Institute of Ideas; 2002.
41. Furedi F. *Paranoid Parenting*. London: The Penguin Press; 2001.
42. Harker L, Kendall E. *An Equal Start*. London: IPPR; 2002.
43. Lee E, Ingham R, Clements S, Stone, N. *A Matter of Choice? National Variation in Teenage Pregnancy, Abortion and Motherhood*. York: Joseph Rowntree Foundation; 2004.
44. Murray I. Abortion rise for first time in 5 years'. *The Times*, 23 July 1997.
45. BBC News on line. 'Abortions continue to rise'; 16 February 1999 [http://news.bbc.co.uk/1/hi/health/280722. stm].
46. Carvel J. Abortion at record level, despite better contraceptive services. *The Guardian*, 28 August 2004.
47. National Statistics. *Health Statistics Quarterly*. London: TSO; Winter 2004.
48. Matheson J, Summerfield C. Household and families. In: Matheson J, Summerfield C, editors. *Social Trends 31*. London: The Stationery Office; 2001.

Chapter 6
Overview of contraceptive methods: a provider's perspective

Diana Mansour

Introduction

There is no question that effective provision of contraception is at the heart of improving maternal and child health. Across Europe, sexual health advice and the prescribing of birth control methods occurs in a variety of settings. Emphasis is placed on accessibility of appropriate up to date information to users, be it in the pharmacy, from gynaecologists, specialists in sexual health, primary care physicians or allied healthcare professionals. In most European countries, a wide variety of contraceptive methods is available. These include:

- combined oral contraceptives (COCs), patches and vaginal rings
- progestogen-only pills (POPs)
- progestogen-only injectables and implants
- copper intrauterine contraceptives (IUDs)
- progestogen-only intrauterine systems (IUS)
- diaphragms and cervical caps
- male and female condoms
- natural family planning kits
- male and female sterilisation.

Many couples in Europe pay for these methods, including associated health provision costs such as the physician's consultation and contraceptive insertion charge. Some health insurance policies reimburse some or all of these costs, depending on the country and the methods chosen.

Most of the focus of this chapter will be based on a provider's perspective of contraceptive methods and their provision in the UK, where contraceptives are available through the National Health Service without a prescription charge. Family planning services are available, free of charge, to men and women. The cost benefit of UK family planning services in primary and specialist services has been estimated at £11 for every £1 spent,[1] yet the emphasis on broadening contraceptive choice and services to 'hard to reach' groups over the last 5 years has not led to a significant fall in teenage pregnancy and abortion rates, which remains unacceptably high.

A number of questions arise from this gloomy picture. If contraception is free in the UK then why are so many couples failing to use birth control or using a method poorly? Are providers of these methods partly to blame? Do providers offer real contraceptive choice to couples or do they fail to acknowledge advances in this field? What governs the healthcare provider's decision-making process and how could it be improved? Are there any recommendations that could alter contraceptive provision and increase contraceptive uptake and continuance?

To understand where contraceptive service provision stands today in the UK it is important to look to the past. The provision of contraceptive methods crosses primary, community and secondary care but gaps in services, restriction of choice and funding issues, together with with 'competing' interests of clinicians are often seated in history. It is hoped that after discussing the history of contraceptive services in the UK, present day commissioning arrangements, funding issues, contraceptive use and provision, training needs and support recommendations for improved service delivery and effective, quality-driven provision of contraceptive methods can be made.

History of contraceptive services in the UK

It is hard to imagine that, up until 1946, few contraceptive methods were available: traditional methods such as fertility awareness, condoms, diaphragms, cervical caps and sterilisation. Men and women had to pay health professionals for this luxury, together with medical appointment fees. With the birth of the NHS in 1946, local health authorities and health boards were tasked with the duty of setting up family planning services but they frequently failed to do so.

Charitable and voluntary services, especially the Family Planning Association (fpa), purchased property (often in city centres) and ran contraception services, with costs for contraceptive supplies and services passed on to their users. These charitable organisations often waived the fee for those in need but still only provided help for 'married' women. It was not until the early 1960s that 'unmarried' women's clinics were established, to local public outcry in many cases. In Newcastle upon Tyne, the clinic, housed in a terraced house on a main road, was picketed on a daily basis when news reached the ears of the press. We are fortunate that times have changed and the local newspapers are supportive, striving to disseminate informed sexual health messages. It is a shame that this cannot be said of the national media, which are all too quick to 'scare' the population with inaccurate facts and fail to explain risk in absolute terms.

In the 1960s, advancements in laparoscopic and surgical techniques led to an increased demand for male and female sterilisation. With the introduction of oral contraception and modern IUDs, more single women requested contraception. Unfortunately, when these methods failed, legal abortions were rarely performed, with the result that women suffered the sequelae of 'back street' procedures. In 1967, the Abortion Act was ratified. However, there were concerns that, if contraceptive provision were poor, the numbers of women requesting an abortion would escalate.

To ensure countrywide contraceptive provision, the National Health Service (Family Planning) Act (1967) and Public Health and Health Services Act in Scotland (1968) stated that local authorities should provide contraception services and charges were permissible. These Acts led local authorities and health boards to make agency arrangements with the fpa, with many women finally receiving free contraception. Up until the middle of the 1970s, the fpa ran over 1000 UK family planning clinics.

By 1973, the National Health Service Reorganisation Act led to free family planning provision in clinics and hospitals. By 1975, this was extended into primary care, with the UK becoming the first country in Western Europe to provide a universally free contraceptive service including abortion and sterilisation.

Commissioning of sexual health services in the 21st century

In 2000, the Department of Health published 'The NHS Plan' outlining the vision of a health service designed around the patient.[2] It signalled the UK Government's intention to tackle unjustified variations and raise the standards in health care. This applies to contraception and sexual health services as much as to any others.

Sexual ill health is not equally distributed across the population. The highest burden is borne by women, gay men, teenagers, young adults and black and ethnic minority groups. Provision of contraception and sexual health services in the UK is in disarray, with many people waiting 2 or more weeks for an appointment and over 3 weeks to have an abortion. Few general practitioners offer real contraceptive choice, with most discussing the three most commonly used methods: condoms, pills or injectables. Only those practices that have staff trained to insert IUDs or implants fully explore the possibility of other long-acting, reversible methods. It is only when couples raise the question of alternative methods that they may be referred on to community services.

Previous funding arrangements have led to suggestions that community services are just duplicating GP contraceptive provision instead of providing accessible drop-in health sessions, often in youth projects or community settings, in evenings and weekends providing a full range of contraceptive methods. Women have voiced their concerns about consulting their GP with sexual health problems. They often confuse important issues of confidentiality being broken in primary care, with a lack of anonymity. The latter cannot always be assured.[3] For the future, services should be commissioned with these problems in mind.

Available data suggest that 85% of GPs in Wales and Northern Ireland will see women for contraceptive services who are not registered but there is no indication that this is borne out in practice.[4] There are no data for England or Scotland but a local survey in Newcastle suggested that, although over 90% of practices said they would see women requesting emergency contraception, they were unlikely to see them on a routine basis for contraceptive advice.

The National Statistics omnibus survey (2004) reported that 81% of women between 16 years and 50 years had seen their own GP or practice nurse in the last 5 years for contraceptive advice, 32% had been to a community clinic, 3% had seen another GP or nurse, 8% had seen a pharmacist and 1% had used a 'walk-in' service.[4]

Some genitourinary medicine services see women who request contraceptive advice but more often than not they will provide hormonal emergency contraception and redirect users to other services. Figures, however, show that the number of contraceptive attendances nearly trebled from 1995 to 2000.[5]

Today, early in the 21st century, government and local sexual health strategies have encouraged partnership working in primary, community and secondary care, across health, education and social services. Commissioning of contraceptive and sexual health services since April 2002 is in the hands of local health boards and primary care organisations. It is hoped that these agencies are aware of the local need and provide funding through the new General and Personal Medical Services contracts for primary care. Also, the new consultant contract focuses on service provision rather than 'item of service payments'.

Changes in contraception and sexual health service provision

The first National Sexual Health and HIV Strategy was published for consultation in July 2001.[6] It was welcomed by many because it indicated that the Department of Health was firm in its aims to:

- reduce the transmission of HIV and sexually transmitted infections (STIs)
- reduce the prevalence of undiagnosed HIV and STIs
- reduce unintended pregnancy rates
- improve health and social care for people living with HIV
- reduce the stigma associated with HIV and STIs

However, it was criticised for being overly descriptive and vague, too 'disease focused' rather than supporting sexual health promotion and having 'no teeth'; commissioners could ignore the strategy, as it failed to have the financial backing of a National Service Framework.

The strategy did look at contraception and sexual health services across the UK, identifying that, although there were areas of good practice, services were patchy and fragmented with poor accessibility. To try to find a remedy for these problems, a new structure in service provision has been proposed. Three levels of service provision are described to provide a comprehensive local sexual health service (Table 6.1).

Table 6.1. Levels of provision of contraceptive services

Level	Provision
One	Sexual history and risk assessment
	STI testing for women
	HIV testing and counselling
	Pregnancy testing and referral
	Contraceptive information and services
	Assessment and referral of men with STIs
	Cervical cytology screening and referral
	Hepatitis B immunisation
Two	IUD insertion
	Testing and treating STIs
	Vasectomy
	Contraceptive implant insertion
	Partner notification
	Invasive STI testing for men (until non-invasive tests are available)
Three	Outreach for STI prevention
	Outreach contraceptive services
	Specialised infection management
	Highly specialised contraception
	Specialised HIV treatment and care

Level one

All general practices should be able to provide level one services, with development of nursing roles and support of community pharmacists in expanding provision of emergency contraception. However, there are concerns that many in primary care do not feel confident about providing this level of contraception and sexual health care. A survey carried out in London identified just eight of 133 GPs with a special interest in sexual health. Just 46 had postgraduate training in taking a sexual health history.[7] Health professionals working in primary care will need specific training to develop and maintain their skills to provide a level one service. Can this training be provided by the limited, overstretched health professionals in this field?

There are opportunities for GPs to opt out and deny their patients contraceptive choice or provision. Those practices unable to provide level one services are now obliged to make this clear in practice information and make explicit alternative arrangements for patients to be seen at other practices or community services. Locally agreed protocols and guidance should be developed to ensure quality standards across primary, secondary and community services in sexual health.

Level two

Some primary healthcare teams may have a special interest in sexual health, linking up with specialist services to provide a comprehensive local service and filling gaps in existing service provision. These GP practices are expected to provide all services listed in level one and two (Table 6.1). Experience so far from the North East of England suggests that few GPs wish to provide such a service.

Level three

Specialist services are expected to provide level three health care (Table 6.1), supporting quality standards and clinical governance in this area. Clinicians in these specialist teams act as a clinical resource to those working in levels one and two services locally, leading on professional training and developing effective pathways of care. The National Sexual Health and HIV Strategy identified that the accessibility and range of contraceptive methods available including NHS funded sterilisations varied widely.[6] It supported community family planning services in providing choice and greater service access to users complementing primary care.

Abortion services were also targeted in this strategy, but only one of the four national targets focuses on contraception and abortion. From 2005, commissioners should ensure that women who meet the legal requirements have access to abortion within 3 weeks of their first appointment with the GP or referring doctor. Commissioners and service providers are tasked with informing the public of local services.

The White Paper on Public Health called *Choosing Health: Making Healthy Choices Easier* was published in November 2004.[8] It sets out a framework for developing services in contraception and sexual health, focusing sexual health promotion on teenagers and young men at the heart of developing service provision. Even with this continuing national support, most areas of the country will fail to reach the targets set by the Social Exclusion Unit in their report on Teenage Pregnancy (1999).[9] These two national targets are:

- to reduce by 50% the 1998 English under 18 years conception rate by 2010, with an interim target of 15% reduction by 2004
- to increase to 60% the participation of teenage parents in education, training or employment to reduce their risk of long-term social exclusion by 2010.

Funding of services in primary care

The majority of men and women requesting contraceptive advice in the UK (about 70%) will seek the help of their local GP or practice nurse. The new General Medical Service (GMS) contract (2003) is aimed at investing in primary care providing a practice-based contract with a quality and outcomes framework to monitor care.[10] Will this change lead to an improvement in primary care contraceptive services and an increased contraceptive choice for patients?

Essential services

The new GMS contract talks about essential, additional and enhanced services. Essential services must be provided by all general practices and include management of patients who are ill, terminally ill or who have a chronic illnesses.

Additional services

Additional services (where primary care have a preferential right to provide this service but they have the ability to opt out on a temporary or permanent basis with appropriate loss of income) covers cervical screening and contraceptive services (Box 6.1).

Box 6.1. Contraceptive service provision in the new General Medical Service contract

1. Provide advice about the full range of contraceptive methods.
2. Where appropriate, examine patients seeking contraceptive advice.
3. Treat patients for contraceptive purposes and prescribe contraceptives or refer for the fitting of intrauterine contraceptive devices or implants.
4. Provide advice about emergency contraception and where appropriate supply or prescribe emergency hormonal contraception. Where the doctor has a conscientious objection to emergency contraception it must be promptly referred to a health professional who has no such objection.
5. Provide advice in cases of unplanned or unwanted pregnancy including advice about the availability of free pregnancy testing in the practice area. Where the doctor has a conscientious objection to termination it must be promptly referred to a doctor who has no such objection.
6. Give initial advice about sexual health promotion and sexually transmitted infections.
7. Refer as necessary for specialist sexual health services including tests for sexually transmitted infections.

Most GP practices will deliver these additional services, thereby providing level one care as outlined in the National Sexual Health and HIV Strategy. However, only 3.5% of their income will be derived from such provision, so some smaller or single-handed practices may take a view not to continue to provide basic cervical cytology, contraceptive and sexual health care, thus further reducing contraceptive provision in the community.

Enhanced services

Enhanced services (national and local) for general practice will be commissioned by primary care organisations and local health boards to meet local need. It is hoped that primary care organisations will discuss the setting up of new services with all key stakeholders. This will ensure that joint protocols between primary and secondary care are in place and efficient care pathways have been developed for patient referral, such as intrauterine contraception, contraceptive implants, male and female sterilisation. The payment for such a national enhanced sexual health service will have to fund:

- HIV counselling and testing
- STI screening and treatment using the most reliable testing methods available
- the general practice to act as a resource for other local primary care health profess-ionals
- training of GPs and registrars, practice nurses and other relevant staff
- effective liaison (with local sexual health services, cytology and microbiology services and other statutory or non-statutory services)
- additional training and continuing professional development for clinicians and staff
- development of comprehensive patient records
- development of electronic register of patients
- appropriate arrangements for patient review
- provision of condoms and same-day pregnancy testing
- treatment of STIs without prescription costs
- effective communication with all young people
- holistic approach to assessment of risk of STI, HIV and/or unplanned pregnancy
- provision of information on testing and treatment of all STIs
- assurance of partner notification
- sound understanding of the role of different professional groups and pathways of care through primary to secondary services, e.g. HIV care patients
- regular annual review by the primary care organisation.

The Department of Health has specified set fees for those in primary care providing sexual health as an enhanced service. Each GP will receive £2,064 a year as a retainer and £206 and £103 for each HIV positive patient and other sexual health patient seen annually (2004/05 rates). It will be interesting to see how many GPs negotiate with their primary care organisation to provide this specialist service in primary care. Initial soundings from GP colleagues suggest that the financial rewards will fail to attract significant numbers of primary care practices. The initial set-up costs to establish a sexual health service in primary care are high. Many GPs are hesitant about making such a step, as long-term funding needs to be guaranteed. However, additional local agreements to cover management of intrauterine and implantable contraceptive methods may increase interest, especially in rural communities or in areas poorly served by community sexual health services.

There is a separate national enhanced service to cover 'IUD fittings'. The aim of this enhanced service is to ensure that a wide range of contraceptive options is available by the practice to patients, including the fitting of emergency IUDs. This enhanced service will fund:

- fitting, monitoring, checking and removal of IUDs and IUS

- keeping of an up-to-date register of those women fitted with a device to be used as an audit tool and to target those requiring additional health checks
- the practice to undertake continual professional development
- provision of adequate equipment for managing IUD/IUS fittings and removals
- chlamydia screening, where appropriate
- provision of condoms
- regular assessment of patients
- provision of written information about IUD/IUS
- keeping appropriate GP records detailing clinical findings at IUD/IUS fitting, etc.
- IUS use to manage menorrhagia using an agreed care pathway developed with the local gynaecology department
- annual review to cover IUD/IUS fits, removals and complications.

National enhanced service costs

The GP practice will receive £77 per IUD insertion and £21 for each IUD annual review (2004/05 rates).

Personal medical services

Personal medical service (PMS) contracts for primary care were piloted in 1998, allowing greater freedom to provide the necessary care to patients. It is centred on a team-based approach, with GPs given an option of being salaried and PMS contracts to support the development of an enhanced role of nurses in primary care. These contracts attracted a skilled workforce to areas without sufficient doctors, which often have high levels of social deprivation.

Contraceptive services within PMS are now remunerated as additional service points.[11] Many feel that this change in payment will encourage PMS practices to concentrate on national priority areas, such as coronary heart disease and mental health (attracting more points and therefore money), rather than cervical screening and contraceptive services. Specialist PMS contracts and practice-based commissioning may give opportunities to primary care organisations and local health boards to extend contraceptive services into primary care, particularly where gaps in provision are identified.

Who will be overseeing the running of these additional and enhanced services? As the primary care organisations or local health boards commission such services then the Quality and Outcome Framework (QOF) review visits will monitor progress. Proposals for the process of national QOF annual review visits have been commissioned. Locally, as yet, contraceptive and sexual health provision is barely examined by visiting QOF teams and this is worrying. Those providing enhanced services have to now submit an annual report, which will inform an annual review process. For those GPs working within a PMS practice, the primary care organisations/local health board may be the provider, so strategic health authorities monitor this activity. Again many strategic health authorities fail to have contraception and sexual health on their priority list for annual monitoring.

It does appear that primary care organisations and local health boards have been discussing the roll out of enhanced services with local 'specialists'. Eligibility criteria for GPs have been clarified and additional local training within community services organised. Wherever possible, practitioners have been encouraged to obtain a recognised qualification such as the Letter of Competence in Intrauterine Techniques.

For those who have been inserting intrauterine contraceptives for years and hold a family planning qualification, most primary care organisations require evidence of continuing medical education in this field to the standard specified by the Faculty of Family Planning and Reproductive Health Care (FFPRHC) and the regular fitting of devices (at least 12 per year). Recertification and continuing medical education must also be demonstrated on a regular basis.

Local enhanced services are optional and are commissioned by primary care organisations and local health boards, depending upon local need. Provision of implantable contraceptives fall into this category and in areas where there is no community contraceptive service primary care organisations may wish to spend some of their enhanced services budget developing a service in primary care to improve contraceptive choice. The FFPRHC, together with the Royal College of Nursing, the fpa and the Royal College of General Practitioners' Sex, Drugs and HIV Task Group, have developed a recommended framework for the commissioning of contraceptive implants as a locally enhanced service.[12] This is available on the Faculty's website.

All funding for enhanced services comes from a primary care organisation-administered budget for GMS/PMS contracts. This is a ring-fenced allocation with a spending floor set by the UK Technical Steering Committee for these contracts. The enhanced services floor is the minimum amount that must be spent on enhanced services although primary care organisations are free to spend more using other funding streams. For many cash-strapped areas, this may mean that no local enhanced services are developed or that one provider may be chosen, for example to manage intrauterine contraceptives, if primary care fails to identify specialist practices.

There are some real concerns that in the new world of practice-based commissioning, payment by results and foundation hospitals joint working across primary and secondary care will be destroyed with a return to the dark age of 'fundholding'. Individual community services and practices will be fighting once more over the same pot of money and excellent initiatives such as GPs with a special interest in contraception and sexual health will become a thing of the past. It will be up to commissioners to establish budgets covering streams of care across provider trusts to ensure contraceptive choice in accessible locations for users.

Contraceptive methods

Having explored, from a provider's perspective, the history of contraceptive service provision in the UK, the commissioning and funding of contraceptive services in the 21st century, it is now time to discuss the contraceptive methods available and what governs a provider's prescribing choice.

It has been estimated that at least 60% of women requesting an abortion report that they used a method of contraception at the time of conception.[13] This has invariably been a pill or condom imperfectly used. Evidence suggests that long-acting contraceptive methods are highly effective, even in the first year of use, requiring little forethought or adherence to daily regimen. Unfortunately, it is often only after an unplanned pregnancy that women reassess their contraceptive needs and choose more effective methods.

Ideally at the first contraceptive consultation the health professional should:

● ascertain the importance of contraceptive efficacy and reversibility for the couple. This allows the provider to concentrate on discussing more effective, contraceptive methods (Table 6.2).[14]

Table 6.2. Women experiencing an unintended pregnancy during the first year of use and the first year of perfect use of contraception[14]

Method	Women experiencing an unintended pregnancy within 1st year of use (%)	
	Typical use[a]	Perfect use[b]
No method	85.0	85.0
Spermicides	29.0	18.0
Withdrawal	27.0	4.0
Periodic abstinence:		
calendar		9.0
ovulation method		3.0
symptothermal		2.0
postovulation		1.0
Cap:		
parous woman	32.0	20.0
nulliparous woman	16.0	9.0
Diaphragm	16.0	6.0
Sponge:		
female	21.0	5.0
male	15.0	2.0
Condom:		
female	21.0	5.0
male	15.0	2.0
COC/POP	8.0	0.3
Combined patch	8.0	0.3
Combined vaginal ring	8.0	0.3
Progestogen injectable	3.0	0.3
Combined injectable	3.0	0.05
Intrauterine device:		
copper T	0.8	0.6
intrauterine system	0.1	0.1
Progestogen implants	0.05	0.05
Sterilisation:		
female	0.5	0.5
male	0.15	0.1

[a] among typical couples who initiate use of this method (not necessarily for the first time); [b] among couples who initiate use of a method (not necessarily for the first) and who use it perfectly.

- ask if the client had a particular interest in a contraceptive method
- take a comprehensive medical and sexual history. The reporting of dysmenorrhoea or heavy menstrual loss, for example, may lead the provider to offering contraceptive methods with certain therapeutic benefits
- dispel any contraceptive myths, e.g. pills makes you put on weight, injectables cause infertility
- address the client's worries and concerns before a final decision is made

- explore the reasons why contraceptive methods have been discontinued in the past
- discuss the contraceptive options available. There are 13 contraceptive methods now available in Europe, ranging from pills to patches to implants and intrauterine contraceptives
- explain how individual methods work, the advantages of each method and how it is used
- explain in an unbiased way any nuisance adverse effects that may occur and how they may be resolved
- provide accurate and up-to-date advice
- make contingency plans if adverse effects are experienced, e.g. telephone help lines to improve access to practice nurses or other help from other health professionals
- arrange follow-up appointments, as appropriate

Hormonal contraception

Combined hormonal contraception

About three million women in the UK take the COC as their main method of contraception with more than 90% of sexually active women having used the pill by the time they reach 30.[15] It can be used from menarche to the time of the menopause as long as there are no risk factors or co-existing illnesses present to contraindicate its use.

Are all COCs the same? Some would argue that as COCs have the same mode of contraceptive action and similar efficacy then little choice is required. Providers should therefore choose the cheapest preparation. However, in practice, users report nuisance adverse effects with some pills and 'feel better' and suffer less breakthrough bleeding with others.[16,17] Comparative studies do suggest that some COCs improve skin conditions, such as acne[18,19] and seborrhoea, and fluid retention.[20] This may lead to better continuation rates even when such improvements are small.[21] Therefore one could argue that formularies should specify first and second choices but leave room for providers to be able to prescribe other COCs for women with acne or those who 'fail to settle' on a standard-dose, low-cost COC.

In the recent past, a combined hormonal contraceptive patch has become available and in certain European countries a combined hormonal vaginal ring is also licensed. The patch needs changing every 7 days, with a patch-free week every fourth week. The vaginal ring is worn for 3 weeks out of every four. Apart from these dosing regimens, Table 6.3 describes the advantages and disadvantages apply to all combined hormonal methods.

Progestogen-only pill

The POP is taken by about 8% of women in the UK, although is not so popular in European countries.[4] Ovulation may be suppressed in 15–40% of cycles and only partly contributes to the POP's mechanism of action. A POP containing 75 microgrammes of desogestrel inhibits ovulation in 97–99% of cycles.[22,23] Initial studies suggest that it may be as effective as a COC, although no direct comparative studies have been undertaken. This POP differs from others, as no extra contraceptive cover is required until 12 hours after forgetting the last pill rather than 3 hours in the case of other POPs.[23,24]

Table 6.3. Advantages and disadvantages of combined hormonal contraceptives[43]

Advantages	Disadvantages
Reliable, reversible, convenient, non-intercourse related	Effectiveness depends upon comprehensive instruction and correct usage
Under the user's control	Minor adverse effects may occur in some women when first starting these preparations, such as headaches, weight gain, breakthrough bleeding (although these tend to settle within the first 3 months or so)
Regulate and reduce menstrual loss, thereby decreasing the incidence of dysmenorrhoea, iron-deficiency anaemia; often relieve ovulation pain and premenstrual symptoms	
	Potential drug interactions decrease the efficacy of these methods, e.g. liver enzyme inducing agents
May help with acne	
Helps protect against ectopic pregnancies as they inhibit ovulation	No protection against transmission of sexual transmitted infections
Lower incidence of benign breast disease	May be associated with an increased risk of breast cancer; re-analysis of available data published in 1996 reported that current use of COC increased the risk of developing breast cancer by 24% but this fell back to background level 10 years or more after discontinuing the pill
Long-term users are less likely to develop fibroids and functional ovarian cysts	
Protect against pelvic inflammatory disease caused by gonococcus, reducing the risk of hospitalisation for the disease	May increase the incidence of cervical cancer after 5 years of use; there are a number of other factors that are associated with an increase in preinvasive and invasive cervical cancer particularly high-risk types of human papillomavirus
Reduce incidence of endometriosis in COC users	
Possible reduction in the risk of developing rheumatoid arthritis	May almost double the risk of thrombotic stroke in users; incidence in young women is rare with only 1–2 thrombotic or haemorrhagic strokes occurring per 100 000 women each year
Reduce the risk of epithelial ovarian cancers by about 50%; protection increases with duration of use, with this effect lasting for at least 15 years after COC is discontinued	Increases the risk of venous thromboembolism (VTE) in women taking the COC, although only 1–2% of these women die as a result of this event; incidence of VTE in European women taking COCs has been shown to be 6–7 per 10 000 women each year; obesity, surgery and immobility have increased VTE rates in prospective studies[44]
Protects against endometrial cancer by about 50%; protection continues for at least 15 years after COC is stopped	
Appears to offer some protection against large bowel cancer	
No increase in the risk of myocardial infarction in women at low risk who do not smoke	
No increase in the risk of haemorrhagic stroke in women at low risk who do not smoke	

Providers have frequently marginalised POPs for those women who have contra-indications to taking the COC or for breastfeeding women. However, users from all age groups are interested in POPs, particularly if they have a similar 'forgiveness window' to the COC. Table 6.4 shows the advantages and disadvantages of POPs.

Table 6.4. Advantages and disadvantages of progestogen-only contraceptive preparations (POPs)

Advantages	Disadvantages
Non-intercourse-related contraceptive	Excluding the desogestrel POP, are thought to be less effective than combined pills
Simple and convenient to use	
	Reliant on the user taking it at the same time every day to achieve optimum effectiveness (excluding the desogestrel POP)
Ideal for women who suffer from oestrogenic adverse effects, e.g. breast tenderness, headaches or nausea, when taking combined contraceptives	
Suitable for women over 35 years who smoke[45]	Possible increase in ectopic pregnancy in the event of failure
Can be used in grossly obese women	
Can be taken by women with medical illnesses contraindicating the use of synthetic oestrogen in the COC, e.g. those with hypertension, migraine with focal aura or a previous personal history of VTE[45]	Can alter ovulation in some women, thereby disrupting the menstrual pattern, with users reporting increased spotting, breakthrough bleeding or amenorrhoea
No evidence of an increased risk of cardiovascular disease, thromboembolism or stroke in users of progestogen-only methods[45]	Functional ovarian cysts may develop in a small number of women however these tend to be transient and rarely require surgical intervention[15]
Minimal alteration in carbohydrate and lipid metabolism, so women who have diabetes, even with neuropathic or nephropathic complications, may choose this method[45]	

Injectable contraception

One of the first long-acting hormonal contraceptive preparations to be used was an intramuscular progestogen-only depot that gave contraceptive cover for 2–3 months. Its safety record covers 30–40 years of prescribing.

About 3% of women in the UK use a progestogen-only injectable as their method of contraception,[4] with more than 20 million women worldwide in over 130 countries having used it.[15] There are two injectable contraceptive methods available in the UK:

- depot medroxyprogesterone acetate (DMPA)
- norethisterone oenanthate, (NET-EN).

DMPA and NET-EN inhibit ovulation by suppressing luteinising hormone (LH) and, to a certain extent, follicle-stimulating hormone (FSH). They are therefore helpful for women with menstrual problems, including ovulation pain and painful, heavy periods.

A number of women receive their first DMPA injection and fail to return for the second. This is often because of prolonged and erratic bleeding during the first injection cycle or progestogenic adverse effects. Counselling prior to the first injection is most important to give a realistic picture of this contraceptive and advise that progestogenic adverse effects, such as bloating, will improve with the subsequent one or two injection cycles. About one-third of women experience prolonged bleeding (more that 10 days) after receiving their first injection but 55% are amenorrhoeic by 1 year and 68% by 2 years.[25] Table 6.5 shows the advantages and disadvantages of progestogen-only injectables. Advice from the Committee on Safety of Medicines advises:

- In adolescents, DMPA may be used as first-line contraception but only after other methods have been discussed with the woman and considered to be unsuitable or unacceptable.
- In women of all ages, careful re-evaluation of the risks and benefits of treatment should be carried out in those who wish to continue use for more than 2 years.
- In women with significant lifestyle and/or medical risk factors for osteoporosis, other methods of contraception should be considered.[26]
- There is no evidence that routinely giving 'addback' oestrogen to DMPA users or addition investigations are warranted.

Table 6.5. Advantages and disadvantages of progestogen-only injectable contraceptives

Advantages	Disadvantages
Effective, reversible method of contraception with little dependence on the user	Cause irregular, prolonged vaginal bleeding and amenorrhoea
Non-intercourse related method	Given intramuscularly, therefore cannot be removed if adverse effects occur
Safe, with no reported attributable deaths	Weight gain is commonly reported (women may gain up to 2 kg in the first year)
Breastfeeding mothers can use it	
Helpful for women with premenstrual symptoms, ovulation pain and painful, heavy periods	Some women may complain of progestogenic adverse effects, including mood changes, lassitude, loss of libido, bloatedness, breast tenderness
Can be used in women with sickle cell disease, with evidence suggesting a reduction in crises in these women	Causes a short delay in the return to the woman's normal fertility
Possess most of the non-contraceptive benefits of COCs, including protection against pelvic inflammatory disease, extrauterine pregnancies, endometriosis, functional ovarian cysts, fibroid formation, and reduction in the risk of endometrial cancer[15]	Concern that DMPA may adversely affect bone mineral density (BMD); data suggest that BMD at the lumbar spine and femoral neck are reduced in DMPA users compared with controls but in adults BMD loss is recovered when DMPA is stopped[26]
Minimal metabolic effects occur, with one study reporting no increase in the risk of acute myocardial infarction, venous thrombosis or stroke[46]	

Contraceptive implants

A contraceptive implant offers an alternative way of delivering hormones providing long-acting, low-dose, reversible contraception. Norplant® (Hoechst Marion Roussel), the levonorgestrel implant, was the first to be launched in Europe with more than 54 000 women using Norplant in the UK. Its popularity fell with the increased adverse media coverage given to implant removal and adverse effect problems. Much of the dissatisfaction with Norplant lay with untrained or inexperienced service providers giving poor pre-insertion counselling, coercing women to keep their implants and then attempting Norplant removals without the necessary training/ supervision. Norplant distribution in the UK was discontinued in October 1999.

Lessons were learned from this experience, with implant providers recommended to undertake recognised training, such as the Letter of Competence in subdermal contraceptive implant techniques of the FFPRHC (LoC SDI). In 1999, a single progestogen-only implant, Implanon® (Organon), was launched in Europe. It superseded the multi-rod devices as it was easier to insert and remove and lasts for 3 years instead of 5 years. Table 6.6 shows the advantages and disadvantages of contraceptive implants.

Table 6.6. Advantages and disadvantages of contraceptive implants

Advantages	Disadvantages
Long-lasting (3–5 years depending on the implant), effective, reversible, with no effect on future fertility	Irregular bleeding and other reported adverse effects (similar to other progestogen only contraceptives); most women, after counselling, will accept periods of amenorrhoea or infrequent bleeding but a significant minority (10–20%) will complain of frequent and/or prolonged vaginal blood loss[47]
Non-intercourse related	
Free from oestrogenic adverse effects	
High user acceptability following pre-insertion counselling with continuation rates for Implanon® reported between 67–78% at 12 months[48]	Insertion of implant requires a minor operative procedure, with removal being complicated if the implant is inserted incorrectly
Requires little medical attention other than at insertion and removal	Some women report mild discomfort following insertion or removal of the implants
Can be used by those where synthetic oestrogen is contraindicated	Infection at insertion or removal site, migration of the implants and scarring are rare
Reduced incidence of dysmenorrhoea in Implanon® users	For some women, contraceptive implants may not be a suitable method as they may feel that discontinuation is not under their control
Reduced total menstrual blood loss in Norplant® and Implanon® users	
No evidence to suggest that either Norplant® or Implanon® have an effect on oestrogen levels or bone mineral density[45]	

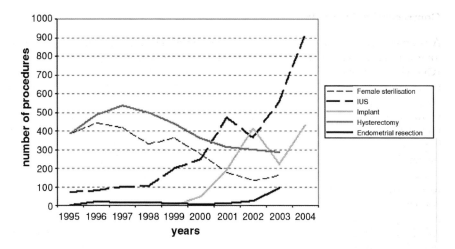

Figure 6.1. Change in gynaecological procedures performed in Newcastle, 1995–2004[27]

Levonorgestrel-releasing intrauterine system

The levonorgestrel-releasing intrauterine system (LNG-IUS) has been available in the UK since May 1995. More than six million women worldwide have used the LNG-IUS for contraception since its launch. It is licensed as a contraceptive lasting for 5 years. It is also licensed for the treatment of primary menorrhagia and for use as the progestogen component of hormone replacement therapy. It exerts its contraceptive action locally, altering the cervical mucus and uterotubal fluid, which inhibits sperm migration. It also causes the uterine endometrium to atrophy and may suppress ovulation in a small number of users in the first year by possibly reducing the preovulatory luteinising hormone surge.

These effects have led to providers offering the LNG-IUS for the treatment of menstrual disorders and an alternative to female sterilisation (Figure 6.1). Local hospital episode figures in the UK are now showing a reduction of gynaecological surgery in units using the LNG-IUS widely.[27] Table 6.7 shows the advantages and disadvantages of the LNG-IUS.

Intrauterine contraceptive devices

Over 110 million women use IUDs worldwide, with nearly 50% of these users in China.[15] In the UK, only 6% of women use this form of contraception, probably because of concerns and myths attached to these methods.[4] The available IUDs in the UK are small copper-containing devices, with most having a central frame made of polyethylene. These come in varying shapes and sizes, with a frameless device (Gyne-Fix®, Family Planning Sales Ltd) launched in 1998. Most devices now contain more than 300 mm² of copper making them a highly effective, reversible, inexpensive contraceptive option for women.

Table 6.7. Advantages and disadvantages of the levonorgestrel-releasing intrauterine system

Advantages	Disadvantages
Highly effective (as effective as female sterilisation), with an immediate return to fertility after removal	Can cause irregular bleeding in the first 3 months of being fitted, with 20% of users experiencing prolonged bleeding (more than 8 consecutive days in the first month) settling to 3% during the third month
Reduces menstrual blood loss (97% after 12 months); can be used to treat primary menorrhagia, with about 20% of women being amenorrhoeic (no evidence of hypo-oestrogenism)	May be expelled or displaced in about 4–6% of cases Fitting may be painful and seen by women as an invasive procedure
Reduces dysmenorrhoea	Like other IUDs there is a small increased risk of pelvic infection immediately after fitting, particularly in young women
Reduces the risk of ectopic pregnancy and can be used in women with a past history of extrauterine pregnancies	A small number of women may develop functional ovarian cysts but rarely require surgical intervention
Long-acting (lasts 5 years) and independent of intercourse	Other rare complications, e.g. perforation of the uterus/cervix (less than 1/1000 device fitted)
Reduces the incidence of pelvic inflammatory disease	Some progestogenic symptoms, such as breast tenderness, bloating or acne may occur in the first few months but these tend to settle
It can be used as the progestogen component of hormone replacement therapy	Small risk of ectopic pregnancy in the event of failure, although overall incidence of ectopic pregnancy is lower than in the general population
May protect against endometrial hyperplasia and fibroid formation	
May be a good maintenance therapy for those with endometriosis and adenomyosis	Cannot be used as an emergency form of contraception[49]
High user acceptance rate with 3-year continuation rates of 75–82%[49]	Non-hormonal contraception

All types of IUDs increase the number of leucocytes in the endometrium and uterotubal fluid, producing a typical foreign-body reaction. Copper enhances this reaction and the copper ions may be toxic to sperm and blastocysts. The main long-term contraceptive effect is, therefore, to prevent fertilisation rather than disrupt blastocyst implantation. As providers, it is all-important to explain the mode of action of an IUD, as many still see it as an abortifacient. The advantages and disadvantages of IUDs are shown in Table 6.8.

Female barrier methods

Diaphragms and caps

Barrier methods are becoming more popular as the increasing incidence of STIs in the community is highlighted. Diaphragms and caps are often thought to be messy and difficult to use. The ease of use and lack of interference with intercourse often come as a surprise to new users, yet this method is used by only a small number of women in the UK. Diaphragms sit between the posterior fornix and behind the pubic bone to cover the cervix. Vault caps suit women with fairly flat cervices and lax pelvic floors. These are dome shaped, fitting over the vault and held in place by

Table 6.8. Advantages and disadvantages of copper intrauterine contraceptive devices

Advantages	Disadvantages
Long term (up to 10 years), highly effective, reversible contraception	May cause menstrual irregularities with intermenstrual bleeding and spotting
Effective immediately after fitting	Periods may become heavier, longer and more painful, especially at first
Non-intercourse related method of contraception	
	IUD may be expelled or displaced leading to unplanned pregnancies (4–6%)
When used in the long term, a copper IUD's main contraceptive action is pre-fertilisation	
Requires no daily action or remembering	Some women may develop a pelvic infection, especially within the first 20 days following IUD insertion; may be prevented by screening for sexually transmitted infections prior to IUD fitting
Low morbidity, with a mortality rate of 1:500 000	
Non-hormonal contraceptive method so will not cause weight gain or give hormonal adverse effects	Risk of ectopic pregnancy in the event of IUD failure, although incidence is lower than the general population in users of IUD containing 300 mm^2 or more of copper
Effective as an emergency contraceptive[50]	Other extremely rare complications, e.g. perforation
High acceptability and continuation rates, with IUDs being ideal for family spacing and as a contraceptive method once a family is compete	

suction. Cervical caps fit directly over the cervix by suction and are ideal for women with long cervices and are a useful option in women who complain of recurrent urinary tract infections when using diaphragms. The advantages and disadvantages of diaphragms and caps are shown in Table 6.9.

Female condom

The female condom is a lubricated, loose fitting, polyurethane sheath with two flexible rings. The closed end with the loose ring is inserted into the vagina and the outer ring covers the vulva. The first female condom, Femidom® (Chartex), was first marketed in the UK in 1992. It can be bought in pharmacies and is acceptable to some women, although complaints of it being 'noisy' and 'intrusive' are often made. The advantages and disadvantages of the female condom are shown in Table 6.10.

Spermicides

Spermicides are one of the oldest forms of contraception known to man and are chemical compounds in the form of foams (contained in aerosols), jellies, creams, films or pessaries. They are also the active component of vaginal sponges. Many different substances have been used in the past but preparations available in the UK are now based on nonoxynol-9. There is active research investigating the viricidal potential of spermicidal substances in the hope of discovering a contraceptive that will help to protect against HIV. The advantages and disadvantages of spermicides are shown in Table 6.11.

Table 6.9. Advantages and disadvantages of diaphragms and caps

Advantages	Disadvantages
Effective with careful, consistent use (about 4% failure rate)	High failure rates
Inserted at any convenient time before having intercourse	Many users suffer more vaginal infections, particularly *Candida albicans*
Theoretical suggestion that diaphragms and caps protect against cancer of the cervix, some sexually transmitted infections and pelvic inflammatory disease, although there is no published evidence to support this	Require careful use on all occasions of intercourse to be effective
	May become dislodged during intercourse
No established health risks or systemic adverse effects	May increase the risk of cystitis or contracting a urinary tract infection
Direct control of the woman[15]	Requires application of a spermicide, making it appear 'messy' for some users
	Needs to be fitted by a health professional
	Users must follow instructions for use carefully[15]

Table 6.10. Advantages and disadvantages of female condoms

Advantages	Disadvantages
No known adverse effects	High failure rate
Acts as both a contraceptive and protects against sexually transmitted infections, including HIV	Requires thought before use
Theoretical benefit to help protect against cancer of the cervix and pelvic inflammatory disease	Requires careful insertion and use for it to be effective
Effective with careful use	Can interrupt intercourse
Under direct control of the user	Can be noisy and intrusive[15]
Can be inserted at any time before sexual intercourse	
No additional spermicide required	
Can be used with oil-based products	
Polyurethane is stronger than latex	
No need for male erection before use[15]	

Table 6.11. Advantages and disadvantages of spermicide

Advantages	Disadvantages
No serious adverse effects	Not effective alone, therefore must not be used as sole contraceptive in most circumstances
Widely available in pharmacies and simple to use	
	Messy
Provides lubrication	
	Intercourse-dependent
Enhances efficacy of barrier methods	
	Waiting time after use of pessaries, foaming tablets
Useful during the perimenopause (women over 45 years with irregular cycles and some vasomotor symptoms)	Those available may damage the vaginal epithelium[15]
Can be used during breastfeeding (until menstruation returns and weaning begins)[15]	

Permanent forms of contraception

Female sterilisation

About 23% of all couples in England and Wales rely on either male or female sterilisation as their main method of contraception.[4] As yet, reversing male or female sterilisation requires performing a surgical procedure, which may not be 100% successful. It is therefore seen as a permanent contraceptive method. All female sterilisation techniques block the path of the sperm, preventing fertilisation, and are normally performed laparoscopically as a daycase procedure.

Providers should counsel women to use effective contraception prior to surgery following evidence suggesting that 2.6% women are pregnant at the time of sterilisation.[28] Many units now perform urinary pregnancy tests on the morning of the procedure.[28,29] It is not good practice to sterilise women routinely immediately postpartum, post-abortion or where other reversible contraceptive options have not been fully considered.[29]

Table 6.12. Advantages and disadvantages of female sterilisation

Advantages	Disadvantages
Highly effective	Involves a surgical procedure and normally a general anaesthetic
Immediately effective	
	Not easily reversible; reversal rarely provided by the NHS
Fear of unplanned pregnancy removed	
	Other hormonal contraceptive methods are equally effective, with additional non-contraceptive benefits
Permanent method	
Does not cause weight gain or heavy periods	Associated complications in 0.9–1.6/100 cases,[51] with clips having the lowest complication rate of 0.47/100 cases (Table 6.13)
May protect against ovarian cancer (unexplained)	

Table 6.13. Complications of female sterilisation

Duration	Type of complication	Comments
Short term	Anaesthesia	Overall mortality is very low
	Perforation of bowel, blood vessels, bladder, at the time of the procedure[51] Wound infection	Risk of laparotomy as a result of a serious complication is about 1.9/1000 procedures[51]
	Abdominal discomfort and shoulder tip pain	From intraperitoneal gas remaining in the abdominal cavity. This slowly improves over 24–48 hours
Long term	Late recanalisation of fallopian tubes	Failure rates with Filshie clips are now quoted as 2–3/1000 procedures.[29] Occurs even up to 10 years following surgery with a cumulative ectopic pregnancy rate being as high as 31.9/1000 procedures, depending on the method used[52]
	Complaints of menorrhagia leading to hysterectomy	Women often stop hormonal methods of contraception that have controlled their menstrual loss and pain; with advancing age, menstrual problems also increase and can lead to requests for treatment
	Regret	Regret is not uncommon with 3–10% of couples reporting this.[29] More common when the operation has been performed in those under 30 years old and within 1 year of the birth of a child

Table 6.14. Advantages and disadvantages of vasectomy

Advantages	Disadvantages
Safe and effective, with a failure rate of about 1/2000 in a lifetime quoted	Not easily reversible; couples can regret taking this decision, especially if they are young (under 30 years)
Permanent method	Not effective immediately, with two negative semen analyses required before other contraceptive methods can be abandoned
Fear of unplanned pregnancy is removed	
Minor operation normally performed under local anaesthesia, taking 10–15 minutes	Involves a surgical procedure with associated complications[29] (Table 6.15)
Can be done at a doctor's surgery or clinic	
Studies have not yet shown an increased risk of testicular or prostate cancer following vasectomy	
Studies have not yet shown an increased risk of coronary heart disease following vasectomy[29]	

Table 6.15. Complications of vasectomy

Complication	Occurrence
Short term:	
Local complications	Bruising and swelling with some discomfort or pain for a short time following the procedure
	Scrotal haematoma formation occurs in 1–2% of men
Wound infection	Can occur in up to 5% of men and may require treatment with antibiotics
Failure to achieve azoospermia	In about 0.5% of men azoospermia is not achieved and further surgery may be required[29]
Long term:	
Sperm granulomas	Small lumps that form at the cut ends of the vas (leakage of sperm into the tissue from the cut ends of the vas deferens leading to local inflammation); can be palpable and painful and can be resolved by excision
Chronic scrotal pain	0.9–5.2% of men see their doctor about chronic scrotal pain following vasectomy; may be made worse by sexual arousal or ejaculation; local scar tissue formation and induration may be the cause; in some cases, further surgery to remove the epididymis and occluded vas may be indicated
Sperm antibodies	Occur in about 60–80% of vasectomised men; their presence may affect the success of a reversal procedure
Late recanalisation	May occur even up to 10 years after the vasectomy operation
Regret following operation	Not uncommon, particularly in countries with high divorce rates

Over the last 10 years or so, with the introduction of highly effective, long-acting, reversible, contraceptive methods, the numbers of women requesting female sterilisation have fallen. Department of Health data reported that 55 000 female sterilisation procedures were performed in 1993 compared with 28 000 in 2003.[30] There was no change recorded in men undergoing vasectomies. The advantages and disadvantages of female sterilisation are shown in Table 6.12 and the complications involved in Table 6.13.

Male sterilisation (vasectomy)

In the UK, about 12% of couples rely on male sterilisation as their chosen method of contraception. Approximately 50% of all sterilisation procedures are performed on men. In other parts of the world this ratio is different, with women ten times more likely to be sterilised compared with their male counterparts. The advantages and disadvantages of vasectomy are shown in Table 6.14 and the complications involved in Table 6.15.

Table 6.16. Advantages and disadvantages of fertility awareness

Advantages	Disadvantages
Can be used to plan pregnancy as well as prevent conception	Requires commitment of both partners Needs to be taught in order to use successfully
No known physical adverse effects	Requires careful observation and record keeping, which may take time to learn
Non-intercourse related method	
No mechanical devices or hormones used	Users must have high motivation, requiring long periods of abstinence from intercourse
Acceptable to all religions	Does not protect against sexually transmitted diseases
Once the methods has been learned by the user, no further follow-up is necessary	

Natural family planning

The traditional terms 'rhythm' and 'safe period' to designate family planning based on the detection of ovulation have been replaced over the last decade by the terms 'natural family planning' or 'fertility awareness'.

Natural family planning is effective if couples abstain from penetrative sex during the fertile period of the menstrual cycle. Normally, 3–12 months of menstrual cycle data are needed to accurately predict the fertile phase. In the UK, only 2% of couples use fertility awareness as their method of contraception but many more use these methods to space their family worldwide. The advantages and disadvantages of fertility awareness are shown in Table 6.16.

Lactational amenorrhoea method

Breastfeeding is a natural way to space children. Suckling during breastfeeding induces a reduction in gonadotrophin releasing hormone, leading to low levels of LH and FSH. This results in amenorrhoea and stimulation of prolactin secretion and milk production. The World Health Organization has confirmed the validity of lactational amenorrhoea as an effective contraceptive method offering 98% protection against pregnancy when the following conditions exist:

- a woman is fully or almost fully breastfeeding (feeding with no substitutes and at regular periods on demand, day and night)
- The baby is less than 6 months of age
- Menstruation has not returned.[15]

Coitus interruptus or 'withdrawal'

Coitus interruptus is the oldest method of birth control and it is still one of the most popular natural contraceptive methods worldwide. In the UK, 4% of couples use this method and it can be practised by any couple at any time. Advantages and disadvantages are listed in Table 6.17.

Table 6.17. Advantages and disadvantages of coitus interruptus

Advantages	Disadvantages
Free of charge	High failure rate
Requires no prescription	Intercourse is incomplete
Does not cause nausea or weight gain	Unsatisfying to both partners
Acceptable to many users	Partial ejaculation of semen can occur
	Does not protect against sexually transmitted diseases

Emergency contraception

Emergency contraception involves methods that can be given in the event of unprotected intercourse to prevent pregnancy.

Hormonal methods

Initial research began in the 1960s but it was not until the early 1980s that a licensed preparation was available in the UK. Combined hormonal emergency contraception has now been withdrawn from the UK as studies have shown fewer adverse effects with progestogen-only emergency contraception and also that it may also be more effective.[31]

In 2003–04, about 600 000 packets of hormonal emergency contraception were issued in England, with over 33% sold in pharmacies.[30] Emergency contraception needs to be easily accessible and, in 2003–04, 41% of women went to their GPs, 21% to a community clinic, 27% to a pharmacy and 16% to an accident and emergency department or walk-in centre to obtain emergency contraception.[4] Over the years,

Table 6.18. Advantages and disadvantages of hormonal emergency contraception

Advantages	Disadvantages
Effective, with low failure rate	Only effective for 72–120 hours after unprotected sexual intercourse
Easily available from GPs, nurses, community settings, pharmacies	Some women complain of nausea and vomiting; up to 25% of women complain of feeling sick but less than 5% of vomiting
Easy to take in tablet form	
Can be taken up to 72 hours after unprotected intercourse with some evidence that it has some effect even up to 120 hours	Other adverse effects include breast tenderness, dizziness, headaches, tiredness
Treatment can be repeated in the same menstrual cycle if required[32]	Can cause disturbance of menstruation, although majority of women will have their next period within 5 days of the expected time
	Does not protect against sexually transmitted infections[32]

since hormonal emergency contraception became a pharmacy-only drug, there has been a move away from GP and community services issuing it to women. Many are now either buying or obtaining it via patient group directions at their local pharmacy.[4]

Hormonal emergency contraception's exact mode of action is unknown but it does not appear to work post-fertilisation. Research fails to support the theory that it prevents implantation of the blastocyst and growing evidence suggests that it prevents or delays ovulation.[32] Providers should inform users of its mode of action, so as to dispel some of the myths that hormonal emergency contraception 'causes abortions', contains 'dangerous hormones' and can affect future fertility. The advantages and disadvantages of hormonal emergency contraception are shown in Table 6.18.

Non-hormonal emergency contraception

The copper IUD is a highly effective emergency contraceptive, particularly if the first episode of unprotected sexual intercourse is more than 72 hour prior to the consultation. Copper-containing IUDs rather than the LNG-IUS are recommended. Copper IUDs reduce the viability of the ova, decrease sperm numbers reaching the fallopian tubes and may also prevent implantation by inducing changes in the endometrium.

An IUD should be offered to all women requesting emergency contraception, as it is the most effective choice. If the provider has to refer the woman to other health professionals or delay fitting, they should prescribe hormonal emergency contraception where appropriate (Table 6.19). This will ensure that women have received a method of emergency contraception if an IUD cannot be successfully inserted or she fails to attend her appointment.

Table 6.19. Advantages and disadvantages of using intrauterine devices (IUDs) for emergency contraception

Advantages	Disadvantages
Can be used when there have been multiple episodes of unprotected sex but the woman presents within 5 days after the earliest calculated time of ovulation	Similar to using IUDs as a long-term method of contraception
Can be used when vomiting has occurred following administration of progestogen-only emergency contraception	Can cause pain at insertion particularly in nulliparous women
Ideal choice if an IUD is requested as a long-term contraceptive method	Can increase the risk of pelvic infection; if an IUD is inserted as an emergency, it is good practice to perform a screen for sexually transmitted infections prior to fitting; some authorities also recommending antibiotic cover in high-risk groups
Is the most effective emergency contraceptive (almost 100% effective), especially if unprotected sex occurs close to the time of ovulation	An emergency IUD is normally removed at the time of the next menses in women choosing alternative long-term methods of contraception, especially if young or nulliparous; some may forget to have the IUD removed, thus increasing their chance of upper genital infection if they contract a sexually transmitted infection
Is the most effective method after 72 hours of unprotected sex[31]	

Who attends community and primary care contraceptive services?

Up-to-date figures for users of community and primary care contraceptive services are not available for all countries within the UK. Approximately four million people used English family planning services each year[30] and it has been estimated that over six million women use services throughout the UK.[5] Roughly 75% see a GP and the remainder attend specialist family planning clinics. What is not evident from these figures is the proportion of women who attend both services. Collation of figures from UK community family planning services is statutory, with services completing annual returns on standardised KT31 forms. However, data on contraceptive services provided in general practice or emergency contraception issued by community pharmacies are far more difficult to ascertain. At the present time, the only inform-ation available is prescribing data and these national figures cannot be broken down into local practices.

The most recent attendance figures from KT31 forms are available for 2003–04 in England.[30] The increasing use of contraceptive services by men and young people is mirrored throughout the UK. In English community contraceptive services during 2003–04:

- there were about 2.7 million attendances at family planning clinics, about 2% more than in 2002–03
- 1.20 million women attended clinics, about the same as in 2002–03
- 106 000 men attended clinics, about 14% more than in 2002–03
- the peak age for clinic attendance was 16–17 years; an estimated 23% of women in this age group visited a clinic during the year.

What contraceptive methods are being issued from primary care and community services?

From the National Statistics Omnibus Study questioning 7258 people (including women below 50 years of age from Great Britain) in 2003–04, 25% of women aged between 16–49 years currently used oral contraception as their main contraceptive method followed by 23% who used condoms.[4] The IUD was used by 4% of women and 2% stated that they used the diaphragm or cervical cap. Just under 25% of women interviewed relied on sterilisation, with 11% of women having been sterilised and 12% of their partners.

Fourteen percent of women were not in a relationship and a small number were pregnant, had surgery that had rendered them infertile or wanted to become pregnant. There were 2%, however, not using any method and who did not want to become pregnant.

Community and primary care services provide contraceptive services for the British population but do they offer the same choice? This is a difficult area to investigate, as there is no national dataset for contraceptive attendances in primary care. One survey published in 1993 suggested that the majority of women use oral contraception but that community clinics provided a more diverse range.[33] To investigate this further I have used data that are available for community clinics and compared these data with prescribing data held by the Department of Health.[30] It may unearth continuing differences in contraceptive provision and therefore highlight areas for improvements in contraceptive choice.

English data are used as recent figures are available and attendances are highest. Available data for Wales, Scotland and Ireland show similar trends. It is recognised that there are regional variations in contraceptive provision across community services. Prescribing data for general practice do not offer a direct comparison to contraception provided to individual women, as different methods require a variable number of prescriptions over the year. It is also noted that GPs cannot prescribe condoms for users, although there are now local distribution schemes through primary care services that will not be picked up from national prescribing data.

Using KT31 2003–04 data for England, 41% of attendees used oral contraception as their main method with 10–12% of these choosing POPs. Thirty six percent used condoms as their main method and 5–6% used IUDs, 1.1% the IUS, 1% diaphragms or caps, 8% injectables and 1.3% relied on implants for contraception.[30] Comparing these data with prescribing data available for England in 2003–04, approximately 8 229 000 prescriptions were written with 74% for combined pills, 13% for POPs, 12.6% for injectables, 0.6% for IUDs, 0.75% for the IUS, 0.2% for diaphragms/caps and 0.2% for implants.[30] Alternative methods are infrequently chosen in primary care because the COC:

- is a well-accepted, effective, reversible contraceptive method
- is inexpensive
- is simple to prescribe and requires no practical expertise on the part of the provider
- has additional noncontraceptive benefits
- is one of a few methods immediately available via prescription.

For a potential user long-acting methods may require another GP to insert or fit the device. Potential users may need a referral to another practice or community service. Often these obstacles result in GPs failing to discuss these methods in detail.

These data confirm the findings of the Manchester survey of 1993.[33] Most couples choose oral contraception as their main method but younger users choose to attend community services, particularly with dedicated young people's sessions.[30] Community clinics appear to offer a greater variety of methods with more emphasis on longer-acting methods. Perhaps this is not surprising, as intrauterine contraceptives and implants require a greater expertise to fit and, in the case of implants, to remove. These data support the continuing development of community services to offer a wide range of contraceptive choice.

Training needs and issues

A survey undertaken by the Contraceptive Education Service run by the fpa and Health Education Authority identified that 88% of GPs had some training in family planning but two-thirds had family planning qualifications issued in the 1970s.[5] Just 12% had recent training, with practice nurses more likely to have attended update training courses. There are no training data available for health professionals working in community services. However, job descriptions for staff grade, associate specialist and consultants specify that candidates should hold either the diploma, membership or fellowship of the Faculty of Family Planning (DFFP and MFFP) or an equivalent qualification with evidence of recertification if appropriate.

For nurses working within community services, a recognised RCN family planning qualification or equivalent is required. Training for both nurses and doctors involves a theoretical component and practical placement. Trainees in genitourinary medicine now need to obtain the DFFP as part of their specialist registrar training but in obstetrics and gynaecology candidates for the membership examination are just required to receive instruction at eight family planning clinics. There is no requirement by the Royal College of Obstetricians and Gynaecologists for specialist registrars to attend a DFFP theory course, which is regrettable, as the level of contraceptive knowledge among trainees is often poor.

Most of the practical, hands-on training takes place in community services but with pressure from increasing patient attendances and referral of complex medical cases training resources are stretched to their limits.

Further obstacles to maintaining and increasing practical placement numbers include:

- poor terms and conditions of employment for senior doctors who are leaving or returning to general practice
- poor support and funding of training by the postgraduate deaneries
- changes to DFFP practical training requiring trainers to spend more time with trainees developing competency-based, learning objectives.

These issues need to be discussed as a matter of urgency locally, regionally and nationally, so that the future workforce is adequately equipped to provide level one services in primary care and accurate contraceptive advice in secondary care.

The Faculty of Family Planning and Reproductive Health Care

The Faculty of Family Planning and Reproductive Health Care of the RCOG was established on 26 March 1993. It has over 11 000 members who either hold a diploma (DFFP), membership (MFFP) or fellowship (FFFP). These are postgraduate medical qualifications that require recertification every 5 years. The Faculty recognises equivalent specialist knowledge and skills in family planning and reproductive health care welcoming nonmedical associate members. No other country has a college or faculty devoted to promoting academic status to the discipline of family planning and reproductive health care.

The Faculty works closely with the Royal College of Nursing, the RCOG and the Royal College of General Practitioners. This network develops and maintains standards of clinical care and training to ensure that all providers of such services give high quality contraceptive care within the framework specified in the Sexual Health Strategy.[6]

FFPRHC workforce planning

The FFPRHC undertakes an annual census of doctors working in family planning and reproductive health care to document staffing levels, service provision and training details for each district in the UK. This informs the Department of Health about the importance of such services but also is a useful tool for local health boards and primary care organisations to maintain staffing levels, develop local medical training programmes and succession plans for medical staff retirement. The number of training centres for career-grade and sub-specialty training in the specialty has grown, as a response to staffing needs.[34]

It is imperative that this data collection process continues ensuring that each region can provide training for health professionals and be an effective resource for local health providers.

Prescribing guidance

Medicines and Healthcare Products Regulatory Agency

The Medicines and Healthcare Products Regulatory Agency (MHRA) is an executive agency of the Department of Health that:

- ensures that medicines for human use, sold or supplied in the UK, are of an acceptable standard of safety, quality and efficacy
- ensures that medical devices meet appropriate standards of safety, quality and performance
- promotes the safe use of medicines and devices.

Committee on Safety of Medicines

The Committee on Safety of Medicines (CSM) is one of the independent advisory committees that advises the UK Licensing Authority on the quality, efficacy and safety of medicines in order to ensure that appropriate public health standards are met and maintained. The Committee provides advice to the Licensing Authority on whether new products should be granted a marketing authorisation and monitors the safety of marketed medicines. Neither the MHRA nor the CSM advises the use or avoidance of specific products or devices unless there is a safety issue.[26]

National Institute for Clinical Excellence and the Scottish Medicines Consortium

The National Institute for Clinical Excellence (NICE) is part of the NHS. It is an independent organisation responsible for providing national guidance on treatments and care for people using the NHS in England and Wales. Its guidance is intended for healthcare professionals, patients and their carers, to help them make decisions about treatment and health care. NICE guidance is developed using the expertise of the NHS and wider healthcare community, including NHS staff, healthcare professionals, patients and carers, industry and the academic community.

No guidance for contraception had been published since NICE was first established but, in November 2005, guidance on the effective and appropriate use of long-acting reversible contraception was published. It is hoped that this will pave the way to improving and developing contraceptive choice across the country.

In Scotland the Scottish Medicines Consortium (SMC) provides advice to NHS Boards and their Area Drug and Therapeutics Committees about the status of all newly licensed medicines, all new formulations of existing medicines and any major new indications for established products. So far the SMC have published statements on the combined contraceptive patch, a new progestogen–only pill and a new combined oral contraceptive.

These two bodies do guide national contraceptive provision by presenting published evidence to support or restrict prescribing or use of certain contraceptive methods. Much of this guidance is driven by cost to promote and provide inexpensive contraceptive methods to the UK population.

Table 6.20. Cost of contraceptive methods in the UK (excluding value added tax)[35]

Method	Cost (£)[a]	Quantity sold (*n*)
Spermicides	2.40–2.65	
Cap/diaphragm	5.68–8.20	
Sponge	2.00	
Female condom	42.85	30
Male condom	28.95	14
COC	2.46–14.70	
POP	1.89–8.8.5	
Combined patch	23.23	
Combined vaginal ring	Not available in UK	
Progestogen injectable	3.59–5.01	
Combined injectable	Not available in UK	
Intrauterine device	7.13–24.75	
Intrauterine system	98.18	
Progestogen implants	90.00	

[a] Cheapest and most expensive given if there are several products

Cost of contraceptive methods in the UK

Cost effectiveness of contraceptives

When looking at Table 6.20 for the first time, healthcare commissioners will immediately calculate the cost of providing each contraceptive method over a period of a month or perhaps even a year.[35] This is rather a simplistic view. In order to understand how cost effective a method actually is, there are a number of other pieces of information required. How effective is each contraceptive method, focusing on the first year of use when user-dependent methods have a learning curve and efficacy is at its lowest? There is a cost to the health service for caring for a child, performing an abortion or operating on a woman with an ectopic pregnancy. Is the contraceptive method acceptable to the user? Copper IUDs are inexpensive and highly effective but many women view the fitting of such a device as being invasive and the associated menstrual problems may make it unsuitable for some. Inconsistent use of the pill (for fear of weight gain) or condoms (as they interrupt sex) leads to increased unplanned pregnancies and decrease the cost effectiveness of that method.

Are there any non-contraceptive health benefits that may reduce visits to healthcare professionals and perhaps even surgery? Data presented have shown that combined pills reduce the risk of ovarian and uterine cancer and the IUS decreases menstrual loss and may lead to a fall in gynaecological surgery. All these factors need to be included in any meaningful cost effectiveness calculation and provide powerful information for those designing sexual health services for the future.

In 1995, McGuire and Hughes[1] calculated cost effectiveness against direct costs of pregnancies avoided. Two US papers looked at the economics of providing contraception. The first examined, from the healthcare services payer perspective, the economic consequences of contraceptives available to women using a Markov model constructed to compare effectiveness and costs among nine commonly used contraceptive methods (vasectomy was excluded).[36] The results showed that the least expensive methods (accounting for all costs) were the IUS, IUDs containing 300mm^2 or more of copper and 3-month injectables.

Sonnenberg *et al.* extended the cost–benefit analysis to comparing 13 methods of contraception with nonuse of contraception with respect to healthcare costs and quality-adjusted life years. Using a Markov model evaluated by Monte Carlo simulation and discounting of future costs and health effects, the following was found.[37] Compared with use of no contraception, contraceptive methods of all types result in substantial cost savings over a 2-year period but, more importantly, even a modest increase in the use of the most effective methods such as the IUS, IUD or implant result in financial savings and health gains.

Supportive educational tools for health professionals

Keeping up to date and providing accurate contraceptive advice is difficult for most healthcare professionals, particularly if reproductive health is not their special interest. There are a number of tools available to help clinicians.

Throughout this chapter, I have quoted from guidance produced by the Clinical Effectiveness Unit (CEU) of the FFPRHC. Every quarter, new CEU articles appear in the *Journal of Family Planning and Reproductive Health Care*. The CEU was established in 1997 and publishes short clinical guidelines, responses to members' enquiries about clinical practice and informed information about new contraceptive methods, to help clinicians make a reasoned choice when prescribing contraceptive methods. These articles are available to everyone on the faculty website in the publication's section.[38]

The World Health Organization (WHO) has led the way in producing guidance for healthcare professionals working across the world in the field of contraception. WHO Medical Eligibility Criteria for Contraceptive Use[39] and WHO Selected Practice Recommendations for Contraceptive Use[40] have been published on their website: www.who.int/reproductive-health/publications. The first document gives a guide to the provider as to who can use the different methods of contraception safely and the second advises how to use these methods safely and effectively. These documents are comprehensive but may provide different guidance when compared with the CEU publications. This is because WHO focuses on developing countries where maternal mortality is high and effective contraception, even when used by women with certain medical conditions, is safer than pregnancy and childbirth. These documents are being modified for the UK and will be distributed to health professionals.

Prodigy guidance is available online and offers advice on the management of conditions and symptoms that are commonly seen in primary care.[41] The guidance has been developed to assist healthcare professionals, together with patients in making decisions about their healthcare management. It is regularly updated and its advice helps to inform providers of contraceptive choices for patients. It also provides useful patient information leaflets that are immediately available for users.

The Scottish Intercollegiate Guidelines Network (SIGN) was formed in 1993 and its aim is to improve the quality of health care for people in Scotland. This network hopes that the development and dissemination of national clinical guidelines containing recommendations for effective practice based on current evidence will reduce variation in practice and achieve better outcomes for patients. At the present time, there are no guidelines covering any aspect of contraception.

One of the most useful resources for providers of health care is the National Electronic Library for Health programme.[42] It is working with NHS Libraries to develop a digital library for NHS staff, patients and the public and has links to sites such as Prodigy, the National Prescribing Centre and the Healthcare Commission. It also guides the user to helpful publications such as Bandolier, the Cochrane Library and Medline.

Conclusion

I started this chapter with a series of questions and I hope that some answers have emerged by examining published evidence. The first and second questions were that, if contraception is free in the UK, then why are so many couples failing to use birth control or using a method poorly? Are the providers partly to blame? These areas are highly complex with a number of solutions being found when looking at contraceptive methods from the user's perspective. From a provider's perspective, it appears we are not offering contraceptive choice because not all health professionals discuss or provide effective, reversible methods. Their ignorance falls at the door of continuing medical education. Local commissioners for health have also failed to provide accessible, comprehensive services to the community, especially for those with the greatest needs. As a result, the commonly held myths and misconceptions relating to contraception still prevail and there is continuing reliance on contraceptive methods with high user dependency.

What governs the healthcare provider's decision-making process and how could it be improved? Not wishing to sound too cynical but, up until 2004, financial rewards in terms of 'items of service' payments for providing contraceptive services in primary care was the main driver. The new GMS and PMS contracts may help to broaden and improve contraceptive provision for the 70% or so who attend their GP practice for contraceptive advice but this extra funding may not be enough. Instead of primary care taking a bigger role in providing a level one service, pressure will be placed on crumbling community contraceptive services that have failed to attract new money for service improvement.

Are there any recommendations that could alter contraceptive provision and increase contraceptive uptake and continuance? Although I have taken a negative view of changes within the NHS to date, there is hope for the future. Local commissioning of services does provide an opportunity to re-evaluate contraceptive needs in the community and it is possible that extra funding might come from the Department of Health in England to improve community contraceptive services. Emphasis must also be placed on extending the nurse's role and increasing NHS contraceptive dispensing to other healthcare professionals, such as pharmacists. Terms and conditions of employment of community medical staff and 'Agenda for Change' for nursing and administration staff are currently being reviewed. It is hoped that these changes will improve recruitment and retention of a highly skilled and dedicated workforce. Local level three services, national colleges and faculties need to support continuing education of all staff counselling couples about contraception with greater emphasis on providing the most effective contraceptive method that is acceptable to users.

References

1.   McGuire A, Hughes D. *The Economics of Family Planning Services. A report prepared for the Contraceptive Alliance.* London: fpa; 1995.

2. Department of Health. *The NHS Plan.* London: The Stationery Office; 2000.
3. Dixon-Woods M, Stokes T, Young B, Phelps K, Windridge K, Shukla R. Choosing and using services for sexual health: a qualitative study of women's views. *Sex Transm Infect* 2001;77:335–9.
4. Office for National Statistics on behalf of the Department of Health. *Contraception and Sexual Health, 2003. A report on research using the ONS Omnibus survey produced by the Office for National Statistics.* London: The Stationery Office; 2004.
5. Family Planning Association. Use of Family Planning Services. Factsheet number 2. London: Sexual Health Direct; 2002.
6. Department of Health. *Better Prevention, Better Services, Better Sexual Health. The National Strategy for Sexual Health and HIV.* London: Department of Health; 2001.
7. Humphery S, Nazareth I. GPs' views on their management of sexual dysfunction. *Fam Pract* 2001;18:516–18.
8. Department of Health. *Choosing Health. Making Health Choices Easier.* London: Department of Health; 2004.
9. Social Exclusion Unit. *Teenage Pregnancy.* London: Department of Health; 1999.
10. Department of Health. *Delivering Investment in General Practice. Implementing the New GMS Contract.* London: Department of Health; 2003.
11. Department of Health. *Sustaining Innovation Through New PMS Arrangements.* London: Department of Health, March 2004.
12. Faculty of Family Planning and Reproductive Health Care. Recommended Local Enhanced Service Framework for Contraceptive Implants. London: FFPRHC; 2004 [www.ffprhc.org.uk].
13. Garg M, Singh M, Mansour D. Peri-abortion contraceptive care: can we reduce the incidence of repeat abortions? *J Fam Plann Reprod Health Care* 2001;27:77–80.
14. Trussell J. Contraceptive failure in the United States. *Contraception* 2004;70:89–96.
15. Guillebaud J. *Contraception. Your Questions Answered.* Third Edition. London: Churchill Livingstone; 1999.
16. Rosenberg MJ, Waugh MS, Higgins JE. The effect of desogestrel, gestodene and other factors on spotting and bleeding. *Contraception* 1996;53:85–90.
17. Loudon NB, Kirkman RJE, Dewsbury JA. A double-blind comparison of the efficacy and acceptability of Femodene and Microgynon-30. *Eur J Obstet Gynecol Reprod Health* 1990;34:257–66.
18. Thorneycroft H, Gollnick H, Schellschmidt I. Superiority of a combined contraceptive containing drospirenone to a triphasic preparation containing norgestimate in acne treatment. *Cutis* 2004;74:123–30.
19. Worret I, Arp W, Zahradnik HP, Andreas JO, Binder N. Acne resolution rates: results of a single-blind, randomized, controlled, parallel phase III trial with EE/CMA (Belara) and EE/LNG (Microgynon). *Dermatology* 2001;203:38–44.
20. Foidart JM, Wuttke W, Bouw GM, Gerlinger C, Heithecker R. A comparative investigation of contraceptive reliability, cycle control and tolerance of two monophasic oral contraceptives containing either drospirenone or desogestrel. *Eur J Contracept Reprod Health Care* 2000;5:124–34.
21. Mansour D, Lister S. A study to compare continuation rates between Yasmin and existing COCs in UK clinical practice. *Eur J Contracept Reprod Health Care* 2004;9 Suppl 1:190.
22. Faculty of Family Planning and Reproductive Health Care, Clinical Effectiveness Unit. Desogestrel-only pill (Cerazette). *J Fam Plann Reprod Health Care* 2003;29:162–4.
23. Korver T, Klipping C, Heger-Mahn D, Duijkers I, van Osta G, Dieben T. Maintenance of consistent ovulation inhibition with the 75 mcg desogestrel-only contraceptive pill Cerazette after scheduled 12-hour delays in tablet taking. *Eur J Contracept Reprod Health Care* 2004;9 Suppl 1:43.
24. Organon Laboratories. User package leaflet for Cerazette, June 2004.
25. Pharmacia Ltd. Depo-Provera patient information sheet, July 2001.
26. Committee on Safety of Medicines. Updated prescribing advice on the effect of Depo-Provera contraception on bone. London: MHRA; 2004 [http://medicines.mhra.gov.uk].
27. Mattinson A, Mansour D. Unpublished data.
28. Kasliwal A, Farquharson RG. Pregnancy testing prior to sterilisation. *BJOG* 2000;107:1407–9.
29. Royal College of Obstetricians and Gynaecologists. Male and Female Sterilisation. National evidence-based clinical guideline Number 4. London: RCOG; 2004.
30. Department of Health. *NHS Contraceptive Services, England: 2003–2004.* London: DoH; 2004.
31. Faculty of Family Planning and Reproductive Health Care, Clinical Effectiveness Unit. Emergency Contraception. FFPRHC Guidance, April, 2003. *J Fam Plann Reprod Health Care* 2003;29:9–15.
32. Croxatto HB, Ortiz ME, Muller AL. Mechanisms of action of emergency contraception. *Steroids* 2003;68:1095–8.
33. Vickers JE, Greatorex IF. Differences between women who use general practice and health

authority family planning clinics. *Br J Fam Plann* 1993;19:184–6.

34. Faculty of Family Planning and Reproductive Health Care. Census of the Family Planning Workforce in the United Kingdom 2003. Provisional data [www.ffprhc.org.uk].

35. British Medical Association, Royal Pharmaceutical Society of Great Britain. *British National Formulary*. BNF 48. London: BMA & RPS; 2004.

36. Chiou CF, Trussell J, Reyes E, Knight K, Wallace J, Udani J, *et al*. Economic analysis of contraceptives for women. *Contraception* 2003;68:3–10.

37. Sonnenberg FA, Burkman RT, Hagerty CG, Speroff L, Speroff T. Costs and net health effects of contraceptive methods. *Contraception* 2004;69:447–59.

38. Faculty of Family Planning and Reproductive Health Care. Publications [www.ffprhc.org.uk].

39. World Health Organization. *Medical Eligibility Criteria for Contraceptive Use*. 3rd ed. Geneva: WHO; 2004.

40. World Health Organization. *Selected Practice Recommendations for Contraceptive Use*. 2nd ed. Geneva: WHO; 2004.

41. PRODIGY guidance [www.prodigy.nhs.uk].

42. National Electronic Library for Health [www.nelh.nhs.uk].

43. Faculty of Family Planning and Reproductive Health Care, Clinical Effectiveness Unit. FFPRHC Guidance (October, 2003). First Prescription of Combined Oral Contraception. *J Fam Plann Reprod Health Care* 2003;29:209-22. Erratum in: *J Fam Plann Reprod Health Care* 2004;30:63.

44. Heinemann LA, Dinger J. Safety of a new oral contraceptive containing drospirenone. *Drug Saf* 2004;27:1001–18.

45. Faculty of Family Planning and Reproductive Health Care, Clinical Effectiveness Unit. Contraception for women aged over 40 years. FFPRHC Guidance, January 2005. *J Fam Plann Reprod Health Care* 2005;31:51–64.

46. Cardiovascular disease and use of oral and injectable progestogen-only contraceptives and combined injectable contraceptives. Results of an international, multicenter, case-control study. *Contraception* 1998;57:315–24.

47. Varma R, Mascarenhas L. Endometrial effects of etonogestrel (Implanon) contraceptive implant. *Curr Opin Obstet Gynecol* 2001;13:335–41.

48. Smith A, Reuter S. An assessment of the use of Implanon in three community services. *J Fam Plann Reprod Health Care* 2002;28:193–6.

49. Faculty of Family Planning and Reproductive Health Care, Clinical Effectiveness Unit. The levonorgestrel-releasing intrauterine system (LNG-IUS) in contraception and reproductive health aged over 40. FFPRHC Guidance, April, 2004. *J Fam Plann Reprod Health Care* 2004;30:99–109.

50. Faculty of Family Planning and Reproductive Health Care, Clinical Effectiveness Unit. The copper intrauterine device as long-term contraception. FFPRHC Guidance, January, 2004. *J Fam Plann Reprod Health Care* 2004;30:29–42.

51. Jamieson DJ, Hillis SD, Duerr A, Marchbanks PA, Costello C, Peterson HB. Complications of interval laparoscopic tubal sterilization: findings from the United States Collaborative Review of Sterilization. *Obstet Gynecol* 2000;96:997–1002.

52. Peterson HB, Xia Z, Hughes JM, Wilcox LS, Tylor LR, Trussell J. The risk of ectopic pregnancy after tubal sterilization. U. S. Collaborative Review of Sterilization Working Group. *N Engl J Med* 1997;336:762–7.

Chapter 7

Contraception: users' perspectives and determinants of choice

Toni Belfield

> CHOICE: act, power, right . . . of choosing; what is chosen;
> variety of choice from
>
> *Oxford Illustrated Dictionary*

Introduction

Contraception and sex are passionate subjects. Both are about people: what we think, what we think people do, what we might like to do, what we actually do and what we do not do. Understanding how and why people make contraceptive choices is important because minimising the likelihood of unintended pregnancy depends on maximising user satisfaction, user effectiveness and continuation of use, by providing a contraceptive method that is truly the method of choice.

The past 50 years have seen a large change in the availability and provision of contraceptive methods. Research shows that people are knowledgeable about contraception. Substantial research and opinion throughout the world, however, continue to demonstrate that women and men do not know about the range of contraceptive choice. They lack knowledge about how methods work, they do not understand how to use methods or know what to do if a contraceptive method's effectiveness is compromised. Contraception enables people to choose whether and/or when to have children. It is inextricably linked with emotional and sexual wellbeing. It is impossible to discuss contraception without addressing sexuality: the two are inseparable. Sexual behaviours are complex, however, and their outcomes have wide practical implications. In developed countries, people are starting their sexual activity earlier, have more sexual partners and use contraception more but not consistently. As a consequence, the numbers of unintended pregnancies, abortions and sexually transmitted infections remain high. Findings from the National Survey of Attitudes and Lifestyles in Great Britain[1-3] illustrate that there is a wide variability in sexual lifestyles by age, gender, relationships and residence and this is normal. Research continues to confirm that people do not always behave rationally or in an organised and planned manner with their sex lives. People do experiment (and not just the young) and sometimes will take risks intentionally or unintentionally. Importantly, sexual lifestyles relate directly to factors such as knowledge and education, employment, deprivation and inequalities.

Harmonised, objective information

Obtaining harmonised, objective information on reproduction and fertility is not only a need, it is a right. Such knowledge provides an understanding of how health, emotions and behaviours relate to fertility. It enables an unravelling of myths, misconceptions and misinformation that exist and can minimise the embarrassment and anxieties that surround this often taboo subject. Knowledge and choice in contraception provide empowerment and confidence, which in turn enables improved reproductive decisions and choices to be made.[4]

'Patients', 'consumers', 'users', 'clients' are all terms for women and men who receive contraceptive and sexual health services. We talk about 'users' as if they are different people to ourselves but all of us are users, past users or potential users of sexual health services, directly or as a partner or friend. Importantly, whatever we call people we see for information, support or treatment, without them we would have no role. Recognising this fact is important. It is central to providing a service that knows and understands what people like or dislike and one that addresses people's expectations, needs, worries and concerns. People accessing contraceptive services are 'well' people and as such should not be called 'patients' who are seen in the context of ill health. This is not just semantics. The way we refer to people in relation to healthcare services affects how we communicate and share knowledge. It has the potential to shift the balance of power between provider and user to one of shared discussion and decision.[5]

Factors involved in choice

Women's and men's contraceptive needs, expectations and choices are influenced by many factors: knowledge, information, lifestyle need, age, religion, ethnicity, perceptions (their own and others), anxiety and embarrassment.[6–8] Provider preference and service delivery contribute to limiting or improving acceptability and choice and can have considerable impact on contraceptive decisions.[7,9] Attempts to categorise people's needs simplistically by, for example, age, parity or social class, is unhelpful and does not reflect the complexity of people's lives or the many factors which influence sexual relationships and reproductive choices. People today are involved much more in the management of their health and have access to enormous amounts of information from a variety of sources. However, sorting out fact from fiction is not easy. While contraceptive methods have become more sophisticated, safer and highly effective, public perceptions have not developed in the same positive way. Research continues to confirm that most women and men still perceive contraceptive choice as a matter of finding the 'least worst' option, balancing effectiveness and ease of use with perceptions and expectations of adverse effects and health risks.[6,10,11] There is a still a lack of clarity regarding the concept of acceptability, how to understand it, how to measure it and what it means. Although contraception is commonplace and affects large numbers of people and their lives, there are still too few qualitative data on users' perceptions and attitudes to contraception. Research continues to focus on clinical adverse effects and safety. This is, of course, important. Contraceptives, particularly oral hormonal contraceptives, are among the most thoroughly researched drugs of all time: rightfully so for a product that is used by young, healthy women for potentially long periods of time. However, while this is vitally important it must be recognised that it does not matter how safe or effective a method is, if it is not liked it will not be used. A review carried out for the World Health Organization in 1997 addressed users' perspectives on contraception and the conclusions are as valid now as then:[8]

- Contraceptive users lack complete information about both methods and services.
- Women and men's needs and preferences for contraception change over time, and vary with the person's stage of life.
- Universally, women and men would like a method that is safe and effective but it is not clear what these concepts mean. Adverse effects and health concerns (particularly with respect to hormonal methods) and method failure (particularly with respect to barrier methods and natural family planning) are the major reasons why women discontinue or do not use contraception.
- Individual perspectives and preferences vary widely and defy generalisation.
- The limited range of methods available in many developing countries necessarily limits people's perceptions and preferences.
- Research on people's reactions to a hypothetical method does not usually yield information predictive of subsequent use or behaviour with the method.
- There is limited information about the perspectives of men, adolescents, women having an abortion, especially repeat abortion, and women in the postpartum period.

Understanding and confusion

The ability to control fertility relates directly to the amount of information an individual has, coupled with feelings of self-worth and self-determination. Sexual adequacy and sexual identity relate directly to choice of contraceptive method. For example: using the pill requires daily acknowledgment of sexual intentions; using contraception, particularly barrier methods, requires affirmation of sexuality before every sexual act.

Comfort and knowledge about one's body and knowledge of how it works is fundamental to understanding how contraception works and why it can fail. Research continues to show that women and men lack accurate or good knowledge about reproduction and fertility. fpa helpline and information services handle over 100 000 enquiries annually from the public and professionals. The enquiries illustrate, on a daily basis, people's poor understanding of reproductive physiology and anatomy, confusion and misinformation about the menstrual cycle and menstruation, how and why ovulation occurs and about conception and pregnancy. How can informed decisions about contraceptive choices and sexual health be made if there is so little basic understanding? Some typical questions to fpa are shown below:

- Where does period blood come from?
- What it ovulation?
- Where does the egg go?
- What happens to sperm inside the body?
- How does a cap (tampon etc.) stay in?
- Can the IUD get lost inside me?
- How does the pill/intrauterine system/intrauterine device work?

fpa enquiries also illustrate the difficulties women and men have in accessing good information about reproduction and sexual health. The media provide an endless stream of information, sometimes providing accurate and up-to-date information but more often providing inaccurate, misleading and sometimes sensationalist information that focuses on victims, plays on emotions and has lasting negative effects.

Bad news is always considered more newsworthy than good news and reports seldom address 'risk' within any overall context. Troughs in oral contraceptive usage following 'pill scares' are a classic example.

Difficulties in accessing or discussing information are compounded by feelings of anxiety or embarrassment that surrounds anything to do with sex and contraception and applies to both users and providers. This has implications for uptake, use and provision of contraception. Increased knowledge and confidence depend on identifying and countering misinformation and promoting the benefits of use through accurate, complete, consistent and memorable information about the method of choice.[12]

Choice is therefore based on many variables and is seldom based on rationale or objective information. The fact that a friend has had a 'dreadful' time with an intrauterine device will have far more influence than any amount of statistics that say otherwise. Snowden wrote in 1990 that 'while it may be argued that the prevention of pregnancy is beneficial, the use of contraception is not pleasant for most people, which is in marked contrast to the sexual behaviour which prompts its need'.[13]

Research findings

Research addressing contraceptive decision making and perceptions has largely focused on women. Women are more directly affected by unintended pregnancy than men and it is more commonly women who experience use and possible consequences of using contraception. Historically then, information, health education programmes, services, research and development of methods have focused more on women's needs than men. Contraceptive choices in the future will include male hormonal contraception. As well as addressing men's general sexual health, there is a need to improve our support of men's involvement in contraceptive decision making and to remove the myth that it is not wanted or that men 'will not be trusted'.[14–16]

Choice of contraception is not a static, 'one-off' decision. People change methods throughout their reproductive lives and decisions are often prompted at different times. Research shows that this has not changed over the years; choice tends to relate to particular life stages or certain events, rather than to characteristics such as age, social class or family size.[7,17–19] Decision to use or change a method relates to:

- the beginning of sexual experience
- an unplanned pregnancy or pregnancy 'scare'
- specific life change, such as illness or career change
- a planned birth, between children (spacing)
- when a family is considered complete
- at the end of a relationship, at the beginning of a new relationship
- the presence of problems or perceived problems with a contraceptive method
- cost (outside the UK: contraception is free in the UK).

Most people have realistic expectations about contraception and understand that there is no single perfect, reversible and totally risk-free method that offers 100% efficacy. There are, however, fears, worries and doubts about potential, perceived and perhaps unknown adverse effects, especially relating to oral contraception.[20] These concerns have consequences for initial use and uptake and for confidence in continuing with a method. The factors that users consider 'important' when choosing contraception are:

- effectiveness: will it work? (emphasis on failure rather than success)
- risk/harm and uncertainties: serious or 'trivial' (who defines 'trivial'?)
- how to use a method: ease of use (the 'bother' factor), intercourse related or non-intercourse related?
- suitability of a method: how it fits into personal lifestyle
- non-contraceptive benefits: protection from sexually transmitted infections, 'help with periods'
- effect on future fertility: will it make me infertile?
- a friend/relative's positive use of a method
- known or 'trusted' brand
- control: ability to stop, start a method without medical intervention
- ease of obtaining it: do I have to see a doctor?

Understanding how choices are made and acknowledging users' concerns are vital. How contraception is considered, and discussed and importantly delivered relates directly to how well methods are accepted and used. fpa enquiries, research and statistics about unintended pregnancy suggest that we are not good at providing full, accessible, objective information. Most importantly, myths are well promoted and as a result are well known. How do myths originate and how good are we at dispelling them? Some common examples include:

- Hormonal contraception
  'the pill' is the most talked about and the most worried about contraceptive method. 'We talk about **the** pill', yet in the UK there are currently 31 brands and, of these, 22 are different; there are 25 combined oral contraceptive pills (18 are different) and six progestogen–only pills (four are different). Women have no idea that there are so many choices and are often deterred from using any pill when they have a problem with one type.

- 'The pill is not safe: it should only be used for short periods and requires regular breaks from taking it'
  There is no evidence for such practice but professionals regularly recommend it.

- 'The pill causes cancer'
  Research is complex and contradictory with regard to any possible association with cancer. Providing women with balanced information that enables them to weigh up harm, benefit and, importantly, uncertainty requires professionals to thoroughly understand the research and be able to discuss it confidently.

- 'All pills have high doses of hormones'
  Today's pills are low in oestrogen and progestogen. One pill taken in the 1960s is equivalent to 1 week's worth today. Many women and professionals are confused around terms such as 'high dose' or what 'first, second, third or fourth generation' mean in relation to the different progestogens in combined oral contraceptive pills. The fact that using the pill is safer than pregnancy and childbirth when it is appropriately prescribed is generally not known or promoted. If we do not unravel these myths how can women choose any hormonal method with confidence?

- 'The IUD causes infection and pain. It cannot be used by women who have not had children, it moves around body and it works by causing abortion'

These are just some of the myths that fpa helplines hear everyday. Perhaps it is not surprising when IUDs are still discussed as 'coils'. The term 'coil' derives from the IUD called the Saf-t-coil® used in the 1960s and early 1970s. Although it is no longer available, the terminology lives on. How can women feel enabled to use modern IUDs, vastly different, with safer profiles when outdated language is used? Professionals suggest that women cannot understand or use terms such as 'intrauterine contraception or IUD'. However, if we can discuss DVDs and CDs this is unlikely.

Choice relates directly to how methods are discussed and promoted. When caps and diaphragms are discussed as messy, who would want to use them? Male condoms come in many varieties, different colours, types, shapes and materials, yet choice is seldom available on the NHS, where cheapest is considered best. The female condom is never discussed other than: 'it's noisy' but sex can be noisy. Fertility awareness and natural family planning are still discussed as 'rhythm methods' or 'Russian roulette', yet method failure rates for natural family planning are as good as male condoms.

Emergency contraception, often wrongly termed the 'morning after pill', which negates its use for 'more than the morning after' and omits any discussion of postcoital IUDs, is still considered 'risky'. Many professionals accuse women of 'abusing use' but what does this mean? Does it mean that a woman making a responsible choice to prevent a possible pregnancy may be using emergency contraception more than her clinician might like? Fear of being disapproved of, judged or 'told off' deters women from seeking early help when they have been at risk of unplanned pregnancy.

Difficulties in accessing services

Choosing and using contraception is complex. It relates not only to how information is given but also to where contraception is made available. fpa experience illustrates the many difficulties people have in knowing about contraception and sexual health services and in accessing services. Many women and men have concerns about attending services: embarrassment, anxiety and concerns over confidentiality are common points discussed by users. Women and men are clear what they want to know. This includes:

- What services are available?
- Where are services available?
- When are they available?
- How do I access services?
- Who will I see?
- Can I choose who I see?
- How will I be treated?
- Will it be confidential?
- What information will I be given?
- What if I do not understand?
- How do I get more information if I need it?
- Can I bring anyone with me?
- How do I provide comment or feedback on the service I have attended?

How people are provided with information must also address the context in which people are involved in making decisions, and on how any information given is understood. It is not what you say but how your say it. For users to participate fully in decision making, they need first of all to be authorised to ask questions, 'to make demands', to make fully informed decisions and must be able to consent. Providing good contraceptive and sexual health information requires training, knowledge, skills and sensitivity by professionals. The facilities in which services are offered are important in determining where people want to go to receive their contraception. However, there is little information on the way in which professionals inform or advise users, and so affect decisions to start, continue or stop a contraceptive method. Communication skills have a major influence on the adequacy of a contraceptive consultation: questioning, listening, nonverbal communication and care given during physical examinations. They relate to user satisfaction, lack of friendliness, poor communication and require use of appropriate or suitable language.[5,21] Lack of communication skills contributes to failure to understand or remember what has been said. Many professionals make assumptions, often underestimating a person's degree of motivation, ability or needs. They 'censor' or limit information, and some 'pressure' women into using certain methods. Because of this women (quite rightly) express feelings of anger, frustration and powerlessness because they feel they are not listened too, not spoken to on equal terms and not given time or permission to voice fears or anxieties. Research shows clearly that women want *more* information not less. This is in direct contrast to many professionals who feel that women cannot 'deal' with 'too much' information. Informed choice is vital for enabling valid consent. Hatcher[22] illustrates the importance of consent in family planning and reproductive health as having three bases: pragmatic; ethical; and legal. Pragmatically, a person who clearly understands their contraceptive method or procedure will be more likely to use it safely and effectively. Ethically, every person has a right to information about methods or procedures that can affect their health. Legally, information must be provided so that an informed decision can be made.

Baraitser[23] addresses how choice can be influenced by the power, knowledge and different experiences of both doctors and users during contraceptive consultations:

- doctor's knowledge from formal training
- doctor's knowledge from observation of users' experience with different contraception
- doctor's knowledge of contraception from their own or partner's personal experience
- contraceptive users' knowledge from own experience
- users' knowledge from experience with friends or relatives
- knowledge from the public domain.

The fpa hears everyday examples of women and men's experiences when trying to access services or information about contraception and sexual health:

- not wishing to be stereotyped, criticised or judged ('foolish', 'feckless', 'promiscuous', 'irresponsible', 'too young', 'should know better')
- the wish to be treated properly and with respect
- to be listened too *and* understood – not interrogated
- to be given permission to voice fears or anxieties
- to be given empathy with the situation

- to receive confidential services and *know* they are confidential
- to be given time
- to be given more information.

Recognising the complexities around contraceptive choices, a number of strategies can be introduced to support good contraceptive services and the contraceptive decision process:

- Contraceptive service provision:
  - provide accessible, flexible services that address the diversity of sexual and reproductive healthcare needs of the community
  - provide services that are designed, developed and delivered on the basis of needs assessment – involve users, potential users and past users of services[24,25]
  - provide up to date information on the services you offer – so that people know about them, what you offer, and how they are offered. Use leaflets, websites, practice leaflets, local directories, posters to inform
  - ensure that all staff (clerical, clinical, medical and nonmedical) are appropriately trained, updated and properly resourced – use different professional skills, strengths and interests to best advantage
  - ensure confidentiality in visits, communication and record keeping – display a confidentiality poster
  - practice an ethos of equality regarding age, gender, race, sexual orientation and disability
  - know your service policies, practices and attitudes are nonjudgemental, friendly and supportive
  - provide, where possible, a choice of female or male practitioners, advocacy workers and interpreters when needed
  - ensure that premises are welcoming, pleasant and accessible for all abilities
  - provide sufficient time for visits – especially a first contraceptive consultation.
- Information, support and counselling:
  - recognise that issues to do with sex can be embarrassing and may cause anxiety to both users and professionals
  - always provide appropriate, accessible, evidence-guided information – recognise the need to not limit or censor information or overwhelm with too much
  - always discuss harm/risk, benefit and uncertainties about any contraceptive method or procedure – not as a 'tick' box for litigious reasons but to enable shared decision making and improved choices
  - provide 'back-up' written information to support verbal advice.[26] Use fpa leaflets on contraception and sexual health
  - use suitable, up to date language that enables and informs. Understand the meaning of value-laden words such as 'serious', 'small', 'large', 'significant'. Use statistics that can be understood[27,28]
  - be a catalyst and facilitator, not an 'educator' who tends to tell what needs to be done. Check out information needs by asking questions
  - understand that people need 'permission' to ask questions – listen and respond
  - pay attention to the adverse effects of contraceptive methods or treatments mentioned by the client (whether real or perceived) – this can say a lot about a person's concerns or need
  - increase motivation – be prepared to offer solutions to problems such as difficulties in pill taking, safer sex issues

    ○ be accessible through telephone support if more information is wanted.[29]

Contraception, sexual and reproductive health are areas where a partnership between users and professionals providing services is vital. Communication and user satisfaction are integral. Research illustrates clearly that dissatisfaction, myth and misinformation are widespread and this has huge outcomes for women and men. Ley[30] wrote more than 20 years ago that we need to discover the issues that contribute to dissatisfaction and do something appropriate about it. Users' views are clear, and they are powerful, they demand not just to be listened to but heard and acted upon.

References

1. Johnson A, Mercer CH, Erens B, Copas AJ, McManus S, Wellings K, et al. Sexual behaviour in Britain: partnership, practices and HIV risk behaviours. *Lancet* 2001;358:1835–42.
2. Wellings K, Nanchahal K, Macdowall W, McManus S, Erens B, Mercer CH, et al. Sexual behaviour in Britain: early heterosexual experience. *Lancet* 2001;358:1843–50.
3. Fenton KA, Korovessis C, Johnson AM, McCadden A, McManus S, Wellings K, et al. Sexual behaviour in Britain: reported sexually transmitted infections and prevalent genital Chlamydia trachomatis infection. *Lancet* 2001;358:1851–4.
4. Belfield T. The contraceptive decision: information and counselling. In: Kubba A, Sanfilippo J, Hampton N, editors. *Contraception and Office Gynecology*. Choices in Reproductive Healthcare. London: WB Saunders; 1999,159–64.
5. Belfield T. 'What we say and how we say it.' *J Fam Plann Reprod Health Care* 2004;30(1):11.
6. Belfield, T. Contraception: consumer perceptions of family planning. *Br J Fam Plann* 1988;13(4):46–53.
7. Oddens BJ. Determinants of contraceptive use among women of reproductive age in Great Britain and Germany. II: Psychological factors. *J Biosocial Sci* 1997;29(4):437–70.
8. Ravindran Sundari TK, Berer M, Cottingham J. Beyond acceptability: users' perspectives on contraception. *Reproductive Health Matters for World Health Organisation*. Geneva: WHO; 1997.
9. Belfield T. Problems of compliance in contraception. *Br J Sex Med* 1992;19(3):76–8.
10. Snowden R. *Consumer Choices in Family Planning*. London: Family Planning Association; 1985.
11. Walsh J, Lythgoe A, Peckham S. *Contraceptive Choices: Supporting Effective Use and Methods*. London: Family Planning Association; 1996.
12. Belfield T. A standardised patient information leaflet on oral contraception for Europe: just around the corner or never-ending circles? In: Hannaford PC, Webb AMC, editors. *Evidence-guided Prescribing of the Pill*. London: Parthenon; 1996.
13. Snowden R. The 16th Jennifer Hallam Memorial Lecture. Fertility regulating behaviour. *Br J Fam Plann* 1990;15 Suppl 1:3–7.
14. Grady RW, Klepinger DH, Nelson-Wally A. Contraceptive characteristics: the perceptions and priorities of men and women. *Fam Plann Perspect* 1999;31(4):168–75.
15. Heinemann K, Saad F, Wiesemes M, White S, Heinemann L. Attitudes towards male fertility control: results of a multinational survey in four continents. *Hum Reprod* 2005;20:549–56.
16. Belfield T. It takes two: men and contraception. *J Fam Plann Reprod Health Care* 2005;30:3–4.
17. Allen I. *Family Planning, Sterilisation and Abortion Services*. London: Policy Studies Institute; 1981.
18. Cartright A. *How Many Children?* London: Routledge & Kegan Paul; 1986.
19. Kember Associates. Talk choices: Women's Choices in Contraception. 2004. Unpublished.
20. Mishell DR, Westhoff CL, editors. The power of the pill. *Contraception* 1999;59 Suppl 1:1s–39s.
21. Williams N, Ogden J. The impact of matching the patient's vocabulary; a randomised control trial. *Fam Pract* 2004;21:630–5.
22. Hatcher RA, Trussell J, Stewart F, Nelson AL, Cates W, Guest F, et al. editors. *Contraceptive Technology*. 18th ed. New York: Ardent Media; 2004.
23. Baraitser P. Power and knowledge in family planning consultations: can a reanalysis of doctor–patient interaction improve client satisfaction? *Br J Fam Plann* 1995;21:18–19.
24. Royal College of Obstetricians and Gynaecologist. *Patient Involvement in Enhancing Service Provision*. Clinical Governance Advice No. 4. London: RCOG; 2002 [www.rcog.org.uk/index.asp?PageID=479].
25. Chambers R, Drinkwater C, Baoth E. *Involving Patients and the Public: How to do it better*. 2nd ed. Oxford: Radcliffe Medical Press; 2003.

26. Little P, Griffin S, Kelly J, Dickson N, Sadler C. Effect of educational leaflets and questions on knowledge of contraception in women taking the combined contraceptive pill: randomised control trial. *BMJ* 1998;316:1948–52.
27. Calman K, Royston G. Risk language and dialects. *BMJ* 1997;315:939–42.
28. Godwin K. Consumers' understanding of contraceptive efficacy. *Br J Fam Plann* 1997;23:45–6.
29. Belfield T. Sexual Health: Learning from Consumers. In: Carter Y, Moss C, Matthews P, Weyman A, Belfield T, editors. *Sexual Health in Primary Care*. London: fpa; 2005.
30. Ley P. Satisfaction, compliance and communication. *Br J Clin Psychol* 1982;21:241–4.

Chapter 8
Patterns of contraceptive use: cross-sectional surveys

Stephen R Killick

Introduction

This review brings together various published studies about the way in which contraception is provided for and used by different communities within Europe, with a particular emphasis on UK practice. Comparisons are made between different European countries and, briefly, with other parts of the world. Some general trends are explored and comment made on the way in which methods of healthcare provision and other factors influence contraceptive use.

Types of information available

The Office for National Statistics publishes yearly information about the patterns of contraceptive use throughout Britain. The information is obtained from two continuing population-based surveys. The General Household Survey has gathered data on contraceptive use as part of its extensive dataset since 1971 and the Omnibus Survey has duplicated these data and added some additional information since 1997. The methodology for both these surveys is carefully controlled, using face-to-face interviews of individuals from households chosen randomly by postcode. Each yearly dataset for the family planning component of each of these surveys is the result of between 3000 and 6500 interviews and the duplicated results are virtually identical, vouching for their accuracy.

No other country publishes population-based information on contraceptive use on the same scale. A number of market research companies collect data from various groups of contraceptive users, primarily for the use of the pharmaceutical industry but also, from time to time, on behalf of a European government agency. There are also publications on patterns of use from individual academic research groups, although these tend to be from smaller study populations and designed to answer specific questions, rather than to record general patterns and trends in use.

In general, the use of different study populations (for example, women in different age groups, only married women, only couples using contraception, only couples at risk of conception) and vastly different methodologies (for example, telephone and face-to- face surveys; general population studies and studies of specific subgroups) make it impossible to compare one study with another. Even if we restrict ourselves to large population studies there can be large variations. For example, condom use may have been recorded when used in combination with the pill or only when used as the sole method of contraception.

A word of caution is also appropriate with regard to cross-sectional studies in general, which only examine the situation at one point in time and are therefore less effective in demonstrating the frequent changes in contraceptive use by some groups. This review concentrates on large cross-sectional population surveys but uses other published data to make relevant points.

Overall use of contraception

Britain and most of Northern Europe have high levels of overall contraceptive use when compared with other parts of the world. Three-quarters of all the women in Britain aged between 15 and 49 years are using some form of contraception.[1-3]

A number of studies[3-10] have consistently highlighted the lower overall contraceptive use in Southern European countries, such as Spain and Italy, with the higher use in Northern European countries, such as France, UK and the Netherlands (Table 8.1). These differences have become less marked in recent years, mainly because of increasing use of effective methods in Southern Europe, so that the rates in those countries are now closer to those of the UK,[3,7] which have remained static.[2]

Risk of unplanned pregnancy

The fact of not using contraception does not necessarily mean that a woman is at risk of unwanted pregnancy. Current British data suggest that the majority of women not using contraception have a reason for not doing so, such as pregnancy or that they were trying to conceive, that they had no heterosexual partner or believed themselves

Table 8.1. Comparative proportions of women aged 18–40 years using any reversible contraception and the popularity of different reversible methods in different European countries

	Proportion of population using any contraception (%)	Proportion of reversible contraceptive users choosing different methods (sterilisation excluded) (%)					
		Pill	Condom	IUD	LNG-IUS	Injection or Implant	Ring
Britain[a]	75	51	38	4	1	5	0
France[b]	73	71	5	21	1	1	0
Netherlands[b]	67	78	30	1	4	6	1
Germany[b]	59	65	13	8	6	6	0
Spain[b]	53	34	60	6	0	0	0
Italy[b]	39	55	38	7	0	0	1

[a] Figures calculated from the published results of the 2003/04 Omnibus Survey[2]; [b] Figures from the 2003 TNS NIPO study[10] using an opinion group of 200 000 Europeans (about 450 female contraceptive users in each country)

Table 8.2. Proportions of the population of different European countries using different contraceptive methods (adapted from Skouby[3])

	OC	Condom	Long-term reversible	Sterilisation	Unreliable	Other	None
France	46	10	15	3	3	1	23
Germany	35	14	13	16	5	1	18
Spain	19	33	5	13	3	1	30
Italy	19	33	7	1	18	1	24
UK	28	12	13	22	2	1	26
European average	30	20	11	11	6	1	23

OC = oral contraception

to be involuntarily sterile. However, contraceptive use may not necessarily remove the risk of unwanted pregnancy if, for example, the method used has a high failure rate (such as withdrawal, Persona® (Unipath Ltd), natural methods or even condoms if used incorrectly) or, alternatively, if user compliance with a reliable method is poor.

Estimates of risk of unplanned pregnancy vary enormously. A review of studies from the International Health Foundation during the 1980s suggested that 79% of fertile women in Italy were at risk of unwanted pregnancy compared with 31% in Britain.[4] A more recent European study reported that only 2% of UK women were using 'unreliable' forms of contraception compared with 18% in Italy (Table 8.2).[3] This equates to some 4.7 million European women at risk of unwanted pregnancy and excludes, of course, the risk of user failures from the improper use of reliable methods (although see Chapter 4 for a discussion of the inadequacy of considering contraceptive use as the sole criterion determining unplanned pregnancy).

User failure is by far the most common cause of unplanned pregnancy.[11] Poor compliance is common[12,13] and depends on the user's age and whether she or he has experienced adverse effects. Action taken after a missed pill is unrelated to either general education or specific knowledge of optimal pill use.[12,14] Contraceptive agents with a longer action are, not surprisingly, associated with fewer problems of compliance[15] and a far lower unplanned pregnancy rate.[16]

Use of different contraceptive methods

Table 8.3 shows the pattern of use of different contraceptive methods by British couples and how this has changed over the previous 18 years. The older data are from the General Household Survey[1] but more detail is available from the Omnibus Survey[2] after 1997.

The most obvious feature of these data is their consistency, with a constant 70–75% of the population using some form of contraception. There has been little change in the pattern of contraceptive use over time, except with regard to condom use. Condom promotion in the context of HIV prevention began in 1986, when the British Government delivered the leaflet "Don't Die of Ignorance" to every house-hold in Britain, with information intended to reduce the spread of the virus. Over

Table 8.3. Changes in the pattern of contraceptive use over time in Britain according to the General Household Survey[1] (1986–1995) and the Omnibus Survey[2] (1997–2004)

	From General Household Survey (%)					From Omnibus Survey (%)						
	1986	1989	1991	1993	1995	97/98	98/99	99/00	00/01	01/02	02/03	03/04
COC	23	22	23	25	25	19	19	18	17	21	18	17
POP						5	5	5	5	5	5	5
Male condom	13	15	16	17	18	21	21	23	21	21	20	23
Withdrawal	4	4	3	3	3	4	6	5	3	4	3	3
IUCD	7	5	5	5	4	4	4	4	5	3	5	4
Injection/implant						2	2	3	3	3	3	3
Safe period/rhythm	1	1	1	1	1	2	2	2	1	2	1	1
Cap/diaphragm	2	1	1	1	1	2	1	1	1	1	1	1
Foams/gels/other	1	1	1	1	1	0	1	0	0	0	0	0
LNG-IUS						0	0	1	1	1	1	1
Female condom						0	0	0	0	0	0	0
Female sterilisation	12	11	12	12	12	11	12	12	11	10	11	11
Male sterilisation	11	12	13	12	11	10	12	11	11	12	12	12
Any method	71	69	70	72	73	74	75	76	73	75	74	75

COC = Combined oral contraceptive; IUCD = intrauterine contraceptive device; LNG-IUS = levonorgestrel-releasing intrauterine system; POP = progestogen only pill

the next 13 years, the proportion of couples using male condoms nearly doubled, from 13% to 23%. However, the proportion of couples using any form of reliable contraception hardly changed at all, suggesting that most, if not all, of this increase was attributable to growing use for the purposes of disease prevention rather than contraception alone. Some 12% of UK women currently rely on condoms as their main contraceptive method,[3] the same proportion as in 1986.[2]

The same increase in popularity did not, however, apply to the female condom, which was introduced in 1992 and remained decidedly unpopular, despite being regarded as probably a better barrier to disease than its male counterpart. The introduction of other contraceptive products such as the levonorgestrel-releasing intrauterine system, Mirena® (Schering Health) in May 1995 and the progestogen implant Implanon® (Organon) in November 1999, similarly had little impact on overall patterns of contraceptive use despite their undoubted contraceptive efficacy and physiological advantages. A consistent, but tiny, proportion of women – only 1% – uses Mirena and the proportion is the same even among older women, for whom it might be seen as having greater advantages. The impressive figures for the safety of long-term copper intrauterine contraceptive device (IUCD) use have not changed the popularity of this method from a constant 4% user rate. Combined oral contraceptives, male condoms or surgical sterilisation continue to be the choice for 85% of all couples using any form of contraception, as they have for nearly two decades (Figure 8.1).

Although this appears to be the general pattern throughout Europe, there are notable exceptions. France has a different pattern of contraceptive use with a high proportion of couples using an IUCD (Table 8.1), probably because of the legal uncertainties of sterilisation for social reasons in that country until 2001. Sterilisation rates are also low in Italy (Table 8.2)[3] and in Northern Ireland, where only 12% of

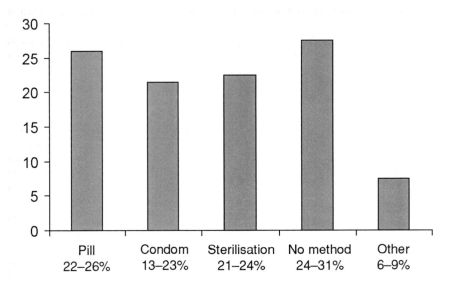

Figure 8.1. Contraceptive use in Britain over the last 18 years (data from 2003/04 Omnibus survey[2])

people 35–44 years of age rely on the method.[17] A similar picture of low sterilisation rates used to exist in Eastern Germany before unification, when communist authorities required a formal application before sterilisation could be sanctioned. Rates in Germany are now midway between those in Italy and in the UK. The UK has the highest rate of sterilisation in Europe and the prevalence is higher among men than women.

Worldwide figures show a much greater reliance on sterilisation (mainly female, which is the single most prevalent method) and the IUCD than in most of Europe (Figure 8.2).[17] IUCD use is favoured in some specific countries, notably Viet Nam,

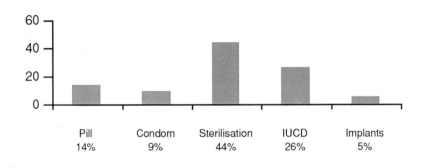

Figure 8.2. Proportion of contraceptive users choosing different methods: worldwide

where it accounts for the vast majority of all contraceptive choices, and China where 90% of the world's IUCDs are inserted. From an economic point of view, the IUCD is by far the cheapest form of contraception. It requires little specialist follow up after insertion, can be left in place for up to 10 years and its user failure rate is virtually zero.

Variation in contraceptive use with age

In recent years, up to 50% of all women in Britain aged 16–17 years of age have been in a sexual relationship, most of whom use some form of contraception. Figures for the use of contraception in the youngest age group of under 16-year-olds are not available. However, 26% of young women have had intercourse before the age of 16 years[18] leading to some 8000 pregnancies,[19] indicating the need for contraceptive services for this age group. Comparative figures for the proportion of sexually experienced under-16-year-olds are 26% for the USA[20] and 15% for Northern Ireland.[21] Among 16–17 year olds, the condom is the most commonly used method of contraception, a pattern which changes in the later teens, so that among 18–19 year olds, the pill supplants condoms as the most widely used method. This pattern continues to 35 years of age, when condom use is once again more common than pill use, although the most prevalent method of contraception is sterilisation.

An abrupt change in use of the pill in women aged over 35 years of age was seen during the early 1990s, coinciding with release of new information about its safety in women of this age. Only 4% of women aged over 35 years relied on the pill in 1986 but by 1995 this had risen to 11% and the proportion has remained constant to date.[1,2]

Figure 8.3 shows clearly the increasing recourse to male or female sterilisation to control fertility with age. Over the last 18 years, the proportion of couples relying on sterilisation has decreased slightly for women in the age group 25–39 years but has increased slightly for the age group 45–49 years, indicating in part that women are now completing their families later in life.

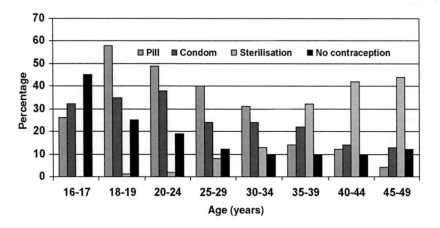

Figure 8.3. Proportion of women in various age groups using the pill, male condom, sterilisation or no contraception in Britain in 2003/04

Men and women have traditionally passed through identifiable phases of contraceptive use, from their first sexual experiences, to established sexual relationships, then to family planning and child spacing and then to family completion. With changing demographic trends, however, this progression may not always be linear, since the breakdown of existing relationships and the establishment of new ones may herald more than one period of childbearing. Studies of different groups illustrate the changing contraceptive needs in different life phases. For example, a study in which pregnant women were questioned about their contraceptive use immediately prior to pregnancy provides information about the way in which couples plan their families. In these groups, there was a higher reliance on oral contraception with up to 60% using some form of pill:[22]

- combined oral contraceptive: 41%
- condom alone: 19%
- condom and another method: 15%
- progestogen-only pill: 5%
- implants or injectables: 3%
- IUCD: 3%
- levonorgestrel-releasing intrauterine system: 1%
- never used contraception: 14%.

It is also interesting to note that, in this study, women who had used contraception for shorter periods of time tended to have used methods promoted for long-term use such as IUCDs, implants and injections. Two-thirds of women using combined oral contraception had done so for more than 2 years. By contrast, two-thirds of those using an IUCD, Mirena, injectables or implants had done so for less than 2 years.

Emergency contraception

Emergency hormonal contraception (EHC) has been available on prescription in the UK since 1984 but its status of supply was changed in January 2001, in order to allow users to obtain it directly from a pharmacy (P status) should they prefer to do so. This change has resulted in one-quarter to one-third of EHC users choosing to obtain their supply directly from a pharmacy without a prescription rather than attend either their GP surgery or family planning clinic (Table 8.4). This has improved access to this method of contraception and reduced the difficulties experienced by some would-be users. It has not, however, increased the overall use of EHC[2] nor have studies shown that the knowledge users have about its use has deteriorated.[23] Less than 10% of women use EHC each year and the proportion does not vary with educational level. EHC users are more likely to be currently using a method of contraception, which temporarily had the potential to fail for whatever reason, than to be using no form of contraception at all.[2] Few individuals use emergency contraception repeatedly and even fewer (less than 1%) request the insertion of an IUCD as an emergency.

Services used to provide health care

In the most recent Omnibus survey, only 57% of women had used any family planning service in the previous 5 years. The vast majority of these had attended their GP or practice nurse but about one-third had attended family planning clinics. Only a few had sought advice from a pharmacist, almost exclusively with regard to emergency contraception (Table 8.4).

The introduction of P status for emergency hormonal contraception achieved, to some extent, the desired objective of allowing some women to obtain treatment more quickly even though the additional number of unplanned pregnancies prevented has been calculated as only five per 10 000 uses.[23] There is also great reluctance on behalf of the public to pay for a service that has traditionally been free at the point of delivery.

Allowing women to keep a supply of EHC for future use when necessary has been shown to have similar effects to P status.[24] Overall use of EHC was not increased and women were able to take their EHC therapy earlier but, again, the overall number of unplanned pregnancies was not appreciably reduced.

The use of patient group directions as a 'half-way house' between having to obtain a prescription and buying the EHC has been successful in a number of situations.[23,25–27] Patient group directions improve accessibility and convenience and have the potential to improve uptake, particularly for groups that might otherwise have difficulty accessing medical care such as the under 16s and those who would have difficulties in meeting the cost.

Factors affecting choice of contraceptive

Cost is an obvious contributing factor to contraceptive choice and national differences in reimbursements of contraceptive cost may be responsible for much of the variation between countries shown in Table 8.1. In the Netherlands and the UK, users contribute minimally, if at all, to the cost, whereas in Spain and Italy not only may the user pay the cost of supply but also the cost of a gynaecological consultation. Higher rates of use may therefore be related to more convenient access rather than simply a less costly supply.[4]

Table 8.4. Use of emergency hormonal contraception (EHC) in Britain 1997–2004 and from where it was obtained compared to where other family planning (FP) services were obtained (data from 2003/04 Omnibus Survey[2])

	Heard of EHC	Used EHC	EHC from own GP	FP usually from own GP	EHC from FPC	FP usually from FPC	EHC from Pharmacy	Difficulty obtaining
	%	%	%	%	%	%	%	%
1997	91	10	68	45	26	16		
1998	93	10	71	45	20	18		P status introduced
1999	91	11	62	45	32	18		
2000/01	92	8	59	48	33	20	0	15
2001/02	94	7	43	48	31	22	20	13
2002/03	93	7	44	47	18	19	33	9
2003/04	94	5	41	46	21	18	27	4

Countries with GPs generally have higher rates of contraceptive use overall but this is mainly with regard to oral contraception, rather than methods that require specific training such as IUCDs or implants (Table 8.1). The relatively low uptake of IUCDs in the UK might reflect the low proportion of GPs promoting and inserting them in preference to referral for sterilisation. Many women who undergo sterilisation have not been counselled about alternative methods.[3]

Although the cost of contraception is quoted as less important than convenience and adverse effects in determining use in other countries in Europe,[10] the situation in the UK is different, as consumers are used to a free system at the point of delivery. Most market research highlights the importance that contraceptive users give to 'nuisance' adverse effects, such as weight gain, or to health risks, such as an increased risk of cancer. Nevertheless, the UK pattern of contraceptive use may be more dependent on cost than initially appears to be the case, since health service providers have a monopoly on contraceptive provision but limited budgets. It is interesting to note the relative uniformity of price of different contraceptives when sold on line directly to the public.[28]

Summary

For almost two decades, the pattern of contraceptive use in Britain has been characterised by high rates of use that have remained remarkably constant over time, despite all attempts to improve both contraceptive agents and sexual and reproductive healthcare provision.

Unplanned pregnancies can result from a number of factors, including not using contraception, using a less effective method or not complying with an effective method. The proportion of young teenagers who do not use contraception when they need to is higher than ideal and it is this group that also has the greatest difficulty accessing contraceptive and sexual health services. P status and patient group directions improve access to services and may be useful systems for future contraceptive provision.

The vast majority of contraceptive users still use oral contraception, condoms or sterilisation, despite the development of modern long-term methods of reversible contraception such as implants, IUCDs, Mirena and injectables, which are underused. We need to look at ways of enhancing the uptake of these methods.

References

1.   Office for National Statistics. General Household Survey 2003.
     [www.statistics.gov.uk/StatBase/Product.asp?vlnk=5756].
2.   Dawe F, Rainford L. Contraception and Sexual Health. Omnibus Survey 2003/04. Office for National Statistics
     [www.statistics.gov.uk/StatBase/Product.asp?vlnk=6988&Pos=1&ColRank=1&Rank=224].
3.   Skouby SO. Contraceptive use and behaviour in the 21st century: a comprehensive study across five European countries. *Eur J Contracept Reprod Health Care* 2004;9:57–68.
4.   Oddens BJ. Evaluation of the effect on contraceptive prices on demand in eight Western European countries. *Adv Contracept* 1992;9:1–11.
5.   Oddens BJ, Visser A Ph, Vemer HM, Everard WAM, Lehert Ph. Contraceptive use and attitudes in Great Britain. *Contraception* 1994;49:73–86.
6.   Oddens BJ, Visser A Ph, Vemer HM, Everard WAM, Lehert Ph. Contraceptive use and attitudes in reunified Germany. *Eur J Obstet Gynecol Reprod Biol* 1994;57:201–8.
7.   Oddens BJ. Contraceptive use and attitudes in Italy 1993. *Hum Reprod* 1996;11:533–9.
8.   Oddens BJ, Milsom I. Contraceptive practice and attitudes in Sweden 1994. *Acta Obstet Gynecol Scand* 1996;75:32–40.

9. Spinelli A, Talamanca IF, Lauria L. Patterns of contraceptive use in five European countries. European Study Group on Infertility and Subfecundity. *Am J Public Health* 2000;90(9):1403–8.
10. TNS NIPO Contraception Study November 2003. Women about contraception. [www.nipo.nl/onderzoek/gratis/persvannipo/pdf/contraceptives04.ppt].
11. Garg M, Singh M, Mansour D. Peri-abortion contraceptive care: can we reduce the incidence of repeat abortions? *J Fam Plan Reprod Health Care* 2001;27(2):77–80.
12. Aubeny E, Buhler M, Colau JC, Vicaut E, Zeatkran M, Childs M. Oral contraception: patterns of non-compliance: The Coaliance study. *Eur J Contracept Reprod Health Care* 2002;7(3):155–6.
13. Rosenberg MJ, Waugh MS, Meehan TE. Use and misuse of oral contraceptives: risk indicators for poor pill taking and discontinuation. *Contraception* 1995;51(5):283–8.
14. Wahab M, Killick SR. Oral contraceptive knowledge and compliance in young women. *Br J Fam Plann* 1997;22:170–3.
15. Archer DF, Cullins V, Creasy GW, Fisher AC. The impact of improved compliance with a weekly contraceptive transdermal system (Ortho Evra®) on contraceptive efficacy. *Contraception* 2004;69:189–95.
16. Luukkainen T, Toivonen J. Levonorgestrel-releasing IUD as a method of contraception with therapeutic properties. *Contraception* 1995;52(5):269–76.
17. United Nations Population Division. World contraceptive use wall chart 2003. [www.un.org/esa/population/publications/publications.htm].
18. National Survey of Sexual Attitudes in Britain. NATSAL 2000 Survey [www.fpa.org.uk/about/PDFs/Factsheet6.pdf].
19. Office for National Statistics. The health of children and young people. March 2004. [www.statistics.gov.uk/cci/nugget.asp?id=721].
20. US National Center for Health Statistics. National Survey of Family Growth [www.cdc.gov/nchs/nsfg.htm].
21. Northern Ireland Health and Social Wellbeing survey 2001 [http://www.nisra.gov.uk/whatsnew/wellbeing/sexual_health/First%20experience%20of%20sexual%20intercourse.PDF].
22. Hassan MAM, Killick SR. Is previous use of hormonal contraception associated with a detrimental effect on subsequent fecundity? *Hum Reprod* 2004;9(2):344–51.
23. Killick SR, Irving G. A national study examining the effect of making emergency hormonal contraception available without prescription. *Hum Reprod* 2004;9(3):1–5.
24. Glasier A, Fairhurst K, Wyke S, Ziebland S, Seaman P, Walker J, Lakha F. Advanced provision of emergency contraception does not reduce abortion rates. *Contraception* 2004;69(5):361–6.
25. Seston EM, Smith I, Cantrill JA, O'Brien K. The impact of the deregulation of emergency hormonal contraception on a patient group direction scheme in the north-west of England. *Int J Pharm Pract* 2002;10 (Suppl):R22.
26. Royal Pharmaceutical Society. Pharmacy for the future [www.rpsgb.org.uk/nhsplan/pgd.htm].
27. Soon JA, Levine M, Ensom MHH, Gardner JS, Edmondson HM and Fielding DW. The developing role of pharmacists in patient access to emergency contraception. *Dis Manag Health Outcomes* 2002;10(10):601–11.
28. Pharma Super Discounts [www.pharmasuperdiscounts.com/health-conditions/contraceptives.asp].

Chapter 9

Longitudinal studies of birth control and pregnancy outcome among women in an urban Swedish population

Ian Milsom

Introduction

Many factors influence birth rates, including, for example, the number of women of childbearing age, social policy, unemployment and immigration rates, accessibility to family planning facilities and the efficacy of contraceptive methods used and childbearing etc.[1] The interaction between these various factors is complex and the importance of single factors difficult to evaluate. The vast majority of studies describing contraceptive use are cross-sectional and often based on selected populations, such as women attending family planning clinics, student health clinics or abortion clinics.[2-5] Such studies provide valuable information but are not truly representative of the total population. In addition, the majority of studies have investigated the prevalence of contraceptive use without relating it to reproductive history.

Conditions in Sweden are extremely favourable for epidemiological studies, in particular longitudinal studies. The Swedish Population Register, with its personal number system, provides up-to-date information on the total population and can be used to obtain random and, in some cases, representative subgroups of the total population for the purpose of longitudinal epidemiological studies. In 1981, we began a prospective longitudinal study of contraception and birth control in a random sample of 19-year-old women resident at that time in the city of Göteborg, Sweden. The initial results were published in 1982 as a cross-sectional study.[6] It was then not possible to assess the impact of time-related factors such as age and parity on the contraceptive habits of the women. A 5-year follow-up study of the same women was published in 1990[7] and, in 1997, we published a 10-year follow-up in the same women, now aged 29 years.[8] As far as we are aware, there are no previous publications describing contraceptive use and pregnancy outcome in the same women from the ages of 19 to 29 years of age. Preliminary data collected from the same women at age 39 years is at present being analysed. Several papers have been published based on this population of women, describing the use of contraception and its association with other medical and social factors, including pregnancy and pregnancy outcome and menstrual disturbances such as dysmenorrhoea.[9-12]

Study design

Every fourth woman born in 1962 and resident in the city of Göteborg was sent a postal questionnaire containing questions on the use of contraception, possible pregnancies and reproductive health. The women were all 19 years of age when the study started. This age was chosen in order to be able to communicate directly with the women themselves (then legally adults in Swedish law) without the necessity of consent from their parents. The first questionnaire was answered by 91% of participants and those who returned the questionnaire in 1981 were contacted again every fifth year, in 1986, 1991, 1996 and 2001.

In 1991, 10 years after the initial longitudinal study was started, a new cohort of women, born in 1972, resident in Göteborg and aged 19 years, was randomly selected. These women answered a similar questionnaire to the one sent to women from the 1962 cohort. This second cohort has also been followed longitudinally every fifth year, i.e. in 1996 and 2001. In 2001, 20 years after the initial longitudinal study was started, a third cohort of women born in 1982 and resident in Göteborg answered a similar questionnaire to the one sent to women from the 1962 and the 1972 cohorts.

With this study design, it has been possible to follow the use of contraception and pregnancy outcome and the prevalence and incidence of gynaecological disorders in the same women over time and to compare them cross-sectionally with women of the same age from different birth cohorts. A summary of the study design is shown in Table 9.1.

The study has created extensive national and international interest, due to its unique design based on a random sample of the total population, with a high participation rate, regular follow-up and the possibility of performing both longitudinal and cross-sectional comparisons.

Material and methods

In 1981, there were 2621 women aged 19 years living in Göteborg, the second largest city in Sweden (approximately 450 000 inhabitants). A random sample of every fourth woman was obtained from the population register ($n = 656$). They were invited by letter to return a questionnaire concerning contraception, reproductive history and related factors. The study design was approved by the Ethics Committee, Faculty of Medicine, University of Göteborg, and the National Data Inspection Board. The

Table 9.1. Summary of study design, permitting longitudinal and cross-sectional comparisons

Cohort	Year of assessment							
	1981	1986	1991	1996	2001	2006	2011	2016
62	19 y	24 y	29 y	34 y	39 y	44 y	49 y	54 y
72			19 y	24 y	29 y	34 y	39 y	44 y
82					19 y	24 y	29 y	34 y
92							19 y	24 y

response rate was 91% (594 women). The first follow-up was performed in 1986 using the same postal questionnaire technique. Addresses were available for 589 of the original 594 responders (one woman had died and four women had emigrated and no forwarding addresses were available). The questionnaire was completed and returned by 487 women, 74% of the original 656 women in the sample.

In 1991, a new attempt was made to contact the responders from 1981, using the same postal questionnaire technique. Addresses were available for 575 of the 594 responders from 1981 (one women had died, two were temporarily living abroad and 16 were no longer available in the Register); 370 of the 575 women were still resident in city of Göteborg.

Reproductive history and pregnancy outcome were also obtained from hospital records. All legal abortions and deliveries in Sweden are carried out in hospitals. Gynaecological complications, defined as the need for readmission or continued hospital care after legal abortion, were obtained from hospital records. There was a good agreement between pregnancy history reported in the questionnaires and information obtained from the hospital records. Only two of the women (0.3%) reported a pregnancy history at odds with available hospital records.

The National Board of Health and Welfare[13] and the state owned pharmacy (Apoteksbolaget)[14] supplied national data on induced abortions and oral contraceptive sales from the same period.

Characteristics of the samples and analysis of nonresponse

The population register includes demographic data, allowing comparison between responders and nonresponders in each sample. By definition, all the women were of the same age and were resident in the city of Göteborg in 1981. There were no differences between responders and nonresponders regarding marital status and foreign extraction at any of the three assessments nor in the proportion of women still resident in Göteborg at the two follow-up assessments (1986 and 1991). For comparison of baseline characteristics, see Table 9.2.

Data analysis and statistical methods

The accuracy of the data entry was checked on an individual basis for each parameter in all subjects. A linear nonparametric test, Student's t-test and Fisher's exact test were used when applicable for comparison of paired data.

Results

The questionnaire was completed and returned by 484 of the 575 women (85%) contacted in 1991, which is equivalent to 74% of the original sample of 656 women contacted initially in 1981. In this paper, only the 430 women who completed the questionnaire on all three occasions (i.e., 1981, 1986 and 1991) are included. They constitute 66% of the original sample of 656 women.

Contraception had been used at some time by 73% of the women by the age of 19 years.. At 24 and 29 years of age, the corresponding figures were 94% and 97%, respectively. Thirty-nine percent of the women were not using contraception at 19 years of age, 26% at 24 years and 25% at 29 years. At 24 and 29 years of age, the majority of women not using contraception were either pregnant, had recently been pregnant or were wishing to become pregnant. In contrast, the majority of women

Table 9.2. A comparison of baseline characteristics in the same women (*n* = 430) at 19, 24 and 29 years of age

	19 years	24 years	29 years
Nationality:			
Swedish citizen	86.0	86.0	86.0
naturalised Swedish citizen	9.2	10.4	11.4
foreign national	4.8	3.6	2.6
Civil status:			
single	93.8	65.5	44.5
married/cohabiting	5.8	25.6	42.3
married, but separated	0.2	4.1	4.2
divorced	0.2	4.8	9.0
widow	0.0	0.0	0.0
Resident in Göteborg	100.0	76.1	77.1
Weight, m, mean (SEM)	58.3 (0.4)	59.9 (0.4)	61.9 (0.4)
range	44–93	44–125	45–100
Height, m, mean (SEM)	167.1 (0.3)	167.4 (0.3)	167.4 (0.3)
range, kg	149–184	149–185	149–185
Menstrual cycle:			
Menarcheal age, years, mean (SEM)	12.9 (0.1)		
range, years	9–17		
Duration of bleeding, days, mean (SEM)	5.3 (0.1)	5.2 (0.1)	5.5 (0.1)
range, days	3–10	1–14	2–14
Cycle length, days, mean (SEM)	28.1 (0.2)	27.2 (0.2)	28.4 (0.3)
range, days	18–80	19–45	20–99
Regular	86.7	93.2	91.0
Dysmenorrhoea	71.1	66.4	69.5

not using contraception at 19 years of age did not wish to get pregnant. Of those using contraception, the most common method was, at all three ages, oral contraception (Table 9.3). The second most popular method was a barrier method, almost exclusively the condom. Intrauterine device (IUD) use became increasingly popular with advancing age. No woman had been sterilised by 29 years of age. The distribution of contraceptive methods among parous compared with nulliparous women is shown in Table 9.4.

The use of IUDs was more common in parous women, whereas oral contraception was more common in nulliparous women at all three ages. Information on natural family planning methods was specifically requested at 29 years of age only and are indicated separately in Table 9.4. Depo-Provera® (Pharmacia) and Norplant® (Hoechst Marion Roussel) were seldom used and are shown in the same column in Table 9.4. The brand names of oral contraception were asked for on all three occasions and the types of oral contraception used at 19 years (1981), 24 years (1986)

Table 9.3. Contraceptive use in the same women ($n = 430$) at 19, 24 and 29 years of age

Method	Use, n (%)		
	At 19 years	At 24 years	At 29 years
Oral contraception only	200 (46.5)	219 (50.9)	95 (22.1)
Oral contraception + condom	5 (1.2)	1 (0.2)	16 (3.7)
Combined oral contraceptive:			
50 micrograms ethinyl estradiol	(21.5)	(10.9)	(8.7)
35–37.5 micrograms ethinyl estradiol	(2.9)	(7.7)	(6.3)
30 micrograms ethinyl estradiol	(70.2)	(34.5)	(41.7)
20 micrograms ethinyl estradiol	(0)	(0)	(0)
Triphasic	(0)	(42.7)	(33.9)
Progestogen-only pill	(1.5)	(4.1)	(8.7)
Type of oral contraception unknown	(3.9)	(0)	(0)
Condom only	47 (10.9)	51 (11.9)	72 (16.7)
IUD	11 (2.6)	48 (11.2)	80 (18.6)
Depot-progestogen	0 (0)	1 (0.2)	2 (0.4)
No contraception	166 (38.6)	110 (25.6)	107 (24.9)

and 29 years (1991) are shown in Table 9.3. The use of oral contraception containing 50 micrograms ethinyl estradiol declined during the 10-year observation period. Triphasic oral contraceptives were not available in Sweden in 1981 when the study was started. In 1986, 35% of the women were using monophasic pills containing 30 micrograms ethinyl estradiol and 43% were using triphasic pills. In 1991, the

Table 9.4. Contraceptive methods (%) in the same women ($n = 430$) at the ages 19, 24 and 29 years, grouped according to parity

	No contraception	Barrier method	IUD	Oral contraception	NFP & other*
19 years:					
nulliparous	37	12	2	49	< 1
parous	53	18	6	23	< 1
24 years:					
nulliparous	24	13	6	57	< 1
parous	31	11	26	32	< 1
29 years:					
nulliparous	30	22	4	29	15/13*
parous	21	14	27	21	17/13*

NFP = Natural Family Planning and rhythm method; * other methods here are depot progestogen methods corresponding figures were 42% for monphasic pills and 34% for triphasic pills. The use of the progestogen-only pill increased from 2% at 19 years of age to 4% at 24 years of age and to 9% at 29 years of age.

Cessation of oral contraception due to menstrual bleeding disorders (10–15%), weight gain (15–20%) and mental adverse effects (15–21%) were equally commonly encountered at all three ages. At 24 and 29 years of age, the desire to become pregnant accounted for a large proportion of oral contraception cessation. Otherwise, at every age, fear of oral contraception was the most common cause of oral contraception cessation. The reasons for IUD removal were more evenly divided (menstrual bleeding disorders 32–50%; pain 29–42%; vaginal discharge 11–32%; desire to become pregnant 22–36%; other reasons 26–44%) and there were smaller, less consistent differences at the three different assessment points.

The prevalence of smoking increased between 19 years (41%) and 24 years (43%) but had declined to 37% at 29 years of age. The differences in oral contraception, IUD and condom use, as well as differences in the history of pregnancy and legal abortion between smokers and nonsmokers at the three different ages are shown in Table 9.5. At 19 years and 29 years, a greater proportion of oral contraception users were smokers than nonsmokers. However, at 24 years of age, in 1986, the situation was reversed and there were more oral contraception users who were nonsmokers. At all three ages, a greater proportion of the women who had been pregnant or women who had undergone a legal abortion were smokers.

At 19 years of age, 5% of the women had one or two children, at 24 years of age 27% of the women had one to three children and at 29 years of age 59% were mothers to one to five children. One woman had a premature child in 1985 that died perinatally. Pregnancies had been experienced by 17.2% at 19 years of age and by 42% and 71% at 24 and 29 years, respectively. Pregnancy outcome is shown in Table 9.6. At 19 years of age, 12% of the women had undergone one or more legal abortions, 3% had experienced at least one miscarriage and one woman had suffered an ectopic pregnancy. At 24 years of age, the equivalent figure for induced abortion was 25%, for miscarriage 8% and five (1%) women had experienced an ectopic pregnancy. At 29 years of age, 30% had undergone one or more induced abortions, 15% had experienced one or more miscarriages and nine (2%) had experienced at least one ectopic pregnancy. On all three occasions, more than 97% of the legal abortions were performed at or before 12 weeks of gestation. The proportion of live births by the total number of pregnancies was 25% at 19 years of age, 45% at 24 years of age and 61% at 29 years of age.

Discussion

Choice of contraceptive method is influenced by many different factors, relating both to the woman herself as well as to the prevailing attitude of her health provider and to the contraceptive techniques available. This study has clearly illustrated several trends in the choice of contraception during the study period 1981–1991. Several of these trends may be attributable to time-related changes in society or improvements in available contraceptive techniques during this 10-year period, while others relate more to the women's life situations and changed with increasing age and parity.

The most commonly used method of contraception on all three occasions was oral contraception. However, there were changes in the type of oral contraception used during this 10-year period. The use of high-dose oestrogen pills, i.e., containing 50 micrograms ethinyl estradiol, decreased during the observation period, illustrating the

Table 9.5. Distribution of method of contraception, history of pregnancy and legal abortion in the same women at 19, 24 and 29 years of age, grouped according to smoking habits (Fisher's exact test)

	Smokers, n (%)	Non-smokers, n (%)	Significance of difference, n (%)
19 years of age (n = 427)	174 (40.8%)	253	(59.3%)
Oral contraception	94 (54.0%)	105 (41.5%)	P < 0.014
Oral contraception + condom	1 (0.6%)	4 (1.6%)	NS
Intrauterine device	5 (2.9%)	6 (2.4%)	NS
Condom	18 (10.3%)	28 (11.1%)	NS
Contraceptive users	118(67.8%)	143 (56.5%)	P < 0.020
History of pregnancy	48 (27.6%)	25 (9.9%)	P < 0.001
History of legal abortion	33 (19.0%)	16 (6.3%)	P < 0.001
24 years of age (n = 419)	178 (42.5%)	241 (57.5%)	
Oral contraception	83 (46.6)	130 (53.9%)	NS
Oral contraception + condom	1 (0.6%)	0 (0%)	NS
Intrauterine device	26 (14.6%)	20 (8.3%)	NS
Condom	19 (10.7%)	31 (12.9%)	NS
Contraceptive users	129 (72.5%)	181 (75.1%)	NS
History of pregnancy	102 (57.3%)	71 (29.5%)	P < 0.001
History of legal abortion	67 (37.6%)	40 (16.6%)	P < 0.001
29 years of age (n =427)	156 (36.5%)	271 (63.5%)	
Oral contraception	42 (26.9%)	107 (18.5%)	P < 0.05
Oral contraception + condom	9 (5.8%)	7 (2.6%)	NS
Intrauterine device	32 (20.5%)	45 (16.6%)	NS
Condom	27 (17.3%)	43 (15.9%)	NS
Contraceptive users	110 (70.5%)	145 (53.5%)	P < 0.001
History of pregnancy	120 (76.9%)	182 (67.2%)	P < 0.036
History of legal abortion	63 (40.4%)	65 (24.0%)	P < 0.001

NS = not significant

acceptance of low-dose pills, and there was also an increase in the use of progestogen-only pills, particularly at 29 years of age. In the mid-80s, government subsidies on oral contraceptives were reduced and the costs increased considerably for individual women. Sales of oral contraception decreased and there was a concomitant increase in the number of legal abortions.

In Sweden, as elsewhere, the media have tended to report the negative consequences of contraceptive methods, e.g., risk of breast cancer and thromboembolic disease, rather than giving a balanced appraisal of the method's advantages and

Table 9.6. Pregnancy outcome (%) in the same Swedish women ($n = 430$) during the three age periods and in all pregnancies at 29 years of age; total number of pregnancies at 29 years = 744

Age (years)	Live birth	Miscarriage	Legal abortion	Ectopic pregnancy	Unknown
≤ 19	25.2	14.7	58.9	1.1	0
20–24	52.3	10.0	36.2	1.5	0
25-29	74.8	10.5	10.0	1.0	3.6

disadvantages.[15,16] Fear of oral contraception was the most common cause of cessation of oral contraception use during this 10-year period. Swedish women have been influenced by periodically occurring alarming reports in the media on potential adverse effects of the pill. This has also been seen in the national sales figures for oral contraceptives, where the number of oral contraception users decreased drastically in the early 1970s, when the first reports of a connection between oral contraception and venous thromboembolism were published. Similar decreases in oral contraception sales occurred in the late 1970s, due to reports on the risk of cardiovascular disease and the pill, and in the mid-1980s, due to reports on a possible connection between breast cancer and oral contraceptive use.

The increase in condom use during the study period is, however, more difficult to interpret. The increase in condom use may simply be a result of changing lifestyle. A greater number of the 29-year-old women were living in a stable relationship and might accept the use of a less effective contraceptive technique and more readily accept a possible pregnancy within the near future. However, it is also possible that the increase in condom use was due partly to information campaigns in the 1980s highlighting the risk of sexually transmitted infections (STI), such as chlamydia, human papillomavirus infection and HIV, and the protective effect of condoms.[5,17] In the early 1980s, 20% of young people in Sweden attending youth clinics were found to be infected with chlamydia. In contrast, the prevalence of chlamydia in the early 1990s was estimated to be less than 5%.[18] This reduction has been achieved by a combination of measures, such as educational efforts directed towards both healthcare staff and young people, screening programmes and treatment policies, including partner tracing. One of the most important measures taken was an attempt to increase the use of condoms.

The use of different contraceptive methods varies considerably between different countries. In Sweden, as in many of the other Scandinavian countries, there is a greater use of IUDs than, for instance, in Great Britain or West Germany.[19,20] In Sweden, the sterilisation rate is extremely low compared with other countries, such as Great Britain and Norway.[19,21] Although postcoital contraception has been well known and well documented for many years,[22] the method was seldom used in Sweden before 1993 (i.e., during the whole of this study period).

Among this cohort of Swedish women, the majority of pregnancies occurring ended in legal abortion. The proportion of women undergoing legal abortion decreased with increasing age, indicating that a greater number of women were prepared to have children. However, even in the age group 25–29 years, about one in seven of the pregnancies ended in an induced abortion. In this group of women, the use of oral contraception had decreased considerably which may have been due to the previously mentioned factors relating to the costs and concerns about the safety of long-term oral contraception. Failure of less effective contraceptive methods or non-use of contraception may thus have contributed.[23]

The prevalence of smoking was almost unchanged between 19 years (41%) and 24 years (43%) but declined to 37% when the women were 29 years of age. Being pregnant will *per se* encourage smoking cessation and health personnel at the antenatal clinics reinforce the wish to stop. Most women who stop smoking during pregnancy, however, will relapse after childbirth.[20] The continuous use of nonsmoking campaigns and more strict legislation on smoke-free public places has certainly also contributed to smoking cessation. The prevalence of smoking has declined in the general population since the 1960s in most Western countries and may obscure the effect that childbirth has on smoking cessation. There was a greater use of oral contraception among smokers compared with nonsmokers at 19 and 29 years of age. However, at 24 years of age, in 1986, the situation was reversed and there were more oral contraceptive users who were nonsmokers. A possible explanation of the lower prevalence of oral contraceptive users who were smokers at 24 years of age in 1986 may also be related to the influence of mass media. In the early 1980s, the potentially harmful effects of the simultaneous use of oral contraception and smoking were frequently highlighted in the media.

Conclusions

Our results reflect the many difficulties that still exist regarding the occurrence of unwanted pregnancies, even though present legislation is liberal and the availability of contraception is satisfactory, at least theoretically. The proportion of legal abortions to live births remains high. Approximately one-third of the legal abortions that are performed in Sweden are performed in women who have previously undergone a legal abortion.[8] Follow-up visits should be offered after induced abortions, something which is not generally available today throughout Sweden. Counselling for contraception and legal abortion in Sweden is still free of charge. However, there are at present economic and political pressures to remove this social benefit that has been available for many years.

Acknowledgements

Important contributions to this longitudinal study, which has now been in progress for over 20 years, have been made by the following persons: Gerd Larsson MD, Björn Andersch MD PhD, Anne Marie Kullendorff MD, Gunilla Sundell MD, Febe Blohm MD, Ingela Lindh and Marianne Sahlén. We also wish to thank Björn Areskoug for his valuable assistance regarding the statistical analysis. The study was supported by grants from the Göteborg Medical Society, Hjalmar Svensson's Fund and the University of Göteborg.

References

1. Guillebaud J. Sex and contraception: yesterday, today and everywhere. In: The Pill, 4th ed. Guillebaud J. Oxford, Oxford University Press. 1991: 15.
2. Mosher WD. Contraceptive practice in the US, 1982–1988. *Fam Plann Perspect* 1990;22:198–205.

3. Rimpelä AH, Rimpelä MK, Kosunen EA. Use of oral contraceptives by adolescents and its consequences in Finland 1981-91. *BMJ* 1992;305:1053–7.
4. Ingelhammar E, Möller A, Svanberg B, Törnbom M, Lilja H, Hamberger L. The use of contraceptive methods among women seeking a legal abortion. *Contraception* 1994;50:143–52.
5. Tydén T, Björkelund C, Odlind V, Olsson S-E. Increased use of condoms among female university students: a 5-year follow-up of sexual behavior. *Acta Obstet Gynecol Scand* 1996;75:579–84.
6. Andersch B, Milsom I. Contraception and pregnancy among young women in an urban Swedish population. *Contraception* 1982;26:211–19.
7. Milsom I, Sundell G, Andersch B. A longitudinal study of contraception and pregnancy outcome in a representative sample of young Swedish women. *Contraception* 1991;43:113–21.
8. Larsson G, Milsom I, Sundell G, Andersch B, Blohm F. A longitudinal study of birth control and pregnancy outcome in a Swedish population. *Contraception* 1997;56:9–16.
9. Andersch B, Milsom I. An epidemiologic study of young women with dysmenorrhea. *Am J Obstet Gynecol* 1982;144:655–60.
10. Milsom I, Andersch B. The effect of various oral contraceptive combinations on dysmenorrhea. *Gynecol Obstet Invest* 1984;17:284–92.
11. Sundell G, Milsom I, Andersch B. Factors influencing the prevalence and severity of dysmenorrhea in young women. *Br J Obstet Gynaecol* 1990;97:588–94.
12. Larsson G, Milsom I, Andersch B, Blohm F. Contraception. A comparison of contraceptive habits and pregnancy outcome at 19 years of age in two cohorts of Swedish women born 1962 and 1972. *Contraception* 1996;53:259–65.
13. National Board of Health and Welfare. Abortion statistics 1995.
14. The sale of oral contraceptives. In: Apoteksbolaget. *Annual Report*. Stockholm; 1995.
15. Escobedo L, Lee NC. Beyond contraception: the health benefits and risks of the pill. *IPPF Med Bull* 1988;22:2.
16. Mishell DR Jr. Medical progress: Contraception. *N Engl J Med* 1989;320:777–87.
17. Aboulkhair M N, Unfer V, Costabile L. An Italian survey on how information campaigns about AIDS have changed contraception in young couples. *Clin Exp Obstet Gynecol* 1995;22:32–5.
18. Persson E. The sexual behaviour of young people. *Br J Obstet Gynaecol* 1993;100:1074–6.
19. Oddens BJ, Visser AP, Vemer HM, Everaerd WTAM, Lehert P. Contraceptive use and attitudes in Great Britain. *Contraception* 1994;49:73–86.
20. Oddens BJ, Visser APh, Vemer HM, Everaerd WTAM. Contraceptive use and attitudes in reunified Germany. *Eur J Obstet Gynecol Reprod Biol* 1994;57:201–8.
21. Skjeldestad FE. Choice of contraceptive modality by women in Norway. *Acta Obstet Gynecol Scand* 1993;72:48–52.
22. Webb A, Morris J. Practice of postcoital contraception - results of a national survey. *Br J Fam Plann* 1993;18:113–18.
23. Savonius H, Pakarinen P, Sjöberg L, Kajanoja P. Reasons for pregnancy termination: Negligence or failure of contraception? *Acta Obstet Gynecol Scand* 1995;74:818–21.
24. Brenner H, Mielck A. The role of childbirth in smoking cessation. *Prev Med* 1993;22:225–36.

Chapter 10
Contraceptive adherence and continuation rates

Carolyn Westhoff

Introduction

Contraceptive success means avoiding unintended pregnancy. Success depends on the intrinsic effectiveness of the contraceptive method, on correct and consistent use and on method continuation throughout times of risk of unintended pregnancy. Most unintended pregnancies are associated with premature discontinuation of a method or incorrect use rather than with method failures.[1] Among 10 683 US women having abortions in 2000–2001, 46% had not used a method in the month they conceived, although most had used contraception in the previous 6 months. Among the 54% of women using a method the month they conceived, most reported condom or oral contraceptive. Fully 75% of the pill users reported inconsistent use, while half of the condom users reported inconsistent use during the month they conceived. This provides strong evidence that incorrect use and premature discontinuation of contraception are major contributors to the many unintended pregnancies that end in abortion. We do not have similar data regarding unintended pregnancies that continue to term. Discontinuation of a method relates to factors that can be categorised according to characteristics of the method itself, characteristics of the user and external factors such as the healthcare system and the social environment. Measured discontinuation rates are highly sensitive to the method of data collection and data analysis.

Sources of data regarding method continuation

Interpreting continuation rates based on data from clinical trials aimed at quantifying effectiveness is problematic. Clinical trials yield much higher continuation rates than the rates seen in community use. This is partly due to the characteristics of women who volunteer for and are accepted into a study. At a minimum in most trials, these women are above the age of legal consent, in good health, in a stable sexual relationship and plan to stay at the same address for the full study period (implying stable housing). They also must subjectively impress the investigator that they will complete the full trial. These highly selected women subsequently benefit from remaining in the trial (and continuing to use the contraceptive) because of improved access to care and direct compensation. Thus, both the initial participant selection process and the incentives for remaining in a trial are biased towards high continuation rates. In addition, regulatory agencies require that data to evaluate tolerability and safety, as well as effectiveness, of new contraceptives be collected over at least 1 year of use. These agencies demand that trials aimed at registration of novel contraceptives include many women who use the product for more than just a few months, reinforcing the biases described above. Moreover, pharmaceutical companies that design clinical trials (both before and after product registration) have a marketing interest in demonstrating high continuation rates of their product and they often will selectively enrol participants who commit to a duration of use, such as 6 or 12 months, that was predetermined by the investigator rather than determined by the woman. The sponsors also have a marketing interest in publishing results of studies with high continuation rates. For all of these reasons, the high continuation rates seen in many trials are biased upward and are not readily able to be generalised to women receiving routine care.

Most clinical trials cannot assess the effects of the healthcare system itself on contraceptive continuation because the routine healthcare system has been replaced by the system available in the trial itself. Another limitation of clinical trials carried out for registration or by pharmaceutical companies after registration is that they often do not collect data regarding psychosocial variables. Finally, continuation rates observed during use of a novel product available only in the setting of a trial may be very different, either higher or lower, than continuation rates of the same product when it has been widely available.

Clinical trials may have limited general applicability but they often have more frequent, detailed data collection and higher rates of follow-up than other studies. In contrast, observational studies carried out among women selecting their own contraceptive method in a clinical setting may have more information about psychosocial variables, a broader spectrum of participants and often less frequent visits. These studies are generally more valuable than clinical trials in identifying patterns and rates of discontinuation in routine use. The results of community-based cohort studies may appear to lack convincing applicability because the population being studied is substantially different from one's own patient population. Nonetheless, well-done cohort studies often have adequate follow-up rates and the observed continuation rates are less likely to be biased upward by efforts of the investigators when compared with data generated in clinical trials. Taken together, several cohort studies done in different populations can illuminate patterns of discontinuation that are widely relevant.

Discontinuation by type of contraceptive

Discontinuation rates are highly variable among the reversible female methods of contraception. In general, methods such as implants or intrauterine devices that require a medical intervention for discontinuation have lower rates of discontinuation. In a New York City clinic population where implants were very popular immediately after their introduction, the 1-year continuation rate in 208 women was 85%.[2] In a cohort of 786 low-income implant acceptors at three widely separated US clinics, the 6-month lifetable continuation rate was 92%.[3] In a cohort of 511 women using Norplant® (now discontinued) implants for up to 5 years, the annual continuation rates were above 80% throughout follow-up.[4] These continuation rates, in a variety of populations, are remarkably similar. In a cohort study of postpartum adolescents, Polaneczky et al. compared those who chose implants to those who chose oral contraceptives.[5] At follow-up (an average of 15 months postpartum) continuation rates were 95% for those with implants and 33% for those who had chosen oral contraceptives. In all of these clinics, implant removal was freely available. Thus, lack of access to removal had little effect on the continuation rates.

In contrast, early discontinuation of oral contraceptives is widely described. Oakley *et al.* described first-year use among 1311 women making an initial visit to a US health department clinic.[6] Among those who used the pill for at least 1 month, almost 50% changed methods or used no method during an average of 8 months of follow-up. In addition, only 42% of users said they took a pill every day. Only 50% of the women who described the pill as their main method used it throughout follow-up; others had complex patterns of contraceptive use that included condom use and episodes of no protection.

In contrast to implants and similar to oral contraceptives, discontinuation of contraceptive injections is a passive act requiring only that the user fail to return as scheduled. In a cohort of 402 low-income depot medroxyprogesterone acetate (DMPA) users, the 12-month lifetable continuation rate was 42%, with 50% of the discontinuers stopping after only one injection.[7] A cohort study of 122 postpartum women aged less than 18 years old found that, after 12 months, 27% oral contraceptive users and 55% of DMPA users were still using the method.[8] This translated into repeat pregnancies within 12 months for 24% of the oral contraceptive group and 3% of the DMPA group. In another cohort study of 161 postpartum adolescents, O'Dell *et al.* compared continuation of the pill versus continuation of a contraceptive injection for at least 1 year.[9] In both groups, the 1-year continuation rates were low and similar (32% versus 34%). Nonetheless, the injection group had significantly lower repeat pregnancy rates (15% versus 36%), presumably because the injection suppresses ovulation for a prolonged time and thus can continue to protect against pregnancy even when the user has 'discontinued' it by not returning for the next scheduled injection. A retrospective cohort study of 494 adolescents compared the continuation of implants, injections and pills, with up to 48 months of follow-up.[10] The 1-year continuation rates were 82% for implants, 45% for DMPA and 12% for the pill. The relative position of the three methods remained constant throughout follow-up. Live births occurred by the end of follow-up among 14% of implant users, 21% of DMPA users and 27% of pill users. These data confirm the relative continuation rates of these three methods reported throughout the literature.

In all of these studies of hormonal contraceptives, participants were not randomised but chose the method they preferred, so unhappiness with an assigned method did not contribute to the high discontinuation rates.

Most of the studies described above relate to method use in deprived populations. Within this social stratum, continuation rates are clearly highest for implant users where discontinuation requires an action by the user and by the healthcare provider. These studies show similar, low continuation rates for pill and injection users where discontinuation is passive. Newer hormonal methods include the contraceptive patch and the contraceptive ring. At this time, there are no published discontinuation data from community use studies. Because these new methods permit passive discontinuation, patterns may prove to resemble those seen for pill and injection users.

There are representative national data from the USA that give an indication of discontinuation or incorrect use by method. Because most pregnancies that occur during use of highly effective self-reversible contraceptives are the result of incorrect or inconsistent use, accidental pregnancy itself can serve as an indicator of either incorrect use or premature discontinuation according to method. The 1995 cycle of the National Survey of Family Growth included data regarding contraceptive use and accidental pregnancies from 10 847 US women aged 15–44 years. Contraceptive failure rates among the commonly used methods were highest for condom users, followed by pill users, followed by injection users; implant users had the lowest rates. This ranking was consistent within strata defined by age, by poverty level and by marital status.[11] This approach cannot distinguish user failure from method failure; the high failure rates reported among condom users are probably a combination of both factors. Less commonly used methods included in this analysis were spermicides, withdrawal and periodic abstinence; all of these exhibited higher failure rates than condoms or the other methods. As with condoms, this analysis cannot distinguish incorrect or inconsistent use of these methods from method failure. Not enough US women used intrauterine devices to include this method in the analysis.

Other data suggest that first-year IUD discontinuation rates are lower than most other reversible methods except the implant. A clinical trial in the USA of 1202 users of the Copper T® 380A IUD yielded 1-year continuation rates of 75% and 2-year rates of 57%.[12] A post-marketing postal study of levonorgestrel-releasing intrauterine system (LNG-IUS) users in Finland (n = 17 360; response rate 75%) yielded a 1-year continuation rate of 94% and a 2-year rate of 87%.[13] An international randomised trial comparing these two devices yielded 1- and 2-year continuation rates of 82% and 69% for the Cu-T380A and 76% and 60% for the LNG-IUS, respectively.[14] There are no published direct comparisons between continuation of these devices versus hormonal methods. The available data regarding IUD discontinuation come largely from clinical trials, not from community-based studies, which may bias the reported rates upwards. Parenthetically, tubal ligation failure rates and discontinuation (i.e., reversal) have not been directly compared with reversible methods in developed countries but, based on other data, tubal ligation discontinuation is lower than for any other method.[15]

Discontinuation by duration of use

Across all reversible methods, discontinuation is greatest during the first months of contraceptive use and during the first episode of method use. In a study of oral contraceptive initiation in inner-city clinics in the USA, among 1021 women aged 25 years or younger, only 61% were current and continuous users at 3 months after initiation. Women in this study who had a previous episode of oral contraceptive use were much more likely to continue than the women starting the oral contraceptive for the first time (adjusted OR 1.6; 95% CI 1.2–2.1).[16] Similarly, among 1657 US women starting the oral contraceptive in a broader range of clinics and practices, at 6 months, 68% of new starts and 84% of women switching from another oral contraceptive were still using the method.[17] This paper notes that "of the women who discontinued, most did so early on, within the first 2 months of use". The only variable in that study that significantly predicted discontinuation was recency of use.

Greater continuation rates over time may be due to several factors. Theories of health behaviour change predict that new health behaviours (such as taking a contraceptive pill) take about 6 months to become habitual.[18] First, this suggests that some women who stop early are having trouble forming the habit of continuing contraceptive use. Just like eating healthy food or quitting smoking, learning to use contraceptives consistently can take more than one try. Second, women unhappy with a new method for any reason may drop out early, leaving only happier users who will be at low risk of a later discontinuation. Absolute continuation rates for any method are thus dependent upon the past experience of the women being studied and the duration of current use. Comparisons of discontinuation rates across methods also need to take into account the previous use of the method. Unfortunately, these data are often either not collected or provided, making comparisons of published continuation rates difficult. Young age is a predictor of discontinuation, in part because the youngest women have little past contraceptive experience, but multivariate analyses show that young age also has an independent effect.[16] Clinical trials all demonstrate higher continuation rates among 'switchers' and 'restarts' compared with new users, supporting the notion that there is a learning period that precedes long-term continuation of a method. Overall, past experience with a method and current duration of use are the strongest predictors of continued use of the same method.

Discontinuation or incorrect use by user characteristics

In many of the studies described above, participants within each study were fairly similar with regard to age and measures of social deprivation. However, these studies do not permit detailed comparisons of discontinuation according to those characteristics. In addition, these studies generally did not report details regarding other user characteristics such as previous method use or measures of motivation to avoid pregnancy.

All cycles of the National Survey of Family Growth include data regarding age, parity, marital status, income and education, as well as contraceptive use and accidental pregnancies. As described in the introduction to this chapter, accidental pregnancy rates can be a proxy for method discontinuation rates or incorrect use rates according to characteristics of the woman. Based on data from the 1995 Survey, contraceptive failure rates were higher for poor women (that is, income less than 200% of the US federal poverty line) using implants, injections, pills and condoms within strata of age and marital status.[11] Similarly, stratified for poverty, marital status and method, contraceptive failure rates were higher for younger women. Failure rates decreased with each 5-year increment of increasing age starting with women 15–19 years old. Women over 30 years of age had substantially lower failure rates than younger women, which may reflect declining fecundity as well as differences in continuation or correct use. Finally, union status affected failure rates within strata defined by method, age, and poverty status. Failure rates were highest for cohabiting women, intermediate for unmarried women who were not cohabiting and lowest for married women. Taken together, poor, young, cohabiting women experienced the highest failure rates regardless of the contraceptive method they used. Conversely, married women over age 30 years with income above the poverty line experienced the lowest failure rates regardless of which method they used. A limitation of these data is that they do not measure discontinuation or inconsistent use directly but rather use accidental pregnancy as a proxy for these. A unique strength of these data, however, is that they come from a large nationally representative survey that collected uniform and detailed information regarding user characteristics.

Discontinuation due to adverse effects and fear of adverse effects

A major reason cited by users for avoidance or discontinuation of a contraceptive method is adverse effects. The topic of adverse effects subsumes actual adverse effects due to the method, coincidental symptoms attributed to the contraceptive and fear of possible adverse effects. Fears are driven by publicity in the media about specific cases of bad outcomes that are possibly related to a method, or about epidemiological studies.

Many prevalent symptoms are widely attributed to oral contraceptives. Several surveys demonstrate that teenagers believe, in the absence of personal experience, that oral contraceptives cause weight gain, nausea, headaches and emotional changes.[19] Such pre-existing beliefs may predispose pill users to early discontinuation. Although this association has not been directly tested in oral contraceptive users, a clinical trial of an experimental drug found that subjects told of possible gastrointestinal adverse effects were more likely to report such effects than subjects did not receive this information.[20]

Large surveys in Europe and the USA describe reasons for discontinuation with particular attention to adverse effects.[17,21] A 1993 survey of 6676 current or past oral contraceptive users aged 16–30 years in Denmark, France, Italy, Portugal and the UK interviewed women identified on the street, not in a healthcare setting.[21] Of these, 51% reported at least one adverse effect while using the oral contraceptive. Women experiencing adverse effects were almost twice as likely to stop using the pill while still at risk of unintended pregnancy as women who did not report the same adverse effect. Women reporting two or three adverse effects were even more likely to discontinue prematurely. In addition, women reporting adverse effects were significantly more likely to miss one or more pills per cycle. A nationwide US study conducted from 1995 to 1996 identified 1657 women initiating or switching to a new pill in several healthcare settings, including both clinics and private practices.[17] Six-month follow-up interviews were available for 54% of women who enrolled in this study. In this study, 293 women discontinued the oral contraceptive during follow-up; 37% of these women cited adverse effects as their reason for discontinuing. The reported adverse effects included bleeding irregularities, nausea, weight gain, breast tenderness and headaches. Adverse effects, however, were not a significant predictor of discontinuation.

Several placebo-controlled trials of oral contraceptive use have reported on adverse effects in both groups.[19,22–24] The study of Goldzieher et al.[22] was specifically designed to examine the frequency of adverse effects and mainly included high-dose pills no longer in use. This study asked specific questions about possible adverse effects and found that oral contraceptive users reported more nausea and vomiting and more breast pain that placebo users. In contrast, there was no difference between oral contraceptive users and placebo users regarding headache or nervousness. Redmond et al.[23] and Coney et al.,[24] in studies of contemporary low-dose pills, used open-ended questions to elicit adverse effects. Overall, reported adverse effects were much less frequent than in the Goldzieher study,[22] and neither study found clinically important differences between oral contraceptive users and placebo users with regard to symptoms including nausea and vomiting, headache and weight gain.[23,24] Redmond et al. found a difference in breast pain between the groups (9% versus 5%).[23]

Data regarding the discontinuation of other methods due to adverse effects are less extensive than data regarding the contraceptive users. Discontinuation of the IUD is mainly attributable to changes in menstrual bleeding. For the LNG-IUS, spotting and amenorrhea are the most common reasons for discontinuation. For the Cu T380A IUD, increased bleeding and pelvic pain are the most common. For both of these devices, discontinuation due to other adverse effects is uncommon. However, the information regarding discontinuation comes primarily from clinical trials rather than from community use.[14] These studies did not report on the frequency of these complaints among women who chose to continue the method.

Among the many women who discontinue DMPA in the first year of use, most cite adverse effects. In a US study, 58% of 402 women with follow-up at 1 year had discontinued DMPA. Of these, 36% stopped because of menstrual changes and 39%

because of other adverse effects: weight gain, headaches, mood changes and acne.[7] In a survey of all adolescents who discontinued DMPA in a single clinic ($n = 35$), 21 cited irregular bleeding, 14 cited weight gain and nine cited increased headaches as the reason for stopping; fatigue and mood changes were each cited by seven participants.[25] These studies, similar to the IUD studies cited above, did not report on these complaints among continuing users.

In contrast, a prospective study of 786 implant initiators compared adverse effects among those who continued and those who discontinued.[3] Adverse effects were prevalent and similar among continuers and discontinuers. At a 6-month telephone re-interview, 76% of all women in the study reported less regular periods, 55% reported increased spotting, 43% reported heavier flow, 43% reported weight gain and 40% reported headaches. Thirty-eight percent reported that the implants were visible and 34% reported hair loss. Regarding these adverse effects, the 58 women who discontinued the implants by 6 months were significantly more likely to report weight gain, headache and hair loss but their experience of the other adverse effects seemed to be similar to the continuing users. This study showed that many adverse effects are highly prevalent but do not lead women to discontinue use of the implant. Across all contraceptive methods we have little information about this phenomenon. The women who discontinue because of an adverse effect may have more severe adverse effects than those who continue; they may have different beliefs regarding the importance of the adverse effect; they may have less motivation to avoid pregnancy or they may have more alternative contraceptive options.

The implant study took place at a time when there was a burst of widespread adverse publicity about the health effects of implants in the US media. Only 5% of the women in this study reported long-term health concerns regarding the implant but fully 37% of those who discontinued reported these concerns.[3] In a logistic regression analysis including 15 subject characteristics, exposure to negative media coverage had the strongest association with discontinuing the implant within 6 months following insertion. The adverse publicity regarding the Norplant implant in 1994 was not associated with any new findings regarding the safety or effectiveness of this product but merely dramatised information regarding well-characterised minor adverse effects and hypothesised more serious adverse effects, which have not been substantiated. This media frenzy led to a dramatic increase in requests for implant removal throughout the USA, together with a collapse in the request for insertions and, subsequently, the voluntary removal of implants from the US market by the manufacturer.[26]

Much better known are the recurring pill scares. The 1995 pill scare in the UK led to documented decreases in oral contraceptive use and an immediate rise in the abortion rate that was documented in the UK and elsewhere.[27–30] Pill scares started in 1969 with the publication of studies linking the pill to cardiovascular disease.[31] Where detailed data were available, pill discontinuation due to media coverage was most common among the youngest users. Similarly, the post-scare increases in abortions were most common in the youngest women. These scares led to immediate discontinuation of the contraceptive being publicised but also have led to long-term health concerns about the method that limit uptake by potential new users.

Other reasons for discontinuation

Ambivalence toward pregnancy would seem to be an obvious risk factor for contraceptive discontinuation or incorrect use but analyses of data from the US National Longitudinal Study of Adolescent Health show this to be a complex subject.[32,33]

Sophisticated analyses yield different conclusions, perhaps demonstrating only that ambivalence is difficult to measure. A simple measure of motivation – the desire to avoid pregnancy in the next few months – is generally associated with increased continuation rates. In a short-term study of women initiating the pill those who would be unhappy if pregnant in the 6 months were 2.3 times as likely to continue the oral contraceptive to the second pack as others. This was an independent protective factor in a multivariable analysis.[34] Similarly, in a cohort study of implant users, those with negative feelings about pregnancy in the next year were much less likely to discontinue the implant by 6 months.[3] A common reason given for method discontinuation is a change in fertility desire.[6,17] Even more frequent is a relationship change, such that the woman stops her method due to lack of sexual activity. This becomes a problem when sexual activity resumes before contraceptive use resumes.[25] Change in fertility desires or change in sexual activity were given as reasons by about 25% of pill discontinuers.[6,8,17]

The influence of partners and mothers on a woman's method continuation is still inadequately studied. Emans *et al.*[35] found that adolescents were significantly more likely to continue the pill at 3 months if their mothers did not know they were using the method. This effect disappeared at later follow-up. We do not know how the mothers' knowledge acted to decrease compliance. In a short-term study of pill continuation, partner knowledge of planned pill use at baseline was the strongest predictor of continuation (adjusted OR 3.43; 95% CI 1.7–7.1).[34,36] In the implant cohort study, partner fertility desires predicted early implant removal in an adjusted analysis accounting for 14 other characteristics; the only stronger predictor of removal was exposure to negative media coverage.[3]

Can we providers influence contraceptive continuation?

Contraceptive continuation, together with correct and consistent use of a recommended regimen, is often poor. We need to appreciate that this problem is not unique to contraception but is common to any type of long-term treatment. Typical adherence rates for many medical regimens are 50% or lower.[37] The World Health Organization (WHO) confirmed that premature discontinuation of medications averages 50% across a wide range of chronic conditions in its 2003 report on improving adherence to long-term therapies.[38] A scientific review of randomised clinical trials identified several interventions that improve adherence to long-term treatments.[39] These studies evaluated specific interventions for chronic medical illnesses. While hormonal contraceptive use has not been studied, these same interventions may prove useful in increasing adherence to contraception.

The evidence-based interventions that may improve contraceptive adherence include using a combination of the following:

- simplifying the regimen (e.g. less frequent dosing)
- instruction and instructional materials
- counselling about the regimen
- support group sessions
- cuing medications to daily events
- reminders (manual and computer) for medications and appointments
- self-monitoring with regular physician review and reinforcement
- involving family members and significant others
- reinforcements and rewards.

Several of these approaches may work in the family planning setting but little explicit evaluation is available. Reducing dosing from four times or twice daily to a single daily dose of oral medications for chronic illnesses is effective in increasing compliance. Testing of simplified regimens has included less frequent dosing of daily oral medications for preventive indications. In contraception, we have moved to weekly, monthly and less frequent dosing of hormonal methods but we do not yet have clear evidence from community-based studies that this increases adherence to self-administered contraceptives. Continuation rates clearly show that certain long-acting methods, implants and intrauterine devices, have substantially higher continuation rates. For instance, direct comparison of daily pills to a long-acting contraceptive implant in cohort studies showed dramatically higher continuation rates at 1 year for those using the long-acting method.[5,8,9] Contraceptives are far ahead of most other classes of medication in providing non-daily regimens.

Information sheets are widely used but data clearly indicate that information sheets have limited value if used alone. When information sheets are combined with specific instructions or counselling, high adherence rates ensue. This approach is already widespread in family planning clinics, together with individual and group counselling about the methods. A challenge outside of the research setting is to identify or develop culturally appropriate educational materials at a suitable literacy level. An aspect of counselling already widely used for oral contraceptives is cuing medications to daily events (e.g. keep your pills with your toothbrush). The use of automated reminders, such as beeping pill packs and text messages, is an area for increasing correct method use and for prompting pick-up of refills. One randomised trial of reminders for DMPA users found no difference in the rate of continuation or on-time injections in the intervention group. However, the intervention was limited to a single letter backed up by telephone call if the appointment was missed.[40] These approaches deserve more systematic study.

Studies of self-monitoring to improve adherence typically included diabetics who measured blood sugar levels or hypertensives who measured blood pressure themselves at home. These situations do not have an analogue in contraceptive practice. Involving family members and significant others in contraceptive adherence may be useful for some users. Observational studies found that partner knowledge of and approval of a contraceptive method is strongly associated with higher continuation rates.[3,34,36] A caveat is that involving partners or other family members may compromise patient privacy and autonomy. Furthermore, if the family or partner disapproves of the contraceptive method, then involving them may have adverse effects on adherence and continuation. We need studies to assess this area of influence. We also lack information specific to contraceptive practice regarding reinforcements and rewards; in studies of chronic illnesses these were often linked to results of self-monitoring, which does not apply to contraception. None of the studies included in the review evaluated increased access to care or increased access to medications. The WHO report emphasises that provider and health system factors have a major effect on adherence and deserve increased attention.[38] Unfortunately, the bulk of existing data regarding contraceptive discontinuation emphasises user-related factors. This reinforces a tendency to blame the user for discontinuation.

Practitioners often assume that the user's desire to avoid pregnancy is sufficient motivation to use a contraceptive method correctly and continuously. Behavioural sciences research reveals this assumption to be incorrect. In fact, in every situation in which patients must self-administer their treatment, even for life-threatening conditions, non-adherence is prevalent. Hence, it is not a surprise that women choosing long-acting contraceptives which do not require self-administration will achieve greater continuation and greater success than women choosing methods that require self-administration. Long-acting methods confer the same benefit to women at high risk of discontinuation; that is, women who are young, poor, unmarried and using a method for the first time.

References

1. Jones R, Darroch J, Henshaw S. Contraceptive use among U. S. women having abortions in 2000–2001. *Perspect Sex Reprod Health* 2002;34:294–303.

2. Gerber S, Westhoff C, Lopez M, Gordon L. Use of Norplant implants in a New York City clinic population. *Contraception* 1994;49:557–64.

3. Kalmuss D, Davidson A, Cushman L, Heartwell S, Rulin M. Determinants of early implant discontinuation among low-income women. *Fam Plann Perspect* 1996;28:256–60.

4. Sivin I, Mishell D, Darney P, Wan L, Christ M. Levonorgestrel capsule implants in the US: a 5-year study. *Obstet Gynecol* 1998;92:337–44.

5. Polaneczky M, Slap G, Forke C, Rappaport A, Sondheimer S. The use of levonorgestrel implants (Norplant) for contraception in adolescent mothers. *N Engl J Med* 1994;331:1201–6.

6. Oakley D, Sereika S, Bogue E. Oral contraceptive pill use after an initial visit to a family planning clinic. *Fam Plann Perspect* 1991;23:150–4.

7. Davidson A, Kalmuss D, Cushman L, Romero D, Heartwell S, Rulin M. Injectable contraceptive discontinuation and subsequent unintended pregnancy among low-income women. *Am J Public Health* 1997;87:1532–1534.

8. Templeman C, Cook V, Goldsmith J, Powell J, Hertweck S. Postpartum contraceptive use among adolescent mothers. *Obstet Gynecol* 2000;95:770–6.

9. O'Dell C, Forke C, Polaneczky M, Sondheimer S, Slap G. Depot medroxyprogesterone acetate or oral contraception in postpartum adolescents. *Obstet Gynecol* 1998;91:609–14.

10. Zibners A, Cromer B, Hayes J. Comparison of continuation rates for hormonal contraception among adolescents. *J Pediatr Adolesc Gynecol* 1999;12:90–4.

11. Fu H, Darroch J, Haas T, Ranjit N. Contraceptive failure rates: New estimates from the 1995 National Survey of Family Growth. *Fam Plann Perspect* 1999;31:56–63.

12. Sivin I, Tatum H. Four years of experience with the TCu 380A intrauterine contraceptive device. *Fertil Steril* 1981;36:159–63.

13. Backman T, Huhtala S, Tuominen J, Luoto R, Erkkola R, Blom T, *et al.* Sixty thousand woman-years of experience on the LN intrauterine system: an epidemiological survey in Finland. *Eur J Contracept Reprod Health Care* 2001;6 Suppl:23–6.

14. Sivin I, El Mahgoub S, ChCarthy T, Mishell D, Shoupe D, Alvarez F, *et al.* Long-term contraception with the Levonorgestrel 20 mcg/day and the Copper T 380Ag intrauterine devices: A five-year randomized study. *Contraception* 1990;42:361–89.

15. Westhoff C, Davis A. Tubal sterilization: Focus on the U. S. experience. *Fertil Steril* 2000;73:913–22.

16. Westhoff C, Robiletto C, Richmond A, Cushman L, Kalmuss D. Three-month continuation rates after immediate initiation of oral contraceptives. *Obstet Gynecol* 2004;103 Suppl:14.

17. Rosenberg M, Waugh M. Oral contraceptive discontinuation: a prospective evaluation of frequency and reasons. *Am J Obstet Gynecol* 1998;179:577–82.

18. Prochaska J, Redding C, Evers K. The transtheoretical model and stages of change. In: Glanz K, Lewis F, Rimes B, editors. *Health Behavior and Health Education.* 2nd ed. San Francisco, CA: Jossy-Bass: 1998. p. 60–84.

19. Davis A, Teal S. Controversies in adolescent hormonal contraception. *Obstet Gynecol Clin North Am* 2003;10:391–406.

20. Flaten M, Simonsen T, Olsen H. Drug-related information generates placebo and nocebo responses that modify the drug response. *Psychosom Med* 1999;61:250–5.

21. Rosenberg M, Waugh M, Meehan T. Use and misuse of oral contraceptives: risk indicators for poor pill taking and discontinuation. *Contraception* 1995;51:283–8.

22. Goldzieher J, Moses L, Averkin E, Scheel C, Taber B. A placebo-controlled double-blind crossover investigation of the side effects attributed to oral contraceptives. *Fertil Steril* 1971;123:878–914.

23. Redmond GP, Olson WH, Lippman JS, Kafrissen ME, Jones TM, Jorizzo JL. Norgestimate and ethinyl estradiol in the treatment of acne vulgaris: a randomized placebo-controlled trial. *Obstet Gynecol* 1997;89:615–22.

24. Coney P, Washnik K, Langley R, DiGiovanna J, Harrison D. Weight change and adverse event

incidence with a low-dose contraceptive: two randomized, placebo-controlled trials. *Contraception* 2001;63:297–302.

25. Harel Z, Biro F, Kollar L, Rauh J. Adolescents' reasons for and experience after discontinuation of the long-acting contraceptive Depo-provera and Norplant. *J Adolesc Health* 1996;19:118–23.
26. Klaisle C, Darney P. From launch to litigation. Norplant in America. *Infertility and Reproductive Medicine Clinics of North America* 2000;11:587–96.
27. Furedi A. The public health implications of the 1995 'pill scare'. *Hum Reprod Update* 1999;5:621–6.
28. Skjeldestad F. Increased number of induced abortions in Norway after media coverage of adverse vascular events from the use of third-generation oral contraceptives. *Contraception* 1997;55:11–14.
29. Williams D, Kelly A, Carvalho M, Feely J. Effect of the British warning on contraceptive use in the General Medical service in Ireland. *Ir Med J* 1998;91:202–3.
30. Dillner L. Pill scare linked to rise in abortions. *BMJ* 1996;312:996.
31. Bone M. The "Pill scare" and fertility in England and Wales. *IPPF Med Bull* 1982;16:2–4.
32. Jaccard J, Didge T, Dittus P. Do adolescents want to avoid pregnancy? Attitudes toward pregnancy as predictors of pregnancy. *J Adolesc Health* 2003;33:79–83.
33. Bruckner H, Martin A, Bearman P. Ambivalence and pregnancy: Adolescents' attitudes, contraceptive use and pregnancy. *Perspect Sex Reprod Health* 2005;36:248–57.
34. Westhoff C, Kerns J, Morroni C, Cushman L, Tiezzi L, Murphy P. Quick Start: a novel oral contraceptive initiation method. *Contraception* 2002;66:141–5.
35. Emans SJ, Grace E, Woods E, Smith D, Klein K, Merola J. Adolescents' compliance with the use of oral contraceptives. *JAMA* 1987;257:3377–81.
36. Kerns J, Westhoff C, Morroni C, Murphy P. Partner influence on early discontinuation of the pill in a predominantly Hispanic population. *Perspect Sex Reprod Health* 2003;35:256–60.
37. Haynes R, McDonald H, Garg A. Helping patients follow prescribed treatment; clinical applications. *JAMA* 2002;288:2880–3.
38. World Health Organization. *Adherence to Long-term Therapies: Evidence for Action.* Geneva: WHO; 2003.
39. McDonald H, Garg A, Haynes R. Interventions to enhance patient adherence to medication prescriptions; Scientific review. *JAMA* 2002;288:2868–79.
40. Keder L, Rulin M, Gruss J. Compliance with DMPA: a randomized, controlled trial of intensive reminders. *Am J Obstet Gynecol* 1998;179:583–5.

Chapter 11

Highly effective contraception and sexually transmitted infections in the Western European context

Charles S Morrison, Abigail Norris Turner, Kathryn Curtis, Patricia Bright and Paul D Blumenthal

Introduction

The negative effects of unprotected sex – unintended pregnancy and acquisition of sexually transmitted infections (STIs) – are usually treated as distinct events, although the same behaviour places individuals at risk for both outcomes. Unfortunately, no single method is superior for the prevention of both pregnancy and STIs. In recent years, women hoping to control their fertility and avoid infection have faced an additional concern, that some highly effective contraceptive methods may increase women's risk of certain STIs.

A possible increase in STI risk as a result of highly effective contraceptive methods is extremely relevant, given the more than 1.5 billion women of childbearing age worldwide.[1] Globally, more than 100 million women use hormonal contraceptive methods and approximately 150 million women use intrauterine devices (IUDs).[1,2] In the late 1990s, 58% of women of reproductive age in developed countries who were married or in informal unions used 'modern' contraceptive methods, including combined oral contraceptive pills, progestogen-only injectable contraception, IUDs, female or male sterilisation, or condoms.[1] However, although the proportion of women using any contraception in Western and Northern Europe and in North America is similarly high (around 70% of married women use modern methods),[1] considerable variation in method preference occurs by region (Table 11.1). Western Europeans have high oral contraceptive pill use (49% of married women) and less frequent use of IUDs (10%) or condoms (6%). Fewer Northern Europeans take oral contraceptives (22%), more use condoms (17%) and a similar proportion choose IUDs (8%) compared with Western Europe. In North America, women also use pills (15%) but female (23%) and male (14%) sterilisation are more common and IUD use is rare (1%).[1]

Europeans and North Americans suffer a large burden of curable STIs. The World Health Organization (WHO) estimates that, in 1999, there were 17 million new cases of curable STIs in Northern and Western Europe and 14 million cases in North

Table 11.1. Percentage of women of reproductive age who are married or in informal unions using modern contraception in two regions of Europe and North America[1]

	Western Europe[a]	Northern Europe[b]	North America[c]
Oral contraceptive	49	22	15
Intrauterine device	10	8	1
Injection	–	2	1
Condom	6	17	13
Female sterilisation	5	10	23
Male sterilisation	2	11	14
Other modern methods	1	1	3
Total modern methods	73	67	71

[a] includes Austria, Belgium, France, Germany, Netherlands and Switzerland, data from 1991–98; [b] includes Estonia, Finland, Latvia, Lithuania and UK, data from 1994–99; [c] includes Canada and USA, data from 1995

America.[3] Reducing STI incidence is a major public health priority, both to directly decrease the STI burden in the general population and to reduce the long-term consequences of untreated infection in women: bacterial STIs are associated with pelvic inflammatory disease (PID), chronic pelvic pain, ectopic pregnancy and infertility. Finally, STIs may increase the risk of acquisition of HIV,[4–6] providing further incentive to understand factors that increase STI susceptibility.

Hormonal contraception could act through several biological mechanisms to facilitate STI acquisition. These include:

- increased cervical ectopy associated with oral contraceptive use[7,8]
- humoral and cell-mediated immunological changes associated with use of exogenous steroids[9]
- direct influence of sex hormones on organism virulence, resulting in enhanced transmission efficiency[9]
- a hypoestrogenic effect associated with depot medroxyprogesterone acetate (DMPA) use resulting in thinning of the vaginal epithelium, reduction in the production of hydrogen-peroxide producing lactobacilli (and thereby decreased vaginal acidity) and irregular uterine bleeding.[10–12]

In addition, substantial behavioural differences may exist between women choosing various methods of contraception, both in underlying risk practices and in changes in risk-taking subsequent to contraceptive initiation. Women choose their regular contraceptive method for varied reasons, including type of partnership, duration of the relationship, frequency of sex, timing of coitus within the menstrual cycle or any combination of these and other factors. In addition, studies suggest that women starting on hormonal contraceptive methods generally decrease their condom use,[13–17] while one study found the inverse effect: consistent condom users were less likely to be compliant takers of oral contraceptive pills.[18]

Even though dual use of condoms, together with highly effective contraception provides the best overall protection against STIs and pregnancy, this practice is not common.[19–21] Several studies in developed countries have demonstrated that individuals choose a method based on the outcome they most fear; for example, although the absolute risk of acquiring an STI may be higher, those who perceive unintended pregnancy as a greater threat may forgo condom use and choose hormonal contraceptive methods instead.[22,23] Greater concern about unintended pregnancy than STIs may be a consequence of low STI knowledge; studies both in the UK[24,25] and the USA[26] have found low levels of understanding concerning the prevalence, symptoms and consequences of STI.

Methods

This paper summarises peer-reviewed research, published between January 1966 and December 2004, on the association between highly effective reversible contraception and the risk of STIs. Our review focuses largely on prospective studies where contraceptive use was assessed prior to infection status, and we have de-emphasised cross-sectional studies where the temporal sequence of contraceptive exposure and STI outcome cannot be determined. We first reviewed articles referenced in the third edition of WHO's *Medical Eligibility Criteria for Contraceptive Use* (MEC).[27] We then searched MEDLINE for all pertinent articles published since the most recent MEC update.

In view of the widespread use of certain hormonal methods and IUDs, and due to the limited data on other methods, we focused on infection risk associated with combined oral contraceptive pills, DMPA injections, progestogen-only implants, and IUDs. No published prospective studies have evaluated STI risk among users of other progestogen-only methods (including progestogen-only pills, injectable norethisterone enantate (NET-EN) or etonogestrel implant, or among users of newer combined hormonal methods such as the patch, the ring or injectables. Since the role of barrier methods, particularly condoms, in preventing STIs has been evaluated extensively in other reports,[28-31] condoms will not be addressed in detail here.

We chose to limit our review to STIs other than HIV and we further focused our discussion on the risk of cervical infections due to *Chlamydia trachomatis* and *Neisseria gonorrhoeae*. Owing to limited prospective data on other STI endpoints, we could not evaluate in depth the effect of contraceptive method on the acquisition of human papillomavirus (HPV), herpes simplex virus (HSV), syphilis or trichomoniasis, although we present data where these are available. We summarise findings from cross-sectional studies where no prospective data exist.

Methodological challenges

Methodological and ethical difficulties are common in designing prospective studies to answer aetiological questions about contraception and STIs. Perhaps most challenging is that, outside the specific context of partner studies of the viral STIs, we cannot directly measure women's exposure to sexually transmitted pathogens. For ethical reasons, we do not intentionally expose women to STIs and compare subsequent disease rates. Several measures of sexual behaviour are used to characterise women's risk of STI exposure but, without biological markers on women's sexual partners, these measures may not be adequate proxies for pathogen exposure.[32] In addition, the quality of sexual behaviour data is highly variable.[33]

Although the randomised controlled trial (RCT) is typically considered the most robust study design to provide an unbiased estimate of an association between exposure and outcome, RCTs have not been widely used to evaluate the effect of contraceptive use on STI risk. Instead, prospective cohort designs have been justifiably employed, where participants choose their preferred contraceptive method and researchers attempt to control bias by collecting in-depth data about risk behaviours and adjusting for these factors in analyses.

However, lack of randomisation introduces several challenges in study interpretation. We cannot assume that study groups are comparable in their underlying characteristics, average protocol adherence, distribution of various risk factors or STI exposure. If the differences between women using various methods are not adequately measured, comparing disease risks among these groups may yield biased effect estimates. Because selection and confounding biases cannot be ruled out, the results of multiple, well-conducted, prospective studies conducted in varying populations should be carefully considered before concluding that sufficient evidence exists of a causal association between contraceptive use and STIs.

Although non-randomised prospective studies have limitations, the RCT may also not be ideal for answering aetiological questions relating to contraception and STIs. One obvious challenge is the ethical difficulty of randomising women seeking highly effective contraception to methods with lower contraceptive efficacy. With multiple contraceptive options and widespread knowledge (or perceptions) about the advantages and disadvantages of each contraceptive method, many women have strong opinions about which method they wish to use, and women who receive their preferred method generally have higher levels of contraceptive continuation.[34] Reduced method switching generally improves the methodological quality of contraceptive research. Therefore, RCTs may not be feasible in settings where women have strong method preferences or where one of the randomisation arms involves an unpopular contraceptive option. Strong method preferences can also result in low study enrolment and can reduce the generalisability of the study results. If volunteers for trials of new contraceptive products are not representative of the larger target population, safety and effectiveness statistics, adherence or acceptability may not be applicable to other groups. Lastly, the typical intention-to-treat analysis of RCTs may fail to capture informative differences in method discontinuation and can result in significant misclassification of contraceptive exposure. For example, discontinuation of DMPA may be 50% or higher after 1 year,[35] whereas IUD users generally have substantially lower 1-year discontinuation rates (approximately 10%).[36,37] If discontinuation between randomisation arms is substantial and differential, effect estimates may be biased either towards or away from the null.

Other shortcomings in study design may further complicate comparisons of infection risk in users of different contraceptive methods. Many studies reviewed here had small samples with findings based on relatively few incident cases of disease (and therefore reduced power to detect an effect). Some studies compare contraceptive groups with unknown STI risks. For example, comparing oral contraceptive users to IUD users may be of limited utility, since the absolute STI risk in each group is unclear. Also, since current clinical guidelines do not recommend IUDs for women with high individual STI risk, differences in the underlying STI risk of each user population may further complicate study interpretation.

Difficulties in measuring both contraceptive exposure and STI endpoints are also frequent. Contraceptive research relies in large part on accurate self-reports of method adherence by research participants. For DMPA users, where providers administer and record injections, researchers may be confident about the dose and timing of contraceptive use. Daily oral contraceptive use, however, is more difficult to monitor. Measurement of the frequency and correctness of use of barrier methods such as condoms and diaphragms may be even more problematic. Also, contraceptive method use and exposure to STIs change over time; failure to account for the time-variable nature of these exposures may lead to exposure misclassification and poor control for confounding. Finally, different diagnostic techniques with varied sensitivities and specificities may lead to some misclassification of disease status. For example, older studies often diagnosed chlamydial infection by enzyme-linked immunosorbent assay (ELISA), whereas newer studies use more sensitive culture or nucleic acid amplification tests. Although diagnostic misclassification should be nondifferential with respect to exposure status, it may bias effect estimates toward the null.[38]

Results

C. trachomatis

Existing prospective studies suggest an increase in cervical chlamydia acquisition associated with both oral contraceptive and DMPA use. Six prospective studies (Table 11.2) have evaluated the association between the use of combined oral contraceptives and risk of C. trachomatis, and three of these present statistically significant evidence of a harmful association.[7,39,40] Three other studies found nonsignificant associations between oral contraceptive pills and chlamydial infection: two reported risks suggestive of a harmful relationship[41,42] while the third study suggested a modest protective association.[43] A meta-analysis that pooled results from 29 cross-sectional studies reported a crude pooled odds ratio of 1.9 (95% confidence interval 1.8–2.1) for the effect of oral contraceptives on the risk of chlamydial infection, compared with non-oral contraceptives users.[44] When the meta-analysis compared pill users to barrier method users, the pooled odds ratio rose to 2.9 (95% confidence interval 1.9–4.6). This increase in risk may be due to the protective effect of condoms and demonstrates the importance of careful selection of a referent group for these studies. Three prospective studies have evaluated the risk of chlamydial infection associated with DMPA use.[40–42] Each found a statistically significant association between DMPA and chlamydial infection with hazard ratios ranging from 1.6 to 4.3.

There is no indication of an association between IUD use and risk of chlamydial infection. One of the studies described above examined chlamydial infection in oral contraceptive users compared with women with IUDs,[39] finding that IUD users were at significantly lower risk of chlamydial infection compared with oral contraceptive users. More than 20 cross-sectional studies have also assessed the association between IUD use and chlamydia. None found significantly increased risks of chlamydia among IUD users compared with either oral contraceptive users or to women using no contraception.

No prospective studies have been conducted on the relationship between chlamydial infection and other highly effective reversible contraceptive methods and thus any relationships cannot be established from existing literature.

N. gonorrhoeae

Fewer prospective studies have evaluated the association between hormonal methods and N. gonorrhoeae. The three studies that assessed the effect of oral contraceptives on risk of gonococcal infection cite mixed results (Table 11.2). One study produced a statistically significant harmful association for the effect of oral contraceptive pills,[7] whereas two other studies found no significant association between oral contraceptive

Table 11.2. Prospective studies on the association between contraceptive use and sexually transmitted infections (STIs)

STI	Reference	Population (n)	Estimate adjustments	Oral contraceptives (OC)	DMPA	IUD	Other methods
C. trachomatis	7	American STI clinic patients (818)	Coital frequency, number of sexual partners, age, gravidity, parity	HR 1.7 95% CI 1.1–2.8 Comparing pill users with IUD users and sterilised women			No prospective studies have evaluated combined oestrogen-progestogen releasing patch, ring, or injectables, or progestogen-only pills, non-DMPA injectables or implants, and chlamydia
	39	Belgian family practice patients seeking contraception (231)	Not adjusted	IRR 8.8 95% CI 1.3–59.0 Comparing pill users with IUD users		IRR: 8.8, 95% CI: 1.3–59.0, comparing pill users to IUD users	
	40	Kenyan sex workers (948)	Age, education, years of sex work, parity, place of work, number of sex partners per week, number of sex acts per week, condom use	HR 1.8 95% CI 1.1–2.9 Comparing pill users with women who were sterilised or using no contraception	HR: 1.6, 95% CI: 1.1–2.4, comparing DMPA users to women who were sterilised or using no contraception		
	43	Swedish teenagers attending 'adolescent clinic' (201)	Not adjusted	RR 0.7 95% CI 0.3–1.7 Comparing OC users with non-users			
	41	American patients seeking reproductive health care (819)	Age, race, site, sexual and reproductive health characteristics	HR 1.9 95% CI 0.7–4.8 Comparing pill users with women not using hormonal contraception	HR: 4.3, 95% CI: 1.7–11.1, comparing DMPA users to women not using hormonal contraception		
	42	HIV-positive Kenyan sex workers (242)	Age, education, duration of sex work, parity, number of partners per week, condom use	HR 2.2 95% CI 0.7–7.3 Comparing pill users with women who were sterilised or using no contraception	HR: 3.1, 95% CI: 1.0–9.4, comparing DMPA users to women who were sterilised or using no contraception		

Table 11.2. Prospective studies on the association between contraceptive use and sexually transmitted infections (STIs) continued

STI	Reference	Population (*n*)	Estimate adjustments	Oral contraceptives (OC)	DMPA	IUD	Other methods
N. gonorrhoeae	7	American STI clinic patients (181)	Coital frequency, number of sexual partners, age, gravidity and parity	HR: 1.7, 95% CI: 1.1–2.8, comparing pill users with IUD users and sterilised women			No prospective studies have evaluated combined oestrogen-progestogen releasing patch, ring, or injectables, or progestogen-only pills, non-DMPA injectables or implants, and gonorrhoea
	40	Kenyan sex workers (948)	age, education, years of sex work, parity, place of work, number of sex partners per week, number of sex acts per week, condom use	HR 1.4 95% CI 0.9–2.1 Comparing pill users with sterilised women or those not using contraception	HR: 1.1, 95% CI: 0.8–1.6, comparing DMPA users to women who were sterilised or using no contraception		
	42	HIV-positive Kenyan sex workers (242)	Age, education, duration of sex work, parity, number of partners per week, condom use	HR 0.6 95% CI 0.3–1.3 Comparing pills users with sterilised women or those not using contraception	HR: 1.0, 95% CI: 0.6–1.7, comparing DMPA users to women who were sterilised or using no contraception		
	41	American patients seeking reproductive health care (819)	Age, race, site, sexual and reproductive health characteristics	Insufficient cases to evaluate risk of gonorrhoea alone HR for either chlamydia or gonorrhoea 1.5 95% CI 0.6–3.5 Comparing pill users with women not using hormonal contraception	insufficient cases to evaluate risk of gonorrhoea alone; HR for either chlamydia or gonorrhoea: 3.6, 95% CI: 1.6–8.5, comparing DMPA users to women not using hormonal contraception		

Table 11.2. Prospective studies on the association between contraceptive use and sexually transmitted infections (STIs) continued

STI	Reference	Population (n)	Estimate adjustments	Oral contraceptives (OC)	DMPA	IUD	Other methods
T. vaginalis	39	Belgian family practice patients seeking contraception (231)	Not adjusted	IRR 4.0 95% CI 0.7–8.9 Comparing IUD users with pill users (protective association for pill users)		IRR: 4.0, 95% CI: 0.7-8.9, comparing IUD users to pill users (harmful association for IUD users)	No prospective studies have evaluated combined oestrogen-progestogen releasing patch, ring, or injectables, or progestogen-only pills, non-DMPA injectables or implants, and trichomoniasis
	40	Kenyan sex workers (948)	Age, education, years of sex work, parity, place of work, number of sex partners per week, number of sex acts per week, condom use	HR 0.9 95% CI 0.7–1.3 Comparing pill users with sterilised women or those not using contraception	HR: 0.6, 95% CI: 0.4-1.0, comparing DMPA users to women who were sterilised or using no contraception		
	45	American STI clinic patients (818)	Spermicide use, sexual activity, age, race	HR 0.6 95% CI 0.4–0.8 Comparing pill users with those using IUDs or who had been sterilised			
HPV	47	American adolescents attending family planning clinics (105)	Time in study	HR 0.5 95% CI 0.3–0.9 Comparing current pill users with non-users	HR: 0.8, 95% CI: 0.2-3.3, comparing current DMPA users to non-users	No prospective studies have evaluated the association between DMPA and HPV	No prospective studies have evaluated combined oestrogen-progestogen releasing patch, ring, or injectables, or progestogen-only pills, non-DMPA injectables or implants, and HPV

Table 11.2. Prospective studies on the association between contraceptive use and sexually transmitted infections (STIs) continued

STI	Reference	Population (*n*)	Estimate adjustments	Oral contraceptives (OC)	DMPA	IUD	Other methods
	46	603, random sample of American university students	New sex partners, condom use with new partners, sex partners' number of other partners, duration of relationship prior to sex, smoking status, cumulative sex partners	HR 1.4 95% CI 1.0–1.8 Comparing pills users with non-users			
	48	253, Canadian patients in selected physician practices	Age, median number of sex partners in the last year, median number of lifetime sex partners, marital status, and smoking status	OR 0.7 95% CI 0.2–2.0 Comparing pill users with non-users			
	49	1425, Brazilian women attending a maternal and child health program	Age	Comparing users with never users *For non-oncogenic subtypes:* < 6 years OC use: OR 1.0 95% CI 0.6–1.9 ≥ 6 years OC use: OR 0.9 95% CI 0.5–1.7 *For oncogenic subtypes:* < 6 years OC use: OR 2.5 95% CI 1.0–5.9 ≥ 6 years OC use: OR: 3.4 95% CI 1.3–8.7			

Table 11.2. Prospective studies on the association between contraceptive use and sexually transmitted infections (STIs) continued

STI	Reference	Population (n)	Estimate adjustments	Oral contraceptives (OC)	DMPA	IUD	Other methods
HSV				No prospective studies have evaluated the association between OCs and HSV	No prospective studies have evaluated the association between DMPA and HSV	No prospective studies have evaluated the association between IUDs and HSV	No prospective studies have evaluated combined oestrogen/progestogen-releasing patch, ring or injectables, or progestogen-only pills, non-DMPA injectables or implants and HSV
T. pallidum	40	948, Kenyan sex workers	Age, education, years of sex work, parity, place of work, number of sex partners per week, number of sex acts per week, and condom use	HR 0.4 95% CI 0.1–1.5 Comparing pill users with women who were sterilised or using no contraception	HR 0.5 95% CI 0.2–1.4 Comparing DMPA users with women who were sterilised or using no contraception	No studies have evaluated the association between IUDs and syphilis	No prospective studies have evaluated combined oestrogen/progestogen-releasing patch, ring, or injectables or progestogen-only pills, non-DMPA injectables or implants and syphilis

CI = confidence interval; DMPA = depot medroxyprogesterone acetate; HIV – human immunodeficiency virus; HPV = human papillomavirus; HR = Hazard ratio; HSV = herpes simplex virus; IRR = incidence rate ratio; OC = oral contraceptive; OR = odds ratio; RR = risk ratio; STI = sexually transmitted infection; IUD = intrauterine device use and gonococcal infection.[40,42] Two of these prospective studies also investigated the effect of DMPA on risk of gonococcal infection and both found virtually null risks,[40,42] suggesting no association between DMPA and *N. gonorrhoeae*. A fourth prospective study evaluated the effect of oral contraceptives and DMPA on acquisition of either chlamydial or gonococcal infection. The authors report a nonsignificant elevated risk for acquisition of either infection due to oral contraceptives and a substantial, significant increased risk for the effect of DMPA.[41] However, the outcomes in this study included more incident chlamydial than gonococcal infections (37 chlamydial infections versus 14 gonococcal infections).

Thirteen cross-sectional studies have assessed the association between IUD use and gonorrhoea. None found significantly increased risks among IUD users compared either to pill users or to women using no contraception.

The relationship between gonococcal infection and other highly effective reversible contraceptive methods cannot be established from existing literature.

T. vaginalis

Studies of highly effective contraception and risk of trichomoniasis are inconclusive. Of the three studies on oral contraceptives and risk of trichomoniasis, one found a nearly null risk,[40] one found a statistically significant protective association[45] and one found a nonstatistically significant protective relationship.[39] This third study compared IUD with oral contraceptive users and although only ten cases of *T. vaginalis* were identified, IUD users appeared to be at substantially higher risk of infection than oral contraceptive users. The single study of DMPA and trichomoniasis yielded a borderline statistically significant protective effect.[40] The relationship between trichomoniasis infection and other highly effective contraceptive methods cannot be established from existing literature.

Human papillomavirus

Both prospective and cross-sectional studies report inconsistent findings about the effect of oral contraceptives on the risk of human papillomavirus (HPV) acquisition. Three prospective studies have evaluated oral contraceptive use as a risk factor for HPV acquisition: one study found a significant harmful effect,[46] a second study reported a significant protective effect[47] and a third study found a nonsignificant protective effect.[48] A case–control study nested within a prospective cohort found the risk of acquisition of oncogenic HPV subtypes was significantly increased both for women using oral contraceptives for less than and equal to or more than six years.[49] A review of 19 largely cross-sectional studies on oral contraceptives and HPV infection found no evidence for a strong negative or positive association.[50] One prospective study has evaluated DMPA as a risk factor for incident HPV, finding a statistically nonsignificant protective effect.[47] In addition, one cross-sectional study found a statistically significant elevated risk of prevalent HPV for current users of DMPA.[51] The same study reported a significantly increased risk of HPV for ever-use of the levonorgestrel-releasing implant, Norplant® (Hoechst Marion Roussel). No studies have evaluated IUD use as a risk factor for acquisition of HPV infection.

Herpes simplex virus

No prospective studies have evaluated the association between oral contraceptive use and herpes simplex virus (HSV) incidence, although several cross-sectional studies have been conducted, with mixed findings.[52-56] In addition, no prospective studies have evaluated the relationship between DMPA use and HSV incidence. One cross-sectional study reported a nearly null association for DMPA users compared with pill users.[52] No prospective studies have evaluated IUD use as a risk factor for acquisition of HSV.

T. pallidum

Almost no studies have explored the associations between highly effective contraception and risk of infection with *T. pallidum*. One prospective study described earlier found statistically nonsignificant protective effects for both oral contraceptives and DMPA on syphilis risk.[40] The relationship between syphilis infection and other highly effective contraceptive methods cannot be established from existing literature.

Discussion

High-quality, prospective research on the link between highly effective reversible contraception and STI risk is limited. Publication bias may have further reduced the pool of studies we were able to evaluate. Additional studies are needed to make valid conclusions related to individual contraceptive methods and specific STI. Nevertheless, the prospective studies reviewed were conducted in various populations (including adolescents, women seeking reproductive health and STI care and sex workers) and used a variety of referent groups. Some preliminary conclusions about infection risk are possible.

The most substantial data relate to chlamydial infection and suggest a possible increase in cervical acquisition of *C. trachomatis* associated with both oral contraceptive and DMPA use. The results of studies of oral contraceptives and DMPA as risk factors for gonococcal infection are inconsistent and given these results, no convincing evidence exists that either oral contraceptive or DMPA use is associated with acquisition of *N. gonorrhoeae*. Current data suggest that IUD use is not associated with increased risk of chlamydial or gonococcal infections. However, most data are drawn from cross-sectional studies and higher-quality prospective studies are needed to confirm this finding. Studies of oral contraceptive and DMPA use and risk of trichomoniasis are similarly inconclusive, although more high-quality prospective studies are needed to investigate a possible protective effect for both hormonal methods on the risk of trichomonas infection. No conclusions can be drawn about the relationship of contraceptive methods to risk of HPV acquisition, since the three prospective studies on oral contraceptive use have yielded mixed results and the only prospective study of DMPA use and HPV risk found a statistically nonsignificant protective effect. Evidence evaluating associations between highly effective contraceptive methods and herpes simplex infection or syphilis is similarly weak.

Future research needs

Our review suggests numerous areas for future research. First, we need to address the methodological difficulties associated with conducting prospective observational (cohort) studies and randomised trials to study contraceptive method use and STI risk. Data from a pilot study suggest that conducting an RCT may be technically and ethically feasible for some contraceptive methods in some settings (P Feldblum, personal communication), but additional research to assess the feasibility of RCTs is warranted.

Second, the generalisability of findings from existing research to other populations should be explored. Some of the studies reviewed here, particularly those carried out in high-risk subgroups (e.g. sex workers) in developing countries appear to have less relevance for general populations in Western Europe. Nevertheless, if any contraceptive method raises biological susceptibility to STIs, lower-risk settings will also be affected. Moreover, particular subgroups exist within Western Europe where the dynamics of STI transmission may be similar to those in developing countries. Also, the behavioural link between use of highly effective contraception and decreased condom use appear to be generalisable to both developed and developing country settings.

Third, some believe that the association between contraceptive method use and the development of PID, one of the most important sequelae of chlamydial and gonococcal infections, should be explored. Previous research suggests that oral contraceptive use may protect women with cervical infections from PID;[57–60] that is, although oral contraceptives may be associated with increased risk of acquisition of cervical chlamydial infection, this method may prevent *C. trachomatis* from ascending into the upper genital tract. However, although the relationship between contraception and PID is an important public health question, PID incidence is generally low (even among women with a known STI)[61] and PID diagnosis is difficult and subjective in most settings.[62–64] Fielding a sufficiently powered study would require many thousands of research participants (due to the low incidence of PID) and costs of such a trial may be prohibitive.

Public health implications

If a given contraceptive method is shown more conclusively to increase STI risk, counselling strategies should be adopted to insure that women understand the association between method of contraception and disease acquisition. In the absence of methods that are highly protective against both pregnancy and STIs, women at risk of infection should continue to be encouraged to use highly effective contraception for pregnancy prevention together with condoms for disease prevention. Clinical trials evaluating the effectiveness of the diaphragm for disease prevention (against HIV and other STIs) are continuing and, if the results are promising, this barrier device may give women another, possibly more acceptable, option for dual method use.

Certainly, increased risk of STIs associated with contraceptive method use is a critical concern. Beyond the direct health and economic consequences of STIs, the epidemiological association between prevalent STI and increased risk of HIV acquisition has been well established.[4–6] Methods that increase STI risk, therefore, may indirectly raise risk of HIV acquisition. However, particularly in the European context, care should be taken to avoid inducing unwarranted concern about risks associated with contraceptive use. Mischaracterisation of any increase in STI risk could persuade women to stop method use without plans to switch to a superior product. To avoid a repeat of the 1995 'pill scare' in the UK,[65,66] in which thousands of women stopped using oral contraceptives because of overstated safety concerns (with associated surges in unintended pregnancies and subsequent abortions), well-balanced messages about the significance of any increased risk of STIs would need to be crafted.

The expansion in the use of injectable contraception, particularly DMPA, has greatly increased women's access to highly effective contraception in many areas of the world. Given its widespread use, if an association between DMPA and STIs (particularly chlamydial infection) is validated by additional studies, reproductive health advocates and policy makers need to consider what changes in counselling and method provision guidelines are in order. For example, should DMPA users be advised to switch to oral contraceptives, IUDs or other highly effective reversible methods? Should cautionary messages be reserved for women in high STI-prevalence areas or for particular subgroups perceived to be at higher STI risk? Would such recommendations be feasible or acceptable? Such questions point to the need for additional high-quality research, particularly on highly effective methods such as the IUD, for which there is little prospective research related to STI acquisition. Further studies are also needed on some of the newer highly effective hormonal methods such as the progestogen-only implant Implanon® (Organon), which does not appear to cause the same hypoestrogenic environment as DMPA.[67]

Clinical implications

The risks and benefits associated with use of any contraceptive method need to be carefully evaluated by users and their providers. For many women, increased susceptibility to STIs may legitimately be of little concern, since their lifestyle, age, or other factors put them at low risk of STI acquisition. Indeed, given both the widely varying mix of methods used in developed countries and the range in STI prevalence by region, potential increases in STI risk associated with specific methods may not be relevant for large segments of the population; in subgroups with low STI incidence, the overall impact of a modestly elevated STI risk will be small. Conversely, changing demographics across Europe, including increased immigration from high STI-prevalence areas, later age at marriage and reduced childbearing may increase the likelihood of disease acquisition, even among individuals who perceive themselves to be at low STI risk. Thus, for women not in mutually monogamous relationships, contraceptive counselling should continue to emphasise the need for condom use and frequent STI screening in addition to highly effective contraception.

Finally, it is worth noting that none of the highly effective reversible contraceptive methods reviewed here was developed with STI prevention in mind. The fact that methods such as oral contraceptives and DMPA were developed over 40 years ago and have not changed substantially since then (despite vast changes in the STI landscape) speaks to the urgent need to develop new methods that will better protect against both unintended pregnancy and STIs.

Conclusion

Existing research on the relationships between highly effective contraceptive methods and risk of STIs is limited and many studies suffer from serious methodological concerns. Further high-quality prospective studies are needed to reach informed conclusions about individual contraceptive methods and the risk of acquisition of specific STIs.

Acknowledgements

The authors thank Ms Lisa Murphy for her preparation of the manuscript and Drs Ward Cates and Paul Feldblum for their insightful review and comments.

References

1. Population Reference Bureau.. Family Planning Worldwide 2002 Data Sheet. Washington, DC: PRB; 2002 [www. prb. org/pdf/FamPlanWorldwide_Eng. pdf].

2. United Nations, Department of Economic and Social Affairs, Population Division. World Contraceptive Use, 2003 Chart. New York: UN; 2003 [www. un. org/esa/population/publications/contraceptive2003/WCU2003. htm].

3. World Health Organization, Department of Communicable Disease Surveillance and Response. Global Prevalence and Incidence of Selected Curable Sexually Transmitted Infections: Overview and Estimates. Geneva: WHO; 2001 [www.who.int/docstore/hiv/GRSTI/who_hiv_aids_2001.02.pdf].

4. Fleming DT, Wasserheit JN. From epidemiological synergy to public health policy and practice: The contribution of other sexually transmitted diseases to sexual transmission of HIV infection. *Sex Transm Infect* 1999;75:3–17.

5. Cohen MS. Sexually transmitted diseases enhance HIV transmission: No longer a hypothesis. *Lancet* 1998;351 Suppl 3:5–7.

6. Corbett EL, Steketee RW, ter Kuile FO, Latif AS, Kamali A, Hayes RJ. HIV-1/AIDS and the control of other infectious diseases in Africa. *Lancet* 2002;359:2177–87.

7. Louv WC, Austin H, Perlman J, Alexander WJ. Oral contraceptive use and the risk of chlamydial and gonococcal infections. *Am J Obstet Gynecol* 1989;160:396–402.

8. Bright PL. A longitudinal investigation of cervical ectopy [dissertation]. Chapel Hill, NC: University of North Carolina at Chapel Hill; 2003.

9. Sonnex C. Influence of ovarian hormones on urogenital infection. *Sex Transm Infect* 1998;74: 11–19.

10. Miller L, Patton DL, Meier A, Thwin SS, Hooton TM, Eschenbach DA. Depomedroxyprogesterone-induced hypoestrogenism and changes in vaginal flora and epithelium. *Obstet Gynecol* 2000;96:431–9.

11. Bahamondes L, Trevisan M, Andrade L, Marchi NM, Castro S, Diaz J, *et al*. The effect upon the human vaginal histology of the long-term use of the injectable contraceptive Depo-Provera. *Contraception* 2000;62:23–7.

12. Mauck CK, Callahan MM, Baker J, Arbogast K, Veazey R, Stock R, *et al*. The effect of one injection of Depo-Provera on the human vaginal epithelium and cervical ectopy. *Contraception* 1999;60:15–24.

13. Yarnall KS, McBride CM, Lyna P, Fish LJ, Civic D, Grothaus L, Scholes D. Factors associated with condom use among at-risk women students and nonstudents seen in managed care. *Prev Med* 2003;37:163–70.

14. Ku L, Sonenstein FL, Pleck JH. The dynamics of young men's condom use during and across relationships. *Fam Plann Perspect* 1994;26:246–51.

15. Sheeran P, Abraham C, Orbell S. Psychosocial correlates of heterosexual condom use: a meta-analysis. *Psychol Bull* 1999;125:90–132.

16. Roye CF. Condom use by Hispanic and African-American adolescent girls who use hormonal contraception. *J Adolesc Health* 1998;23:205–11.

17. Ott MA, Adler NE, Millstein SG, Tschann JM, Ellen JM. The trade-off between hormonal contraceptives and condoms among adolescents. *Perspect Sex Reprod Health* 2002;34:6–14.

18. Weisman CS, Plichta S, Nathanson CA, Ensminger M, Robinson JC. Consistency of condom use for disease prevention among adolescent users of oral contraceptives. *Fam Plann Perspect* 1991;23:71–4.

19. Cates W Jr, Steiner MJ. Dual protection against unintended pregnancy and sexually transmitted infections: What is the best contraceptive approach? *Sex Transm Dis* 2002;29:168–74.

20. Anderson JE, Santelli J, Gilbert BC. Adolescent dual use of condoms and hormonal contraception: Tends and correlates 1991–2001. *Sex Transm Dis* 2003;30:719–22.

21. Wilson TE, Koenig LJ, Walter E, Fernandez I, Ethier K. Perinatal Guidelines Evaluation Project. Dual contraceptive method use for pregnancy and disease prevention among HIV-infected and HIV-uninfected women: the importance of an event-level focus for promoting safer sexual behaviors. *Sex Transm Dis* 2003;30:809–12.

22. Whaley AL. Preventing the high-risk sexual behavior of adolescents: Focus on HIV/AIDS transmission, unintended pregnancy, or both? *J Adolesc Health* 1999;24:376–82.

23. Roye CF, Seals B. A qualitative assessment of condom use decisions by female adolescents who use hormonal contraception. *J Assoc Nurses AIDS Care* 2001;12:78–87.

24. Garside R, Ayres R, Owen M, Pearson VA, Roizen J. "They never tell you about the consequences": young people's awareness of sexually transmitted infections. *Int J STD AIDS* 2001;12:582–8.

25. Macmillan S, Walker R, Oloto E, Fitzmaurice A, Templeton A. Ignorance about Chlamydia among sexually active women–a two centre study. *Hum Reprod* 1999;14(4):1131-5.
26. Clark LR, Jackson M, Allen-Taylor L. Adolescent knowledge about sexually transmitted diseases. *Sex Transm Dis* 2002;29:436–43.
27. World Health Organization, Department of Reproductive Health and Research. Medical eligibility criteria for contraceptive use. 3rd ed. Geneva: WHO; 2004 [www. who. int/reproductive-health/publications/MEC_3/mec. pdf].
28. National Institute of Allergy and Infectious Diseases (NIAID). Workshop Summary: Scientific Evidence on Condom Effectiveness for Sexually Transmitted Disease (STD) Prevention. NIAID; July 2001 [www. niaid. nih. gov/dmid/stds/condomreport. pdf].
29. Holmes KK, Levine R, Weaver M. Effectiveness of condoms in preventing sexually transmitted infections. *Bull World Health Organ* 2004;82:454–61.
30. Wald A, Langenberg AG, Link K, Izu AE, Ashley R, Warren T, *et al.* Effect of condoms on reducing the transmission of herpes simplex virus type 2 from men to women. JAMA 2001;285:3100–6.
31. Warner L, Newman DR, Austin HD, Kamb ML, Douglas JM Jr, Malotte CK, *et al.* Condom effectiveness for reducing transmission of gonorrhea and chlamydia: the importance of assessing partner infection status. *Am J Epidemiol* 2004;159:242–51.
32. Slaymaker E. A critique of international indicators of sexual risk behaviour. *Sex Transm Infect* 2004;80(Suppl 2):ii13–21.
33. Cleland J, Boerma JT, Carael M, Weir SS. Monitoring sexual behaviour in general populations: A synthesis of lessons of the past decade. *Sex Transm Infect* 2004;80(Suppl 2):ii1–7.
34. Pariani S, Heer DM, Van Arsdol MD Jr. Does choice make a difference to contraceptive use? Evidence from east Java. *Stud Fam Plann* 1991;22:384–90.
35. Westfall JM, Main DS, Barnard L. Continuation rates among injectable contraceptive users. *Fam Plann Perspect* 1996;28:275–7.
36. Pinter B. Continuation and compliance of contraceptive use. *Eur J Contracept Reprod Health Care* 2002;7:178–83.
37. Batar I, Kuukankorpi A, Siljander M, Elomaa K, Rauramo I. Five-year clinical experiences with NOVA T 380 copper IUD. *Contraception* 2002;66:309–14.
38. Devine OJ, Aral SO. The impact of inaccurate reporting of condom use and imperfect diagnosis of sexually transmitted disease infection in studies of condom effectiveness: A simulation-based assessment. *Sex Transm Dis* 2004;31:588–95.
39. Avonts D, Sercu M, Heyerick P, Vandermeeren I, Meheus A, Piot P. Incidence of uncomplicated genital infections in women using oral contraception or an intrauterine device: A prospective study. *Sex Transm Dis* 1990;17:23–9.
40. Baeten JM, Nyange PM, Richardson BA, Lavreys L, Chohan B, Martin HL Jr, *et al.* Hormonal contraception and risk of sexually transmitted disease acquisition: Results from a prospective study. *Am J Obstet Gynecol* 2001;185:380–5.
41. Morrison CS, Bright P, Wong EL, Kwok C, Yacobson I, Gaydos CA, *et al.* Hormonal contraceptive use, cervical ectopy, and the acquisition of cervical infections. *Sex Transm Dis* 2004;31:561–7.
42. Lavreys L, Chohan V, Overbaugh J, Hassan W, McClelland RS, Kreiss J, *et al.* Hormonal contraception and risk of cervical infections among HIV-1-seropositive Kenyan women. *AIDS* 2004;18:2179–84.
43. Rahm VA, Odlind V, Pettersson R. Chlamydia trachomatis in sexually active teenage girls. Factors related to genital chlamydial infection: A prospective study. *Genitourin Med* 1991;67:317–21.
44. Cottingham J, Hunter D. Chlamydia trachomatis and oral contraceptive use: A quantitative review. *Genitourin Med* 1992;68:209–16.
45. Barbone F, Austin H, Louv WC, Alexander WJ. A follow-up study of methods of contraception, sexual activity, and rates of trichomoniasis, candidiasis, and bacterial vaginosis. *Am J Obstet Gynecol* 1990;163:510–14.
46. Winer RL, Lee SK, Hughes JP, Adam DE, Kiviat NB, Koutsky LA. Genital human papillomavirus infection: Incidence and risk factors in a cohort of female university students. *Am J Epidemiol* 2003;157:218–26.
47. Moscicki AB, Hills N, Shiboski S, Powell K, Jay N, Hanson E, *et al.* Risks for incident human papillomavirus infection and low-grade squamous intraepithelial lesion development in young females. *JAMA* 2001;285:2995–3002.
48. Sellors JW, Karwalajtys TL, Kaczorowski J, Mahony JB, Lytwyn A, Chong S, *et al.* Incidence, clearance and predictors of human papillomavirus infection in women. *CMAJ* 2003;168:421–5.
49. Rousseau MC, Franco EL, Villa LL, Sobrinho JP, Termini L, Prado JM, *et al.* A cumulative case-control study of risk factor profiles for oncogenic and nononcogenic cervical human papillomavirus infections. *Cancer Epidemiol Biomarkers Prev* 2000;9:469–76.

50. Green J, Berrington de Gonzalez A, Smith JS, Franceschi S, Appleby P, Plummer M, et al. Human papillomavirus infection and use of oral contraceptives. Br J Cancer 2003;88:1713–20.

51. Giuliano AR, Papenfuss M, Abrahamsen M, Denman C, de Zapien JG, Henze JL, et al. Human papillomavirus infection at the United States–Mexico border: Implications for cervical cancer prevention and control. Cancer Epidemiol Biomarkers Prev 2001;10:1129–36.

52. Lavreys L, Chohan B, Ashley R, Richardson BA, Corey L, Mandaliya K, et al. Human herpesvirus 8: Seroprevalence and correlates in prostitutes in Mombasa, Kenya. J Infect Dis 2003;187:359–63.

53. Smith JS, Herrero R, Munoz N, Eluf-Neto J, Ngelangel C, Bosch FX, et al. Prevalence and risk factors for herpes simplex virus type 2 infection among middle-age women in Brazil and the Philippines. Sex Transm Dis 2001;28:187–94.

54. Willmott FE, Mair HJ. Genital herpesvirus infection in women attending a venereal diseases clinic. Br J Vener Dis 1978;54:341–3.

55. Evans BA, Kell PD, Bond RA, MacRae KD, Slomka MJ, Brown DW. Predictors of seropositivity to herpes simplex virus type 2 in women. Int J STD AIDS 2003;14:30–6.

56. Wolinska WH, Melamed MR. Herpes genitalis in women attending Planned Parenthood of New York City. Acta Cytol 1970;14:239–42.

57. Burkman R, Schlesselman JJ, Zieman M. Safety concerns and health benefits associated with oral contraception. Am J Obstet Gynecol 2004;190(4 Suppl):S5–22.

58. Rubin GL, Ory HW, Layde PM. Oral contraceptives and pelvic inflammatory disease. Am J Obstet Gynecol 1982;144:630–5.

59. Wolner-Hansson P, Svensson L, Mardh P, Westrom L. Laparoscopic findings and contraceptive use in women with signs and symptoms suggestive of acute salpingitis. Obstet Gynecol 1985;66:233–8.

60. Wolner-Hansson P, Eschenbach D, Paavonen J, Kiviat N, Stevens C, Critchlow C, et al. Decreased risk of symptomatic chlamydial pelvic inflammatory disease associated with oral contraceptive use. JAMA 1990;263:54–9.

61. Best K. IUD not recommended for increased STD risk. Network 2000;20(1):12–15 [www.fhi.org/en/RH/Pubs/Network/v20_1/NWvol20-1IUDsSTDs.htm].

62. Centers for Disease Control and Prevention. Pelvic Inflammatory Disease Fact Sheet. Atlanta: CDC; 2004 [www.cdc.gov/std/PID/STDFact-PID.htm#diagnosed].

63. Hall MN, Leach L, Beck E. Clinical inquiries. Which blood tests are most helpful in evaluating pelvic inflammatory disease? J Fam Pract 2004;53:326,330–1.

64. Simms I, Warburton F, Westrom L. Diagnosis of pelvic inflammatory disease: time for a rethink. Sex Transm Infect 2003;79:491–4.

65. Furedi A. The public health implications of the 1995 'pill scare'. Hum Reprod Update 1999;5:621–6.

66. Ramsay S. UK 'pill scare' led to abortion increase. Lancet 1996;347(9008):1109.

67. Croxatto HB, Makarainen L. The pharmacodynamics and efficacy of Implanon. An overview of the data. Contraception 1998;58(6 Suppl):91–7S.

Chapter 12
Hormonal contraception update on safety: breast and cervical cancer

Philip C Hannaford

Introduction

Before looking at the specific issue of whether hormonal contraceptives are associated with breast or cervical cancer, it is worth briefly looking at some general points about drug safety. First, when looking at relationships between an exposure and outcome, epidemiologists measure the strength of any association in terms of relative risk (risk ratios from cohort studies and odds ratios from case–control studies). In other words, they try to compare whether the frequency of each outcome in those using the drug is materially higher (or lower) than that in those not using the drug. Large relative risks are more likely to be causal than smaller ones, although other considerations (such as whether bias or confounding might have occurred, consistency of findings, dose or duration effects) need to be taken into account before a firm link can be established. The clinical significance of an association, however, depends on the absolute risk; that is, how much more (or less) disease occurs in the user group over and above that which would have occurred anyway in the nonusers. If a drug or medicine is used by many people, as is the case with hormonal contraception, small relative risks for a common event will result in a large number of people affected; conversely, a large relative risk for a rare event results in few people affected. Knowledge about the background risk of an outcome is essential for putting relative risks into perspective, both for individual users and for public health policy makers.

Second, almost all safety data about medicines come from observational studies. This is especially the case for hormonal contraception. Observational studies are inevitably more prone to bias and confounding than randomised clinical trials. It is crucial, therefore, that the results of observational studies are interpreted carefully and that the totality of the evidence is assessed: looking at overall patterns to inform clinical practice rather than concentrating on the findings of one or two studies.

Third, drug safety is about maximising benefits and minimising risks. Every effective medical intervention has some undesired adverse effects. It is important, therefore, to determine as accurately as possible the size of any risks, so that they can be presented to potential or current users in a way that enables them to make informed decisions. Equally as important, potential or current users should be provided with accurate information about any benefits.

Finally, when assessing possible cancer risks associated with a drug or medicine it is important to consider long-term as well as short-term effects. Most carcinogens have a long latent period before their harmful biological effects can be detected. Thus, effects may not be seen while a drug is being used. Alternatively, some effects seen in current users may persist long after the drug is stopped. For these reasons, ever use of a drug needs to be studied, as well as current or recent use.

Breast cancer

Breast cancer is the most common tumour occurring in women living in both developed and developing countries.[1] In the UK alone, there are about 41 000 new cases of breast cancer diagnosed each year, more than the next three most common cancers in women combined (colorectal, about 17 000; lung, 15 000; ovary, 7000). The incidence of breast cancer rises sharply during the fourth decade of a woman's life (Figure 12.1). It is not surprising, therefore, that the relationship between hormonal contraception and breast cancer has been studied in more than 60 epidemiological investigations. Most of the studies have looked at the effects of combined oral contraceptives, the most widely used type of hormonal contraception.

By the end of the 1980s, the picture was somewhat confused: a few studies had found small but statistically significant increases in the overall relative risk of breast cancer among oral contraceptive users and a number of other studies reported higher risks in certain subgroups of users, such as those using oral contraception for prolonged periods, before full-term pregnancy, or before 25 years of age.[2] Unfortunately, it was difficult to compare studies, partly because the various investigators used different categorisations for aspects of contraceptive use, such as age at first use or duration of use. In order to address this problem, the Collaborative Group on Hormonal Factors in Breast Cancer was established in 1992, with the purpose of bringing together, re-analysing and publishing as much of the worldwide data as possible.[3]

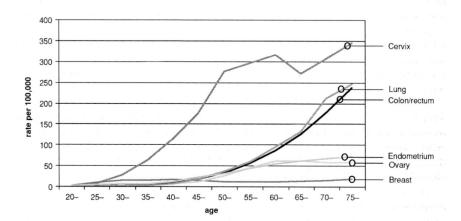

Figure 12.1. Rate per 100,000 women with newly diagnosed cancers in England, 2001

source: http//www.statistics.gov.uk/STATBASE/Expodata/Spreadsheets/D8397.xls (accessed 10.1.05)

Collaborative Group on Hormonal Factors in Breast Cancer reanalysis

The Collaborative Group invited the principal investigators of all epidemiological studies with at least 100 women with breast cancer to supply the coordinating centre in Oxford, UK, with original data in a similar format. Data were made available from 54 studies conducted in 25 countries relating to 53 297 women with breast cancer and 100 239 women without, about 90% of all global information.[3] Data from another 11 studies could not be included because the original information could not be retrieved and one research group declined to participate. What is known about the missing 12 studies suggests that the reanalysis results are unlikely to have been affected by the loss of information.

Similar data about individual women (where possible, about sociodemographic factors, use of hormonal contraceptives and hormone replacement therapy, family history of breast cancer, height, weight, age at menarche, reproductive history, menopausal status, age at menopause, gynaecological surgery and alcohol consumption) was obtained from each included study. Cohort studies were analysed using nested case–control techniques. The assembled data underwent a number of consistency checks before being stratified by study (to ensure that only women from the same study were compared), age at diagnosis, parity and, when appropriate, age when first child was born and age when risk of conception ceased. The stratifications were then combined to produce summary figures of all the data.

The reanalysis provided strong evidence that women have a small increased risk of having breast cancer diagnosed while taking combined oral contraceptives, and for the first 10 years after stopping (Table 12.1). The excess in former users does not persist: there was no evidence of an increased risk of breast cancer 10 or more years after stopping combined oral contraceptives. The pattern of risk was essentially the same, irrespective of type of study, country of residence, ethnic group, family history of breast cancer or other characteristics of the user. In general, once recency of use had been accounted for, similar patterns of risk were seen among women with different duration of use and age at starting use and among those with different dose and type of hormone in their contraceptive. One notable exception was women who started using combined oral contraceptives before the age of 20 years. The relative risk of breast cancer in these women during oral contraceptive use and during the first 5 years after stopping was higher than those observed in women beginning at older ages. For

Table 12.1. Relative risk (RR) and 95% confidence interval (CI) of breast cancer in women taking and stopping combined oral contraceptives, compared with non-users; in a collaborative reanalysis of individual data on 53 297 women with breast cancer and 100 239 women without breast cancer from 54 epidemiological studies (data from Collaborative Group on Hormonal Factors in Breast Cancer[3])

Years since stopping	RR (95 % CI)
0 (never)	1.0
0 (current)	1.24 (1.15–1.33)
1–4	1.16 (1.08–1.23)
5–9	1.07 (1.02–1.13)
10 +	1.01 (0.96–1.05)

instance, the relative risk of breast cancer during current use among women starting oral contraception in their teens (compared with never users of the same age) was 1.59 (95% CI 1.41–1.77), whereas the relative risk in those starting at 20–24 years was 1.17 (95% CI 1.04–1.30).

Intriguingly, the reanalysis found that, if combined oral contraceptive users do have breast cancer diagnosed, it tends to be less advanced clinically than cancer diagnosed in never users, even among women who stopped using oral contraception more than 10 years previously; the relative risk of tumour spread beyond the breast in ever versus never users was 0.88 (95% CI 0.81–0.95).

Some of these findings are difficult to explain in terms of usual understanding of cancer development. A pattern of increased risk soon after starting hormonal contraception, no increase with longer duration of use, and loss of effect by 10 years after stopping does not fit in with the usual model of a carcinogen initiating cancer. Instead, it may reflect the promotion of tumours that have already started to develop. The tendency for oral contraceptive users to have more localised lesions may be due to earlier detection of the disease among ever users than never users, although such an effect would have to persist to account for more localised cancers in ever users who had stopped for more than 10 years. Alternative explanations may be biological effects of oral contraceptives on tumour growth and risk of metastasis (or a combination of explanations).

Important gaps in our knowledge

Overall, the reanalysis results are reassuring, particularly for the first generation of women who used oral contraceptives in the 1960s and 1970s. It would be wrong, however, to assume that we now know everything about the relationship between hormonal contraceptives and breast cancer. Only 14% of women in the data set began using combined oral contraceptives in their teens and, although the reanalysis found no increased risk of breast cancer in this group beyond 5 years after stopping, virtually none of the early starters had reached their late 40s or early 50s, when breast cancer becomes more common. More data are needed about the long-term effects of early use of combined oral contraceptives. Recent studies have produced contradictory results, with some finding weak evidence of extra risk associated with early use of oral contraception[4–6] and others no enhanced risk.[7]

The reanalysis data set contained little information about breast cancer risk beyond 20 years after stopping oral contraception use. Furthermore, most women who had stopped more than 10 years previously had used oral contraceptives for only short periods and tended to use medium- or high-dose preparations (i.e. those containing 50 micrograms or more of oestrogen). A recent large North American case–control study of women aged 35–64 years with breast cancer and which included 1803 women who had stopped oral contraception more than 20 years previously, found no evidence of long-term risk (OR 0.9; 95% CI 0.8–1.0).[8] A similar result was found in a smaller case–control study conducted in Sweden of older women with breast cancer (in women who stopped more than 20 years previously OR 1.02; 95% CI 0.87–1.11).[9] Limited data from three longstanding cohort studies also suggest no long-term risk after stopping oral contraception,[10–12] although a cohort study started more recently in Norway and Sweden observed a continuing elevated risk among former oral contraceptive users who had stopped for more than 15 years.[13] More studies are needed looking at the long-term effects of prolonged oral contraceptive use, particularly of recently introduced preparations containing newer progestogens.

So far there have been few studies that have assessed directly the effects of specific combined oral contraceptives. A North American investigation which assigned hormonal potencies to preparations used before 1993 found an increased risk of breast cancer among users of oral contraceptives with a higher oestrogen content or with higher progestogen or oestrogen potencies.[14] Such studies, however, are fraught with difficulties partly because of problems associated with allocating potency values.[15] Grouping combined oral contraceptives simply by their oestrogen content ignores the biological effects of the accompanying progestogen (and vice versa). Studies looking directly at the risk associated with particular formulations have been difficult to perform because of the large number of preparations on the market, resulting in even very large studies having limited power to examine the effects of less popular products. A recent large Norwegian cohort study that tried to look at the risk of breast cancer associated with combined oral contraceptives containing different progestogens suffered from this problem.[16] Furthermore, it had few data about recently introduced progestogens. At the moment, it is impossible to tell whether any breast cancer risks are combined oral contraceptive 'class' effects, or restricted to particular preparations. It is also impossible to determine the relative contribution of the oestrogen and progestogen components in combined oral contraceptives.

Previous users of oral contraception are more likely than never users to use hormone replacement therapy after the menopause.[17,18] A reanalysis of original data from studies of breast cancer and hormone replacement therapy has found similar effects to those associated with oral contraception (e.g. an elevated risk in current and recent users, which declines within a few years of stopping).[19] Given the high frequency of use of both oral contraception and hormone replacement therapy in many countries, there has been growing interest in examining the combined effects of these products. The few studies so far have tended to examine the combined effects of ever use of oral contraception and hormone replacement therapy, with generally reassuring results. For example, in a North American case–control study of 1030 women with breast cancer, the overall risk associated with exposure to both oral contraception and hormone replacement therapy was the same as that among women not exposed to either product.[20] However, a small subgroup of women who used oral contraceptives for more than 10 years and hormone replacement therapy for more than 3 years had a significantly elevated risk of breast cancer compared with never users of either preparation (RR 3.2; 95% CI 1.4–7.4). A subsequent case–control study of 1847 postmenopausal North American women with breast cancer and with a higher usage of both oral contraception and hormone replacement therapy could not replicate this finding.[18] Furthermore, there was no indication in the later study that long-term use of both oral contraception and hormone replacement therapy increased the risk of breast cancer over and above that which would have pertained if only one product had been used. More studies addressing this issue are needed, particularly with respect to the risk of breast cancer in women who use both classes of exogenous hormones closely together.

More information is also needed about whether the greater likelihood of localised disease in ever users of combined oral contraception is due to the earlier detection of cancer, how long this effect persists for, whether the effect is related to the hormonal content of preparations used and whether it results in improved survival in ever users. Recent studies looking at the relationship between oral contraception and survival after breast cancer diagnosis have produced conflicting results.[21,22]

In the collaborative reanalysis, the relative risk of breast cancer among oral contraceptive users did not appear to be influenced by a family history of the disease.[3]

The results, however, were based on a comparatively small amount of data and no details were available about how family history was ascertained. A historical cohort study of 426 families with breast cancer probands looked more specifically at the risk of breast cancer among oral contraceptive users with a familial disposition to the cancer.[23] In the study, sisters and daughters of the probands who ever used oral contraceptives had a significantly greater risk of breast cancer than first-degree relatives who never used this method of contraception (RR 3.3; 95% CI 1.6–6.7). The increased risk was strongest for oral contraceptive use during or prior to 1975 (when available preparations tended to have higher doses of oestrogen and progestogen), although there was little information about usage after 1975. The risk of breast cancer was not elevated among oral contraceptive users who had a second-degree relative with breast cancer. Oral contraceptive users with a history of breast cancer in a first degree relative also had an increased risk of breast cancer in a large North American case–control study (OR 2.44; 95% CI 1.9–3.1).[24]

Most cases of breast cancer (even among those with a family history) occur in women without mutations on the breast cancer susceptibility genes, *BRCA1* and *BRCA2*. Nevertheless, interest has grown in determining the effects of combined oral contraception in carriers of these mutations.[25–27] This is partly because women with these mutations have a much higher background risk of developing breast cancer, often at a young age, than noncarriers. In addition, women with the mutation have an increase risk of ovarian cancer, which they may wish to reduce through the use of combined oral contraception; these women need to know whether such action increases their chances of developing the more common tumour, breast cancer. A case–control study of 1311 pairs of women with known *BRCA1* and/or *BRCA2* mutations recruited from 52 centres in 11 countries found no increased risk of breast cancer among women with the *BRCA2* mutation who ever used oral contraception (OR 0.94; 95% CI 0.72–1.24).[27] Among *BRCA1* carriers, ever use of oral contraception was associated with a small overall increased risk of breast cancer (OR 1.20; 95% CI 1.02–1.40) and increases in subgroups who used oral contraception: for at least 5 years (but not shorter periods), before age 30 years or before 1975 (but not afterwards). Another two studies have suggested an increased risk of breast cancer among oral contraceptive users with *BRCA* mutations compared with oral contraceptive users without these mutations.[25,26]

Hormonal contraceptives other than combined oral contraceptives

Most of the hormonal contraceptive data in the collaborative reanalysis relate to combined oral contraceptives, reflecting patterns of usage in the general population.[3] Only 0.8% of the women in the dataset had used progestogen-only oral preparations and 1.5% an injectable progestogen. Findings for progestogen-only preparations, therefore, were limited, although broadly in line with those for combined oral contraceptives.[3] A similar pattern of risk among users of progestogen-only oral contraception was found in a case–control study of breast cancer conducted in New Zealand.[28] Other studies have not found an increased risk of breast cancer among users of injectable[29,30] or implantable[30] progestogen-only contraceptives, although the number of women in the studies using either product, particularly implantable devices, was small. Exclusive users of progestogen-only oral contraception in a cohort study of Norwegian and Swedish women did not have an increased risk of breast cancer.[13] On the other hand, women in the same study who were current or recent users of progestogen-only pills after using combined oral contraceptives had a small but significantly elevated risk of breast cancer (RR 1.6; 95% CI 1.0–2.4). This may reflect a hangover effect of the previous use of combined oral contraception. There have been no studies of the breast cancer risk associated with use of the combined contraceptive patch or combined hormonal injection.

Clinical implications

Given that combined oral contraceptives appear to be associated with an increased risk of breast cancer only in current and recent users, the absolute number of women affected will depend on the age at which the method is stopped. Table 12.2 provides estimates of the number of extra cases of breast cancer that would accumulate among women using combined oral contraceptives for 5 years and stopping at different ages. Since most women stop using combined oral contraceptives at an age when the background risk of breast cancer is low (i.e. before their mid-30s), the absolute number of women affected is small. For example, an estimated five extra cases of breast cancer will accumulate by the age of 40 years for every 10 000 European or North American women who stop using combined oral contraceptives at age 30 years. The higher relative risks observed among women starting combined oral contraceptives in their teens (if real) will result in few, if any, extra cases of breast cancer, provided that they stop using this method of contraception at an age when breast cancer is still rare. On the other hand, women using oral contraceptives near their menopause need to be carefully counselled about the extra number of cases of breast cancer that might be expected from such usage.

Based on the available evidence, short-term use of oral contraception has been recommended by some researchers to reduce the risk of ovarian cancer in BRCA carriers.[27] More substantial evidence, however, is needed to put this clinical advice on a firmer footing. More generally, current evidence is insufficient to warrant recommending the avoidance of oral contraception by women with a first-degree family history of breast cancer or advice that they undergo extra screening if they decide to use oral contraceptives. Instead, all users of oral contraceptives, irrespective of their family history, should be informed of the importance of developing and maintaining breast awareness, and of reporting promptly any breast changes to an appropriate healthcare professional.

Table 12.2. Estimated cumulative risk of breast cancer being diagnosed in women who use combined oral contraceptives (COC) for 5 years and who are followed up for 10 years after stopping, compared with non-users (number of cases per 10 000 women from Europe or North America) (data from Collaborative Group on Hormonal Factors in Breast Cancer[3])

Age while using COC (years)	Age at end of follow-up (years)	Numbers of breast cancer cases		Extra number of cases (95% CI)
		Never users	COC users	
16–19	30	4	4.5	0.5 (0.3–0.7)
20–24	35	16	17.5	1.5 (0.7–2.3)
25–29	40	44	48.7	4.7 (2.7–6.7)
30–34	45	100	111.1	11.1 (7.0–15.2)
35–39	50	160	181.0	21.0 (13.9–28.1)
40–44	55	230	262.0	32.0 (22.2–41.8)

Cervical cancer

Invasive cervical cancer is the second most common cancer among women in developing countries, but ranks lower (seventh) in developed countries.[1] In the UK, it is the tenth most common cancer in women, with about 3200 new cases per annum.[1] For many years it has been recognised that the risk of cervical cancer is affected by sexual behaviour and, more recently, by persistent infection with oncogenic types of human papillomavirus (HPV).[31] However, infection of the cervix with HPV is common and usually transient. Thus, on its own, HPV infection does not appear to be a sufficient cause of cervical cancer; cofactors are needed before HPV infection persists and progresses to produce cervical intraepithelial neoplasia (CIN) and invasive cancer. Suggested cofactors include cigarette smoking, high parity and oral contraception.

More than 50 studies have examined the relationship between hormonal contraception and invasive cervical cancer, carcinoma-*in situ* and CIN 3. Many of these studies were brought together in a systematic review of published results.[32]

Systematic review

The reviewers included all epidemiological studies of hormonal contraception and invasive cervical cancer, carcinoma-*in situ* or CIN3, which published age-adjusted or age-matched relative risk estimates, and their corresponding 95% confidence intervals, by duration of hormonal contraceptive use. In studies that measured HPV infection, there had to be at least 50 cases of invasive cervical cancer or carcinoma-*in situ*/CIN3 for inclusion in the review. If HPV infection was not measured, there had to be at least 100 cases of invasive carcinoma, carcinoma-*in situ* or CIN 3 (for cohort studies) and 100 cases of invasive cancer or 200 cases of carcinoma-*in situ*/CIN3 (for case–control studies). Twenty-eight studies met these criteria, comprising at least 80% of the relevant literature worldwide and relating to 12 531 women with invasive or *in situ* cancer. Ten more studies were large enough to be included but were not because they did not publish age-adjusted relative risks for duration of use. Another 13 studies were too small for inclusion in the review. Evaluations of the impact of excluding these 23 studies suggest that loss of the data did not affect the main results of the review.[32]

From the published reports of each eligible study information was collected about: country and year of diagnosis of cases; study design; type of cervical neoplasia; histological type (squamous cell, adenocarcinoma, including adenosquamous carcinoma, or unspecified); measure of HPV infection, if any; whether the relative risks were adjusted for HPV infection, number of sexual partners, previous cervical screening, smoking or use of barrier methods of contraception. The most fully adjusted relative risks for each duration of hormonal contraceptive use were pooled into three main groups: short-duration (generally less than 5 years of use); medium-duration (generally 5–9 years of use); long-duration (generally 10 or more years of use). Almost all of the data about hormonal contraceptives related to combined oral contraceptives.

Taken together, the results showed an increasing risk of cervical cancer with longer duration of use, so that women who used oral contraceptives for 10 years or more had just over twice the risk of cervical cancer than that of never users (Table 12.3; RR 2.2; 95% CI 1.9–2.4).[32] Within each duration of use category, cohort studies consistently found higher relative risks than case–control studies. It is not clear why this was so.

Table 12.3. Relative risk (RR) and 95% confidence interval (CI) of invasive or *in situ* cervical cancer among women using combined oral contraceptives for different duration, compared with non-users; from a systematic review of published results relating to 12 531 women with these conditions (data from Smith JS *et al.*[32])

Duration of oral contraceptive use, years	Type of study RR (95% CI)		
	Any	Cohort	Case–control
0	1.0	1.0	1.0
< 5	1.1 (1.1–1.2)	1.8 (1.4–2.4)	1.1 (1.0–1.2)
5–9	1.6 (1.4–1.7)	2.2 (1.7–2.9)	1.5 (1.4–1.7)
10 +	2.2 (1.9–2.4)	3.3 (2.4–4.5)	2.0 (1.8–2.3)

Most of the studies in the review adjusted, by varying degrees, for factors thought to confound the association between oral contraception use and cervical cancer. These alternative explanations to a real biological effect of oral contraception include: differences between users and nonusers in sexual behaviour (e.g. age at first intercourse, number of sexual partners, number of partners that the male partner had), lifestyle (smoking) and screening.[33] Observed differences might also have been due to a protective effect of barrier methods used by the nonuser group, rather than an adverse effect of oral contraception itself. In the systematic review, similar patterns of increasing risk with longer durations of oral contraceptive use were found among studies that adjusted for different factors (e.g. the 22 studies adjusting for number of sexual partners). This suggests that confounding from these variables is unlikely to fully explain the increasing risk with longer durations of oral contraceptive use.

There has been great debate about how best to allow for HPV status. Analyses in the review restricted to the 12 studies of women who tested positive for HPV found positive trends between cervical cancer and increasing duration of oral contraception. Analyses looking only at studies of HPV negative women and those which adjusted for HPV status found similar trends, albeit possibly with smaller increases with prolonged use among HPV negative women. Studies of HPV negative women, however, may be inappropriate if HPV is associated with all, or almost all, cases of cervical cancer, since women testing negative are probably false negatives. Consistency of results among studies conducted in different countries, and in those looking at different types of cervical cancer, provides further evidence to suggest that the relationship between oral contraception and cervical cancer is real (causal).

The increased risk of cervical cancer among combined oral contraceptive users appears to decline with increasing time since stopping (Table 12.4), although the published data were relatively sparse for women using oral contraceptives for long periods and stopping many years previously. Information about how long effects persist for after stopping combined oral contraception is essential for clearer understanding of the public health significance of these findings. In order to provide such information, a collaborative reanalysis of original (as opposed to published) data is now underway, using variables defined in a similar fashion across each study.

Table 12.4. Relative risk (RR) and 95% confidence interval (CI) of cervical cancer by time since stopping and duration of use of oral contraceptives, compared with non-users; from a systematic review (data from Smith JS *et al*.[32])

Years since stopping	Duration of use in years, RR (95% CI)	
	< 5	**5+**
< 8	1.4 (1.2–1.5)	2.1 (1.8–2.4)
8 +	1.1 (1.0–1.2)	1.4 (1.1–1.9)

Hormonal contraceptives other than combined oral contraceptives

Three studies in the systematic review looked at the effects of different durations of use of injectable progestogen-only contraceptives, and none at progestogen-only oral preparations.[32] Although the data were scanty, there was a suggestion of increasing risk of cervical cancer with longer periods of use of injectable contraceptives.

Clinical implications

If combined oral contraceptive users have an increased risk of cervical cancer after prolonged use, which declines after stopping, the absolute number of women affected in developed countries is probably small. In one of the few cohort studies to provide data on the subject, the Royal College of General Practitioners' Oral Contraception Study observed a four-fold increased relative risk of invasive cervical cancer and a five-fold elevated relative risk of carcinoma-*in situ* among women who had used combined oral contraceptives for 10 years or more (compared with never users).[34] Nevertheless, the estimated absolute excess risk among long-term users was only 34/100 000 woman-years for cervical cancer, and 80/100 000 woman-years for carcinoma-*in situ*. Users of combined oral contraceptives can minimise this risk by making sure that they participate in national screening programmes for cervical cancer. The interval between screens, however, should remain the same as that for users of different contraceptives, since there is little evidence to suggest that oral contraception increases the speed of progression from pre-invasive to invasive cervical cancer.

Balancing risks against benefits

This paper has only considered two important cancers that might be more common in users of combined oral contraceptives. Users of this method of contraception, however, also benefit from important reductions in their risk of endometrial,[34] ovarian[34] and colorectal cancer.[35] The endometrial and ovarian benefits appear to persist for many years after oral contraception is stopped. This could have major public health consequences if the benefits continue in former combined oral contraceptive users until they reach an age when these cancers become more common (Figure 12.1). Users of combined oral contraceptives need to be informed about these benefits when also being told about possible cancer risks. The challenge is to find new ways of conveying this complex message in a balanced, informative and nontechnical manner.

References

1. International Agency for Research on Cancer. Cancer Mondial. Globocan 2000 [http://www-dep.iarc.fr/].
2. Mann RC. Oral contraceptives and breast cancer risk: a problem of consent. In: Mann RD, editor. *Oral Contraceptives and Breast Cancer: the implications of the present findings for informed consent and informed choice.* Carnforth: Parthenon Publishing; 1990. p. 7–33.
3. Collaborative Group on Hormonal Factors in Breast Cancer. Breast cancer and hormonal contraceptives: collaborative reanalysis of individual data on 53,297 women with breast cancer and 100,239 women without breast cancer from 54 epidemiological studies. *Lancet* 1996;347:1713–27.
4. Tryggvadottir L, Tulinius H, Gudmundsdottir GB. Oral contraceptive use at a young age and the risk of breast cancer: an Icelandic, population-based cohort study of the effect of birth year. *Br J Cancer* 1997;75:139–43.
5. Chie W-C, Li C-Y, Haung C-S, Chang K-J, Yen M-L, Lin R-S. Oral contraceptives and breast cancer risk in Taiwan, a country of low incidence of breast cancer and low use of oral contraceptives. *Int J Cancer* 1998;77:219–23.
6. Ursin G, Ross RK, Sullivan-Halley J, Hanisch R, Henderson B, Bernstein L. Use of oral contraceptives and risk of breast cancer in young women. *Breast Cancer Res Treat* 1998;50:175–84.
7. Tavani A, Gallus S, La Vecchia C, Negri E, Montella M, Dal Maso L, et al. Risk factors for breast cancer in women under 40 years. *Eur J Cancer* 1999;35:1361–67.
8. Marchbanks PA, McDonald JA, Wilson HG, Folger SG, Mandel MG, Daling JR, et al. Oral contraceptives and the risk of breast cancer. *N Engl J Med* 2002;346:2025–32.
9. Magnusson CM, Persson IR, Baron JA, Ekbom A, Bergström R, Adami H-O. The role of reproductive factors and use of oral contraceptives in the aetiology of breast cancer in women aged 50 to 74 years. *Int J Cancer* 1999;80:231–6.
10. Hankinson SE, Colditz GA, Manson JE, Willett WC, Hunter DJ, Stampfer MJ, et al. A prospective study of oral contraceptive use and risk of breast cancer (Nurses' health study, United Stated). *Cancer Causes Control* 1997;8:65–72.
11. Beral V, Hermon C, Kay C, Hannaford P, Darby S, Reeves G. Mortality associated with oral contraceptive use: 25 year follow up of cohort of 46 000 women from Royal College of General Practitioners' oral contraception study. *BMJ* 1999;318:96–100.
12. Vessey M, Painter R, Yeates D. Mortality in relation to oral contraceptive use and cigarette smoking. *Lancet* 2003;362:185–91.
13. Kumle M, Weiderpass E, Braaten T, Persson I, Adami H-O, Lund E. Use of oral contraceptives and breast cancer risk: the Norwegian–Swedish women's lifestyle and health cohort study. *Cancer Epidemiol Biomarkers Prev* 2002;11:1375–81.
14. Althuis MD, Brogan DR, Coates RJ, Daling JR, Gammon MD, Malone KE, et al. Hormonal content and potency or oral contraceptives and breast cancer risk among young women. *Br J Cancer* 2003;88:50–7.
15. Sturtevant FM. Breast cancer and oral contraceptives: critique of the proposition that high potency progestogen products counter excess risk. *Biomed Pharmacother* 1984;38:371–9.
16. Dumeaux V, Alsaker E, Lund E. Breast cancer and specific types of oral contraceptives: a large Norwegian cohort study. *Int J Cancer* 2003;105:844–50.
17. Moorhead T, Hannaford P, Warskyj M. Prevalence and characteristics associated with use of hormone replacement therapy in Britain. *Br J Obstet Gynaecol* 1997;104:290–7.
18. Norman SA, Berlin JA, Weber AL, Strom BL, Daling JR, Weiss LK, et al. Combined effect of oral contraceptive use and hormone replacement therapy on breast cancer risk in postmenopausal women. *Cancer Causes Control* 2003;14:933–43.
19. Collaborative Group on Hormonal Factors in Breast Cancer. Breast cancer and hormone replacement therapy: collaborative reanalysis of data from 51 epidemiological studies of 52,705 women with breast cancer and 108,411 women without breast cancer. *Lancet* 1997;350:1047–59.
20. Brinton LA, Brogan DR, Coates RJ, Swanson CA, Potischman N, Stanford JL. Breast cancer risk among women under 55 years of age by joint effects of usage of oral contraceptives and hormone replacement therapy. *Menopause* 1998;5:145–51.
21. Sauerbrei W, Blettner M, Schmoor C, Bojar H, Schumacher M, for the German Breast Cancer Study Group. The effect of oral contraceptive use on the prognosis of node positive breast cancer patients. *Eur J Cancer* 1998;34:1348–51.
22. Reeves GK, Patterson J, Vessey MP, Yeates D, Jones L. Hormonal and other factors in relation to survival among breast cancer patients. *Int J Cancer* 2000;89:293–99.
23. Grabrick DM, Hartmann LC, Cerhan JR, Vierkant RA, Therneau TM, Vachon CM, et al. Risk of breast cancer with oral contraceptive use in women with a family history of breast cancer. *JAMA*

2000;284:1791–8.

24. Brinton LA, Gammon MD, Malone KE, Schoenberg JB, Darling JR, Coates RJ. Modification of oral contraceptive relationships on breast cancer risk by selected factors among younger women. *Contraception* 1997;55:197–203.

25. Ursin G, Henderson BE, Haile RW, Pike MC, Zhou N, Diep A, *et al.* Does oral contraceptive use increase the risk of breast cancer in women with *BRCA1/BRCA2* mutations more than in other women? *Cancer Res* 1997;57:3678–81.

26. Heimdal K, Skovlund E, Moller P. Oral contraceptives and risk of familial breast cancer. *Cancer Detect Prev* 2002;26:23–7.

27. Narod SA, Dube MP, Klijn J, Lubinski J, Lynch HT, Ghadirian P, *et al.* Oral contraceptives and the risk of breast cancer in *BRCA1* and *BRCA2* mutation carriers. *J Natl Cancer Inst* 2002;94:1773–9.

28. Skegg DC, Paul C, Spears GF, Williams SM. Progestogen-only oral contraceptives and risk of breast cancer in new Zealand. *Cancer Causes Control* 1996;7:513–9.

29. Shapiro S, Rosenberg L, Hoffman M, Truter H, Cooper D, Rao S, *et al.* Risk of breast cancer in relation to the use of injectable progestogen contraceptives and combined estrogen/progestogen contraceptives. *Am J Epidemiol* 2000;151:1134.

30. Strom BL, Berlin JA, Weber AL, Norman SA, Bernstein L, Burkman RT, *et al.* Absence of an effect of injectable and implantable progestin-only contraceptives on subsequent risk of breast cancer. *Contraception* 2004;69:353–60.

31. Walboomers JM, Jacobs MV, Manos MM, Bosch FX, Kummer JA, Shah KV, *et al.* Human papillomavirus is a necessary cause of invasive cervical cancer worldwide. *J Pathol* 1999;189:12–19.

32. Smith JS, Green J, Berrington de Gonzalez A, Appleby P, Peto J, *et al.* Cervical cancer and use of hormonal contraceptives: a systematic review. *Lancet* 2003;361:1159–67.

33. Swan SH, Petitti DB. A review of problems of bias and confounding in epidemiologic studies of cervical neoplasia and oral contraceptive use. *Am J Epidemiol* 1982;115:10–18.

34. Beral V, Hannaford P, Kay C. Oral contraceptive use and malignancies of the genital tract. Results from the Royal College of General Practitioners' Oral Contraception Study. *Lancet* 1988;ii:1331–5.

35. Fernandez E, La Vecchia C, Balducci A, Chatenoud L, Franceschi S, Negri E. Oral contraceptives and colorectal cancer risk: a meta-analysis. *Br J Cancer* 2001;81:722–7.

Chapter 13
Hormonal contraception and cardiovascular safety

Kathryn M Curtis and Polly A Marchbanks

Introduction

Combined oral contraceptives (COCs) were first marketed in the early 1960s.[1] In 1961, Jordan published the first article on pulmonary embolism associated with COC use,[2,3] followed by a report of COC use and coronary thrombosis in 1963.[4] Since then, numerous studies have examined the cardiovascular safety of COCs and, to a lesser extent, other combined and progestogen-only contraceptives; many have been large, multicentre, multi-country cohort or case–control studies (Table 13.1). While the incidence of cardiovascular disease among women of reproductive age is low and cardiovascular mortality rare, effects of hormonal contraceptive use on cardiovascular risk may be important as, globally, over 100 million women use COCs[1] and at least 27 million use progestogen-only methods.[5]

A primary goal, as well as a major challenge, of studies of hormonal contraception has been to assess how cardiovascular risk has changed as COCs have been reformulated. The first COCs contained relatively high doses of oestrogen and progestogens compared with today's preparations.[6] As cardiovascular and other health effects of COCs were identified, hormonal doses were lowered and new progestogens were developed. Specifically, desogestrel and gestodene were created to have an advantageous effect on lipid profiles, theoretically decreasing the risk of arterial disease.[7] In 1995, however, three reports appeared that showed an increased risk of venous thromboembolism (VTE) with newer progestogens compared with older progestogens.[8–10] These reports set off a flurry of media and regulatory action, leading to the 'pill scare' of 1995 in the UK and Europe.[11] A series of studies and strong debate followed in the literature regarding the cardiovascular effects of newer progestogens compared with older progestogens. COC formulations are frequently classified by generation, although there is no standard taxonomy and 'generation' may be determined by the timing of market introduction or by chemical structure.[1,6] Generally, COCs containing 50 μg or more of oestrogen are termed 'first-generation' pills, those containing levonorgestrel or norethisterone are described as 'second-generation' pills, while those containing desogestrel or gestodene are considered 'third-generation' pills. Pills containing norgestimate have been classified as either second or third generation, as norgestimate metabolises to levonorgestrel but was introduced at around the same time as desogestrel and gestodene.[6] An additional progestogen,

Table 13.1. Selected studies of combined oral contraceptive use and cardiovascular outcomes

Study	Design	Participants (n)[a]	Location	MI: odds ratio (CI)	Stroke: odds ratio (CI)	VTE: odds ratio (CI)
Mann, 1975[126]	Case–control	MI: 63/189	England and Wales	4.5#		
Collaborative Group for the Study of Stroke in Young Women, 1975[45]	Case–control	IS:140/722, HS:196/722	USA		IS: 4.4 (2.8–6.9)[H], 4.1 (2.6–6.6)[N]; HS: 2.0 (1.3–3.2)[H], 1.9 (1.2–2.9)[N]	
Walnut Creek Contraceptive Drug Study (Petitti, 1978[127]; Ramcharan, 1980[28]	Cohort study, Nested case–control analysis	IS:, VTE: 38/8174	USA		IS: 2.9 (0.6–6.5), 1.9 (0.9–4.1)	
Rosenberg, 1980[14]	Case–control	MI: 156/3120	USA	1.6 (1.0–2.6)#		
Adam, 1981[129]	Case–control	MI: 139/276	England and Wales	1.4 (0.75–2.44)#		
Salonen, 1982[130]	Cohort	MI: 2653 women	Finland	1.3 (0.4–6.9)		
Oxford Family Planning Association (Vessey, 1984[131]; Mant, 1998[31]; Vessey, 2003[132])	Cohort	MI: 310,565, IS: 310,564	UK	1.9 (1.0–3.5) ≤ 8 years of use#, 1.0 (0.6–1.8) < 8 years of use#	IS: 1.2 (0.4–2.9) ≤ 8 years of use#, 2.0 (0.9–4.6), < 8 years of use#	
LaVecchia, 1987[28]	Case–control	MI: 168/251	Italy	1.80 (0.28–11.54)#		
Ananjevic-Pandey, 1989[133]	Case–control	MI: 58/174	Belgrade			
Royal College of General Practitioners (Croft, 1989[16]; Hannaford, 1994[51])	Cohort study (nested case–control analysis)	MI: 158/474, IS: 26/88, SH: 34/126, CH: 9/32	UK	1.8 (0.9–3.6)#	IS: 3.5 (1.1–10.8)#, SH: 1.5 (0.6–3.7)#, CH: 1.1 (0.2–7.1)#	
Thorogood 1991,[18] Thorogood 1992,[64] Thorogood 1992,[134]	Case–control	MI: 161/309, IS: 21/42, SH: 296/592, VTE: 60/115	England and Wales	1.9 (0.7–4.9)[b]	IS: 4.4 (0.8–24.4)[b], SH: 1.1 (0.6–1.9)	2.1 (0.8–5.2)[b]
D'Avanzo, 1994[32] Lidegaard 1993,[60] Lidegaard 1995[56]	Case–control, Case–control	MI: 251/475, CTA: 320/1197	Italy, Denmark	2.0 (0.6–6.7)#, CTA: 1.8 (1.1–2.9)#		

Table 13.1. Selected studies of combined oral contraceptive use and cardiovascular outcomes continued

Study	Design	Participants (n)[a]	Location	MI: odds ratio (CI)	Stroke: odds ratio (CI)	VTE: odds ratio (CI)
WHO Collaborative Study of Cardiovascular Disease and Steroid Hormone Contraception (WHO 1995,[58] WHO 1996,[47] WHO 1996,[63] WHO 1997,[21] Chang 1999,[59] Poulter 1999[53])	Case–control	MI: 368/941 IS: 697/1962 HS: 1068/2910 VTE: 1143/2998	21 centres, 17 countries in Africa, Asia, Europe, Latin America	Europe: 5.01 (2.54–9.90) Developing countries: 4.78 (2.52–9.07)	IS: Europe: 2.99 (1.65–5.40) Developing countries: 2.93 (2.15–4.00) HS: Europe: 1.38 (0.84–2.25) Developing countries: 1.76 (1.34–2.30)	Europe: 4.15 (3.09–5.57) Developing countries: 3.25 (2.59–4.08)
Transnational Study on Oral Contraceptives and the Health of Young Women (Lewis 1996,[67] Lewis 1997,[27] Heinemann 1998,[49] Lewis 1999[35])	Case–control	MI: 182/635 IS: 220/775 VTE: 471/1702	16 centres in 5 countries (Austria, France, Germany, Switzerland, and the UK)	2.26 (1.32–3.86)	IS: 2.86 (2.02–4.04)	4.4 (3.4–5.8)
MICA Study (Dunn 1999,[24] Dunn 2001[36])	Case–control	MI: 448/1728	England, Scotland, Wales	1.40 (0.78–2.52)		
Pooled analysis of Kaiser CA and University of Washington, US (Sidney 1996,[26] Sidney 1998,[20] Schwartz 1998[49])	Case–control	MI: 271/993 IS: 175/1191 HS: 198/1191	USA	0.94 (0.44–2.20)	IS: 1.09 (0.54–2.21) HS: 1.11 (0.61–2.01)	
Lidegaard 1999,[37] Lidegaard 1999[38]	Case–control	MI:94/1041 CTA: 219/1041	Denmark		CTA: 1.75 (1.24–2.47)	
Bloemenkamp, 1999[69]	Case–control	VTE: 185/591	Netherlands			3.2 (2.3–4.5)
Rosenberg, 2001[22]	Case–control	MI:627/2947	USA	1.3 (0.8–2.2)#		
Risk of Arterial Thrombosis in Relation to Oral Contraceptives (RATIO) Study (Tanis 2001,[25] Kemmeren 2002[41])	Case–control	MI:248/925 IS: 203/925	Netherlands	2.0 (1.5–2.8)	2.3 (1.6–3.3)	

Table 13.1. Selected studies of combined oral contraceptive use and cardiovascular outcomes continued

Study	Design	Participants (n)[a]	Location	MI: odds ratio (CI)	Stroke: odds ratio (CI)	VTE: odds ratio (CI)
Lidegaard 2002,[50] Lidegaard 2002[70]	Case–control	CTA:626/4054 VTE: 987/4054	Denmark		CTA: 1.6 (1.3–2.0)[d]	3.4 (2.8–4.2)[†]
Melbourne Risk Factor Study Group (MERFS), 2003[62]	Case–control	IS:234/234	Australia		IS: 1.76 (0.86–3.61)	
Gillum, 2000[40]	Meta-analysis	16 studies	No geographic restrictions		IS: 2.75 (2.24–3.38)	
Spitzer, 2002[38]	Meta-analysis	7 studies	No geographic restrictions	2nd gen: 2.18 (1.62–2.94) 3rd gen: 1.13 (0.66–1.92)		
Khader, 2003[13]	Meta-analysis	23 studies	No geographic restrictions	3.00 (1.70–5.38)		
Chan, 2004[39]	Meta-analysis	20 studies	No geographic restrictions	2.48 (1.91–3.22)#	IS: 2.74 (2.24–3.35) HS: 1.30 (0.99–1.71)	

[a] Cohort studies = total woman-years at risk; case–control studies = cases/controls; [b] Fatal events;; [c] 30–40 microgram pills; # = comparison is never-use (all others are non-use); [d] comparison is never-use; CTA = cerebral thrombotic attack; gen = generation; H = hospital controls; HS = haemorrhagic stroke; IS = ischaemic stroke; MI = myocardial infarction; N = neighbourhood controls; SH = subarachnoid haemorrhage; VTE = venous thromboembolism;

drospirenone, lacks androgenic activity and is sometimes denoted as a 'fourth-generation' pill.[1]

Combined oral contraceptives

Myocardial infarction

The incidence of myocardial infarction among young women of reproductive age is low but rises steeply with age. Estimates of the incidence of first myocardial infarction in Europe and North America range from 0.2 per 100 000 to 0.6 per 100 000 woman-years for those aged 15–19 years and from 9.6 to 33.3 for those aged 40–44 years.[12] The case fatality rate is approximately 30%.[12] A meta-analysis of 23 studies examining COC use and myocardial infarction estimated an overall odds ratio of 2.5 (95% CI 1.9–3.2) for COC users compared with never users.[13] In this meta-analysis, risk dropped with decreasing oestrogen dose: OR 3.6 (95% CI 2.2–5.9) for ≥ 50 µg pills, OR 2.0 (95% CI 1.4–2.7) for 30 µg pills and OR 0.9 (95% CI 0.2–4.1) for 20 µg pills. The effect of COC use on risk of myocardial infarction is restricted to current use. Past use[13–22] and time since last use are not associated with increased risk of myocardial infarction.[13,15,18–20] Duration of use in both current[14,18,20–25] and past[17,20,22,23] users is also not associated with greater risk of myocardial infarction.

Cardiovascular risk factors

Much of the myocardial infarction risk among COC users is due to well-established cardiovascular risk factors, most notably smoking and hypertension. Most studies that have been able to examine COC users without risk factors have found little or no risk of myocardial infarction,[16,21,22,26,27] although one study reported an OR of 3.1 (95% CI 1.0–9.2) associated with COC use among women without hypertension, hypercholesterolaemia, diabetes or smoking.[25]

Smoking is a primary risk factor for myocardial infarction among women of reproductive age, with relative risks comparing smokers with non-smokers ranging from 4.0 to 16.5.[25,28,29] A meta-analysis of COC use and myocardial infarction estimated an OR of 9.52 (95% CI 5.41–16.72) for smokers who used COCs compared with non-smoking, non-COC users, although relative risks of up to 87.0 have been reported.[21] Studies have reported different findings of level of smoking, with some reporting an effect of COC use only among 'heavy' smokers ($\geq 10, \geq 15,$ or ≥ 25 cigarettes per day)[19,22,30,31] and others reporting increased risk at all levels of smoking.[16,21]

Hypertension among non-COC users is associated with a four- to five-fold relative risk of myocardial infarction and several studies have reported higher relative risks of myocardial infarction among COC users with hypertension than in hypertensive non-users.[16,21,24,25,27,32] Investigators from the World Health Organization Collaborative Study of Cardiovascular Disease and Steroid Hormone Contraception reported an OR of 68.1 (95% CI 6.18–751.0) for European COC-users with a history of hypertension compared with normotensive non-users, or a risk 12 times that of hypertensive non-users.[21] Three studies have also reported higher risks of myocardial infarction among women who did not have their blood pressure measured prior to initiating COC use.[21,24,27] A meta-analysis reported a summary OR of 9.30 (95% CI 1.83–53.53) for the combined effect of COC use and hypertension on risk of myocardial infarction.[13]

Overall, risk of myocardial infarction rises with age (more so than for stroke and VTE) but age has not been shown to modify any effect of COC use on risk of myocardial infarction.[19–22,25,33,34] While most studies that have examined other risk factors have been underpowered, some studies have suggested increased risks of myocardial infarction among COC users with diabetes,[25] hypercholesterolaemia[25] and history of hypertension or toxaemia during pregnancy.[16,21]

A remaining question is whether there is a difference in risk of myocardial infarction associated with progestogen type. Newer progestogens have fewer adverse effects on carbohydrate and lipoprotein metabolism than do older progestogens.[35,36] It has been postulated that this could decrease the risk of myocardial infarction associated with use of COCs containing desogestrel and gestodene.[25,37] Two meta-analyses have attempted to resolve this question. The first included eight studies and estimated that users of first- and second-generation COCs had significantly increased risks of myocardial infarction (OR 2.2, 95% CI 1.3–3.8 and OR 2.2, 95% CI 1.8–2.7, for first- and second-generation pills, respectively) but users of third-generation pills did not (OR 1.3, 95% CI 0.96–1.7).[13] The second meta-analysis examined seven studies and estimated an OR of 2.2 (95% CI 1.6–3.0) for second-generation pills and 1.13 (95% CI 0.6–1.9) for third-generation pills, yielding a risk of 0.6 (95% CI 0.4–0.99) for the comparison of third- versus second-generation pills.[38] More careful examination of the individual studies included in the two meta-analyses revealed that none found a significantly increased risk of myocardial infarction with third-generation pills and two found significantly increased risks with second-generation pills. Only two studies had adequate sample sizes to compare progestogen types; one found a non-significant decreased risk (OR 0.5, 95% CI 0.2–1.1)[25] and the other found a non-significant increased risk (1.78, 95% CI 0.66–4.83)[24] for third- versus second-generation pills. Given the inconsistent results and wide confidence intervals, a definitive conclusion cannot be made. However, if there is a difference in myocardial infarction risk between second- and third-generation pills, it is small and the effect on attributable risk most likely negligible.

Ischaemic stroke

The incidence of ischaemic stroke in women of reproductive age is low, albeit somewhat higher than for myocardial infarction. Estimated incidence rates range from 0.6 per 100 000 to 2.8 per 100 000 woman-years for ages 15–19 years, increasing to 1.4–14.1 for women ages 40–44 years.[12] The case fatality rate for ischaemic stroke is about 25%.[12] Two meta-analyses have reported almost identical pooled ORs of 2.7 for the risk of ischaemic stroke with COC use (OR 2.74, 95% CI 2.24–3.35, 12 studies;[39] OR 2.75, 95% CI 2.24–3.38, 16 studies[40]). Two case–control studies that were published after these meta-analyses reported somewhat lower point estimates: OR 2.3 (95% CI 1.6–3.3)[41] and OR 1.76 (95% CI 0.86–3.61).[42]

Past COC use generally has not been associated with ischaemic stroke[31,42–50] but the WHO Collaborative Study reported non-significant increases among women who had stopped using COCs in the past 3 years[47] and past users in the Royal College of General Practitioners study had a significant 2.4-fold risk of fatal stroke.[51] Duration of current COC use,[31,42,47–52] duration of past use[48] and time since last use have not been associated with increased risk.[48,51] Results have conflicted regarding oestrogen dose and ischaemic stroke risk, with some studies reporting no difference[41,47] but other studies and a meta-analysis reporting increased risks with oestrogen doses of 50 μg and above.[40,47,49,50] Most studies have found no difference in stroke risk by progestogen-type.[41,49,53,54] A Danish study, however, found a decreased risk of cerebrothrombo-embolic attack when comparing desogestel- or gestodene-containing pills with levonorgestrel- or norgestimate-containing pills (OR 0.6, 95% CI 0.4–0.9).[50]

Cardiovascular risk factors

Studies that have examined COC users with no other risk factors have not found significant risks of ischaemic stroke with COC use compared with non-use,[47,48,55] with the exception of one study that reported a significantly increased odds ratio among women without other risk factors (OR 3.2, 95% CI 1.5–6.6).[41]

Several studies have examined the risk of ischaemic stroke associated with COC use and hypertension.[41,42,45,47,49,50,56] Odds ratios for ischaemic stroke among COC users with a history of hypertension ranged from 3.1 to 10.7 among populations in the USA and Europe and were somewhat higher in developing countries (14.3–14.5) compared with non-COC users without hypertension. Most of the studies found that hypertensive women who used COCs had between a 1.5- to two-fold risk of ischaemic stroke compared with women with hypertension and no COC use.[41,45,47,50,56] The exceptions were the Royal College of General Practitioners' study, which found no difference in risk between women with hypertension who used COCs and women with hypertension who did not use COCs (both groups had a similar five-fold risk of all stroke combined),[51] and the Transnational study, which reported a higher risk for hypertension alone (OR 9.6, 95% CI 3.25–30.57) than for hypertension and COC use combined (OR 3.07, 95% CI 0.85–11.05).[49] None of these studies reported a statistical interaction between COC use and hypertension. A meta-analysis reported that the overall relative risk of ischaemic stroke in a comparison of COC users and non-users was 1.73 (95% CI 0.83–3.60) among women with hypertension and 2.47 (95% CI 1.80–3.38) among women without hypertension.[40]

Women using COCs who did not have their blood pressure checked before their most recent episode of COC use had about a 1.7- to 2.5-fold risk of ischaemic stroke compared with women who had their blood pressure checked.[47,49]

A meta-analysis of COC use and stroke identified seven studies examining the use of COCs and risk of ischaemic stroke by smoking status.[40] The association between COC use and ischaemic stroke was slightly higher among smokers (RR 3.41, 95% CI 2.51–4.63) than for non-smokers (RR 2.68, 95% CI 2.09–3.43), although not significantly so, suggesting that the effects of smoking and COC use are independent. Of studies that have examined the risk of ischaemic stroke among COC users by level of smoking, two found that increased risk was restricted to COC users who were 'heavy' smokers (≥ 10 or ≥ 15 cigarettes per day)[31,49] but one-third found that risks were similar for light (less than one pack per day) and heavy (more than one pack per day) smokers.[45]

Migraine has been shown to be an independent risk factor for ischaemic stroke, with one meta-analysis reporting an OR of 2.16 (95% CI 1.89–2.48).[57] Migraine with aura has generally been associated with a higher risk of ischaemic stroke than migraine without aura, although confidence intervals generally overlap.[57] Studies have reported that COC users with a history of migraines are two to four times as likely to have an ischaemic stroke as non-COC users with a history of migraine.[45,48,50,56,58–61] No studies have had enough power to examine the risk of stroke by COC use and type of migraine simultaneously. MacGregor et al. estimated that at age 20 years, women with migraine who are also taking COCs have an absolute risk of stroke of ten per 100 000, with eight cases due to migraine and COC use.[62] By age 40 years, the absolute risk rises to 100 per 100 000, with an attributable risk of 80 per 100 000.

Evidence of other cardiovascular risk factors is limited to one study that reported increased risk of ischaemic stroke among COC users with hypercholesterolaemia or obesity.[41]

Haemorrhagic stroke

Information on risks associated with COC use is more limited for haemorrhagic stroke than for ischaemic stroke. Background incidence rates of haemorrhagic stroke range from 0.9 per 100 000 women ages 15–19 years to 10.1 for women ages 40–44 years, with a case fatality rate of about 30%.[12] Most recent studies have found no significantly increased risk of haemorrhagic stroke with COC use.[48,51,63,64] The WHO Collaborative Study found an increased risk among women in developing countries (OR 1.76, 95% CI 1.34–2.30) but not in Europe (OR 1.38, 95% CI 0.84–2.25).[63] This difference may have reflected higher prevalence of other cardiovascular risk factors in the developing countries than in Europe.[63] A meta-analysis estimated the odds ratio of haemorrhagic stroke among COC users to be 1.3 (95% CI 0.99–1.71).[39] The WHO Collaborative Study found no effect of past COC use, oestrogen dose, or progestogen type on risk of haemorrhagic stroke.

Cardiovascular risk factors

The two main sources of information on the interaction between COC use and other risk factors for haemorrhagic stroke are the WHO Collaborative Study and a pooled analysis of two case–control studies from the USA. The WHO study found no increased risk among COC-users less than 35 years old, but a doubling of risk for those 35 years and older; this elevated risk was significant only for developing countries.[63] The WHO study also found odds ratios of 3–4 among COC users who smoked and 10–14 among COC users with a history of hypertension.[63] Risks for haemorrhagic stroke did not differ between COC users with and without a blood pressure check or with different doses or types of progestogens. A pooled analysis of two case–control studies in the USA found no overall risk of haemorrhagic stroke with COC use and no increased risk with COC use among women 35 years and older or among women who smoked, although the number of women who used COCs and had one of these risk factors was small and confidence intervals were wide.[48] This study also found no association with past use, duration of current or past use, and time since last use.

Venous thromboembolism

The incidence of VTE among women of reproductive age, while low, is higher than that of myocardial infarction or stroke. Incidence rates range from 7.1 per 100 000 to 10.9 per 100 000 woman-years for ages 15–19 years to 6.2 to 34.9 among women ages 40–44 years.[12] However, mortality from VTE is much lower than for myocardial infarction and stroke, with case fatality rates of about 2%.[12] COC users have approximately three to six times the risk of VTE as that of non-users and, unlike myocardial infarction and stroke, young women who use COCs are at increased risk of VTE even if they have no other cardiovascular risk factors.[65–67] Increased risk of VTE with COC use persisted in two studies that tried to eliminate diagnostic bias by restricting the study population to women who had been clinically tested for deep vein thrombosis.[68,69] Risk has been shown to be highest in the first year of COC use, although some amount of risk remains with any current use.[9,10,70,71]

Thrombogenic mutations

A primary risk factor for VTE is genetic susceptibility to prothrombotic states. The Leiden Thrombophilia Study (LETS) in the Netherlands was the first to observe that factor V Leiden mutation increases the risk of VTE among women of reproductive age (OR 7.9, 95% CI 3.2–19.4).[72] Compared with non-users who did not have the mutation, COC users with the mutation had more than 30 times the risk of VTE (OR 34.7, 95% CI 7.8–154) and they had four times the risk when compared with non-users with factor V. The authors estimated the background incidence of VTE in the Netherlands to be 0.8 per 10 000 person-years for women aged 15–49 years. The incidence increased to 3.0 among COC users without the mutation, 5.7 among non-COC users with the mutation and 28.5 among COC users with the mutation. Subsequent studies[71,73–79] have shown that COC users with factor V have 2–20 times the risk of non-users with the mutation but confidence intervals have been wide because of the small number of controls with the mutation. Studies of prothrombin and other thrombogenic mutations, such as protein S, protein C and antithrombin deficiency have also found increased risk of VTE among COC users with those mutations but the magnitude is not as great as for factor V.[71,73–76,78–81] While relative risks are high, the prevalence of these mutations is low (about 5% of the white population and less than 2.5% of other ethnicities)[82] and screening for thrombophilias prior to COC initiation has been shown to be not cost effective.[82,83]

COC formulation and VTE

Much of the recent work on COC use and risk of VTE has focused on progestogen type. While the controversy continues in the literature, two meta-analyses have estimated that COCs containing gestodene or desogestrel increase the risk of VTE by about 70% compared with those containing levonorgestrel or norethisterone (OR 1.7, 95% CI 1.3–2.1 for 12 studies[84] and OR 1.7, 95% CI 1.4–2.0 for 7 studies[85]). Meta-analysis is dependent upon the quality of the individual studies included in the analysis and cannot, of itself, account for the biases of independent studies. Both sets of authors, however, methodically examined the potential for bias and concluded that the increase in risk could not be explained completely by bias. If there is a difference in risk between progestogen type, the difference is small and would translate to approximately one to two excess cases per 10 000 woman-years.[12,84,85] Evidence for other new progestogens, including norgestimate, drospirenone[86] and cyproterone acetate[87] is limited. A meta-analysis of six studies concluded that the risk of VTE with cyproterone acetate combined with ethinyl oestradiol was similar to that of other COCs.[87]

Other risk factors

Several studies have shown increased risk of VTE among COC users with an elevated body mass index (generally ≥ 25 or ≥ 30 kg/m²),[70,71,88,89] with one study reporting an interaction between COC use and obesity.[71] In the only study to examine prolonged immobilisation and COC use, there was a four-fold risk of VTE among COC users regardless of immobilisation status. Immobilisation itself, however, conferred an almost six-fold risk of VTE (OR 5.93, 95% CI 4.18–8.41).[71] A study of air travel found a 23.4-fold (95% CI 2.6–211.2) risk of VTE for COC users who travelled by air in the month preceding occurrence of VTE compared with non-users with no air travel.[90]

Other cardiovascular outcomes

While not well-studied, COC use has also been associated with an increased risk of peripheral arterial disease[91] and cerebral vein and cerebral sinus thrombosis.[92,93]

Clinical risk markers for cardiovascular disease

Drawing conclusions from clinical surrogates for the development of cardiovascular disease can be problematic, as the interrelationships among these risk markers and their link with the risk of cardiovascular events are not always clear.[94] However, studies of these markers may help to elucidate possible mechanisms for the observed associations between COC use and cardiovascular disease. A thorough discussion of the effects of COCs on clinical risk markers for cardiovascular disease is beyond the scope of this paper. In general, changes in clinical risk markers, such as blood pressure,[95–97] lipid profiles,[94] haemostasis[98] and carbohydrate metabolism[94] are small, within the normal range, and reversible upon discontinuation of COC use. Effects of COCs on lipid metabolism are dependent upon the dose of oestrogen and the dose and type of progestogen. In general, oestrogens tend to increase levels of high-density lipoprotein (HDL), while progestogens may counteract this effect by increasing levels of low-density lipoprotein (LDL).[94] Overall, COCs containing gestodene or desogestrel are associated with higher HDL levels than those containing levonorgestrel, theoretically conferring less risk of cardiovascular disease.[94] Several, more recently discovered, clinical risk markers are also beginning to be studied. For example, C-reactive protein is a marker of increased inflammatory response and high levels of C-reactive protein have been associated with increased risk of coronary heart disease.[99] Three cross-sectional studies have reported increased concentrations of C-reactive protein among COC users compared with non-users.[100-102] One of these studies found no difference between second and third generation pills,[101] while another found statistically higher levels of C-reactive protein among third generation compared with second generation pills users.[102]

Total cardiovascular morbidity and mortality attributable to combined oral contraceptives

Overall, rates of cardiovascular morbidity and mortality among women of reproductive age are low. Therefore, it is important to examine the absolute risks of cardiovascular events among COC users, and the number of events attributable to COC use, under the assumption that the observed associations between COC use and cardiovascular disease are causal.[103] In 1998, WHO estimated the risk of cardiovascular events attributable to COC use and other risk factors, based on background incidence of events from nationally reported statistics from several countries and from published studies on cardiovascular risks of hormonal contraception (Table 13.2).[12] In the WHO model, incidence of cardiovascular events among non-smoking, non-COC users ranged from 51 per million woman-years for women ages 20–24 years to 143 for women ages 40–44 years. Corresponding cardiovascular mortality rates were 6 and 25

Table 13.2. Estimated incidence of cardiovascular events per 1 000 000 woman-years[a]

	Ages 20–24 years					Ages 40–44 years				
	MI	IS	HS	VTE	Total	MI	IS	HS	VTE	Total
Non-COC users, non-smokers	0.14	6.0	12.7	32.2	51.1	21.3	16.0	46.3	59.3	143.0
COC users, non-smokers	0.34	15.1	12.7	96.7	125.0	53.2	40.1	92.6	178.0	364.0
COC users with blood pressure check, non-smokers	0.20	9.0	12.7	96.7	119.0	31.9	24.1	92.6	178.0	326.0
Smokers, non-COC users	1.1	12.1	25.5	32.2	70.8	170.0	32.1	139.0	59.3	401.0
Smokers, COC users	2.7	30.2	38.2	96.7	168.0	426.0	80.2	232.0	178.0	915.0
Hypertension, non-COC users	0.81	24.1	76.4	32.2	134.0	128.0	64.2	278.0	59.3	529.0
Hypertension, COC users	2.0	60.3	153.0	96.7	312.0	319.0	160.0	556.0	178.0	1213.0
COC use (norgestrel, levonorgestrel, norethisterone or lynestrenol), non-smoker	0.34	15.1	12.7	96.7	125.0	53.2	40.1	92.6	178.0	364.0
COC use (desogestrel or gestodene), non-smoker	0.14	15.1	12.7	193.0	221.0	21.3	40.1	92.6	356.0	510.0
Pregnant women				600.0 –800.0[b]						

[a] Adapted from Farley et al.[12]; [b] All ages[13b]; HS = haemorrhagic stroke; IS = ischaemic stroke; MI = myocardial infarction; VTE = venous thromboembolism

per million woman-years for women ages 20–24 years and 40–44 years, respectively. COC use among women who had their blood pressure checked led to an additional 68 cases, including two deaths caused by cardiovascular disease among women ages 20–24 years and 183 cases, including 21 deaths, among women ages 40–44 years. By comparison, smoking by itself led to an excess of 20 cases, including six deaths, among women aged 20–24 years and 258 cases, including 76 deaths, among women ages 40–44 years. Among smokers, COC users experienced 97 excess cases, including ten excess deaths, for ages 20–24 years and 514 excess cases, including 119 deaths, for ages 40–44 years. For overall cardiovascular morbidity and mortality, hypertension and COC use may be a worse combination. Among women with hypertension, COC use added 178 cases, including 54 deaths, for ages 20–24 years and 684 cases, including 249 deaths, for ages 40–44 years. Use of third-generation pills led to 96 excess cases, including two deaths, compared with second-generation pills among women aged 20–24 years; among women aged 40–44 years, third-generation pills led to an excess of 146 cases but six fewer deaths compared with second-generation pills.

Other combined hormonal contraceptives

Evidence on cardiovascular safety of combined hormonal contraceptives other than COCs is quite limited. Other combined methods include combined injectables (two formulations: 25 mg medroxyprogesterone acetate and 5 mg oestradiol cypionate; 50 mg norethisterone enantate and 5mg oestradiol valerate), the combined hormonal patch (20 μg ethinyl oestradiol and 150 μg norelgestromin) and the combined vaginal ring (15 μg ethinyl oestradiol and 120 μg etonogestrel). Clinical studies have suggested that combined injectables may have less impact on blood pressure, haemostasis and coagulation, lipid metabolism and liver function than COCs.[21,104–108] Limited evidence on the combined patch and ring suggests a pharmacokinetic and safety profile similar to that of COCs.[109–111] The WHO Collaborative Study found no suggestion of an increased risk of cardiovascular disease, except for a non-significant increased risk of VTE, among women using combined injectables.[112] WHO has concluded that, until more method specific information is available, evidence regarding medical eligibility criteria for COCs also applies to the patch and the ring but may allow for less restrictive eligibility criteria for combined injectables.[113]

Progestogen-only contraception

Epidemiological evidence regarding the cardiovascular safety of progestogen-only methods of contraception is limited. Studies of metabolic indices during use of progestogen-only contraception have not found clinically meaningful changes. Progestogen-only pills have negligible effects on lipid metabolism, carbohydrate metabolism (even among women with diabetes), coagulation factors and blood pressure.[114,115] Studies of progestogen-only implants have shown no clinically important changes in blood pressure, glucose tolerance, lipids and lipoproteins or clotting factors.[116] Among depot medroxyprogesterone acetate (DMPA) users, some studies have reported increases in low-density lipoproteins and decreases in high-density lipoproteins but the clinical implications of these changes are unknown.[117] An intriguing study published in 2002 found that arterial endothelium function was impaired in long-term (mean 52 months) DMPA users.[118] How this finding might relate to risk of cardiovascular events is unclear.

In epidemiological studies, progestogen-only pill use has not been associated with myocardial infarction,[18,112,119] stroke[60,112,119] or VTE,[112,119] although a small non-significant increased risk for VTE was observed in one study (OR 1.82, 95% CI 0.79–4.22).[112] The same study also suggested that progestogen-only pills may increase the risk of stroke among women with hypertension but the numbers were small and confidence intervals overlapped (OR 10.0, 95% CI 3.55–33.8 for progestogen-only pill users with hypertension compared with OR 7.21, 95% CI 6.10–8.52 for non-users with hypertension).[112] Two studies found an increased risk of VTE, but not myocardial infarction or stroke, among women using oral progestogens for therapeutic indications (OR 5.92, 95% CI 1.16–30.1 and OR 5.3, 95% CI 1.5–18.7, respectively).[53,54] Whether this increased risk is due to the higher doses of progestogen used for therapeutic indications or the indications themselves was unclear.

Among progestogen-only injectable users, the WHO Collaborative Study found no significantly increased risks for myocardial infarction, stroke or VTE, although the point estimate for VTE was elevated (OR 2.19, 95% CI 0.66–7.26).[112]

Cardiovascular events have rarely been reported among levonorgestrel implants (Norplant®, Hoechst Marion Roussel, now discontinued in the UK) users.[120–122] In the largest comparative study, which followed Norplant users, intrauterine contraceptive device users and women with female sterilisation for 5 years, one haemorrhagic stroke and one ischaemic stroke were identified, both among Norplant users, for an incidence rate of 0.05 per 1000 woman-years for all stroke combined.[123] No myocardial infarctions were reported. One case of deep-vein thrombosis was identified, also in a Norplant user, for an incidence rate of 0.03 per 1000 women years. No studies examining risk of cardiovascular events among users of the levonorgestrel-releasing intrauterine system were identified.

Guidelines

Several evidence-based guidelines exist regarding use of hormonal contraception among women with cardiovascular risk factors, including WHO's Medical Eligibility Criteria,[113] the UK Faculty of Family Planning and Reproductive Health Care (FFPRHC) guidance[124] and guidance from the American College of Obstetricians and Gynecologists.[1,125] Table 13.3 summarises these guidelines for the use of COCs among women with cardiovascular risk factors. Recommendations for use of the combined hormonal patch, combined vaginal ring and combined injectables generally follow those for COCs.[113] However, recommendations for progestogen-only contraceptive methods among women with cardiovascular risk factors are less restrictive than for combined methods and most women with cardiovascular risk factors can safely use progestogen-only contraception, with the exception of women who have already experienced a cardiovascular event.[113,124,125]

Conclusions

Overall, the incidence of cardiovascular disease among women of reproductive age is low and mortality is rare but risk increases with cardiovascular risk factors such as age, smoking, hypertension and adverse lipid levels. Total cardiovascular morbidity and mortality attributable to hormonal contraceptives are low. Risks of stroke and myocardial infarction among COC users are low; these risks may be essentially nonexistent for COC users with no risk factors for cardiovascular disease. COC users have three to six times the risk of VTE as non-users, even among women without cardiovascular risk factors.

Table 13.3. Guidelines for combined oral contraceptive use among women with cardiovascular risk factors

Risk factor:	WHO[113]	UKFFPRHC[124 a]	ACOG[125]
Age:			
Menarche to < 40 years	1	1	
≥ 40 years	2	2	Safe for healthy, non-smoking women older than 35 years
Smoking:			
Age < 35 years	2	2	Age < 30 years: generally can use COCs
Age ≥ 35 years, <15 cigarettes/ day	3	3	Prescribed with caution, if ever
Age ≥ 35 years, ≥15 cigarettes/ day	4	4	Prescribed with caution, if ever
Obesity (≥ 30 kg/m² body mass index)	2	2	Not addressed
Hypertension:			
Adequately controlled hypertension	3	3	Well-controlled and monitored hypertension, age < 35 years: trial of COC appropriate
Systolic 140–159 mmHg or diastolic 90–99 mmHg	3	3[b]	
Systolic ≥ 160 or diastolic ≥100	4	4[b]	
Vascular disease	4	4	
History of high blood pressure in pregnancy, where current blood pressure is normal	2	2	Not addressed
History or current DVT/PE	4	4	Should not use COCs, unless they are currently taking anticoagulants
Family history of DVT/PE	2	2	Not addressed
Major surgery:			
With prolonged immobilisation	4	4	Risks of stopping COCs should be weighed against risks of unintended pregnancy
Without prolonged immobilisation	2	2	Screening may be appropriate in selective circumstances
Known thrombogenic mutations	4	4	Contraindicated.
History of ischaemic heart disease or stroke	4	4	Controlled dyslipidaemia: can use COCs.
Known hyperlipidaemias	2/3†	2/3†	Uncontrolled LDL cholesterol or multiple additional risk factors for coronary heart disease: alternative contraceptives should be considered.
Major surgery:			
With prolonged immobilisation	4	4	Risks of stopping COCs should be weighed against risks of unintended pregnancy
Without prolonged immobilisation	2	2	

Table 13.3. Guidelines for combined oral contraceptive use among women with cardiovascular risk factors continued

Risk factor:	WHO[113]	UKFFPRHC[124 a]	ACOG[125]
Known thrombogenic mutations	4	4	Screening may be appropriate in selective circumstances
History of ischaemic heart disease or stroke	4	4	Contraindicated.
Known hyperlipidaemias	2/3[c]	2/3[c]	Controlled dyslipidaemia: can use COCs. Uncontrolled LDL cholesterol or multiple additional risk factors for coronary heart disease: alternative contraceptives should be considered.
Headaches:			
No migraine	1	1	COCs may be considered
Migraine, without aura, age < 35 years	2	2	Use not appropriate
Migraine, without aura, age ≥ 35 years	3	3	
Migraine, with aura, any age	4	4	
Diabetes:			
Non-vascular disease	2	2	COC use limited to non-smoking, otherwise health women with diabetes , 35 years, no evidence of hypertension, neuropathy, retinopathy, or other vascular disease
Nephropathy/retinopathy/neuropathy, other vascular disease, or diabetes of > 20 years' duration	3/4[c]	3/4[c]	
Multiple cardiovascular risk factors	3/4[c]	3/4[c]	Not addressed.
Progestogen type	Guidelines pertain to COCs containing ≥ 35µg ethinyl oestradiol; progestogen type is not addressed	A monophasic COC containing 30–35 µg ethinyl oestradiol with a low dose of either norethisterone or levonorgestrel is a suitable first-line option	Guidelines pertain to <50 µg ethinyl oestradiol with the lowest progestogen dose; progestogen type is not addressed

1: A condition for which there is no restriction for the use of the contraceptive method.
2: A condition where the advantages of using the method generally outweigh the theoretical or proven risks.
3: A condition where the theoretical or proven risks usually outweigh the advantages of using the method.
4: A condition which represents an unacceptable health risk for the contraceptive method is used.
a The guidance of the UKFFPRHC generally follows that of WHO, with the exception of progestogen type and a clarification for hypertension.
b UK guidance advises consistently measured blood pressure over these thresholds.
c The classification depends on the type and severity of the condition and the presence of other cardiovascular risk factors.
Abbreviations: ACOG = American College of Obstetricians and Gynecologists; DVT/PE = deep vein thrombosis/pulmonary embolism; UKFFPRHC = United Kingdom Faculty of Family Planning and Reproductive Health Care; WHO = World Health Organization

Pills containing desogestrel and gestodene may confer a slightly greater risk of VTE than pills containing levonorgestrel. If so, the absolute risk is likely to be small. Data are inconclusive regarding risk of myocardial infarction, and limited data do not show any difference by progestogen type for risk of stroke.

Among women with some cardiovascular risk factors, use of COCs may further increase risk of cardiovascular events.

Evidence is limited regarding the cardiovascular safety of other combined hormonal methods. It is expected that combined hormonal patches and combined hormonal rings will have the same cardiovascular profile as COCs. Combined injectable contraceptives may confer slightly less cardiovascular risk, given studies that show less adverse effect on metabolic parameters than with COCs. Evidence is also limited regarding use of progestogen-only contraceptives and cardiovascular safety. Limited epidemiological evidence does not suggest increases in risk, except possibly in women with other cardiovascular risk factors.

References

1. Petitti DB. Combination estrogen–progestin oral contraceptives. *N Engl J Med* 2003;349:1443–50 [erratum in *N Engl J Med* 2004;350:92].
2. Jordan WM. Pulmonary embolism. *Lancet* 1961;ii:1146–7.
3. Hannaford P. Cardiovascular events associated with different combined oral contraceptives: a review of current data. *Drug Saf* 2000;22:361–71.
4. Boyce J, Fawcett JW, Noall EW. Coronary thrombosis and Conovide. *Lancet* 1963;i:111.
5. United Nations. World Contraceptive Use, 2003. New York: United Nations [www.un.org/esa/population/publications/contraceptive2003/WallChart_CP2003. pdf]
6. Wallach M, Grimes DA, editors. *Modern Oral Contraception*. Totowa, NJ: Emron; 2000.
7. Oral contraceptives and cardiovascular risk. *Drug Ther Bull* 2000;38:1–5.
8. World Health Organization Collaborative Study of Cardiovascular Disease and Steroid Hormone Contraception. Effect of different progestagens in low oestrogen oral contraceptives on venous thromboembolic disease. *Lancet* 1995;346:1582–8.
9. Jick H, Jick SS, Gurewich V, Myers MW, Vasilakis C. Risk of idiopathic cardiovascular death and nonfatal venous thromboembolism in women using oral contraceptives with differing progestagen components. *Lancet* 1995;346:1589–93.
10. Spitzer WO, Lewis MA, Heinemann LA, Thorogood M, MacRae KD. Third generation oral contraceptives and risk of venous thromboembolic disorders: an international case-control study. Transnational Research Group on Oral Contraceptives and the Health of Young Women. *BMJ* 1996;312:83–8.
11. Furedi A. The public health implications of the 1995 'pill scare'. *Hum Reprod Update* 1999;5:621–6.
12. Farley TM, Collins J, Schlesselman JJ. Hormonal contraception and risk of cardiovascular disease. An international perspective. *Contraception* 1998;57:211–30.
13. Khader YS, Rice J, John L, Abueita O. Oral contraceptives use and the risk of myocardial infarction: a meta-analysis. *Contraception* 2003;68:11–17.
14. Rosenberg L, Hennekens CH, Rosner B, Belanger C, Rothman KJ, Speizer FE. Oral contraceptive use in relation to nonfatal myocardial infarction. *Am J Epidemiol* 1980;111:59–66.
15. Stampfer MJ, Willett WC, Colditz GA, Speizer FE, Hennekens CH. Past use of oral contraceptives and cardiovascular disease: a meta-analysis in the context of the Nurses' Health Study. *Am J Obstet Gynecol* 1990;163:285–91.
16. Croft P, Hannaford PC. Risk factors for acute myocardial infarction in women: evidence from the Royal College of General Practitioners' oral contraception study. *BMJ* 1989;298:165–8.
17. Rosenberg L, Palmer JR, Lesko SM, Shapiro S. Oral contraceptive use and the risk of myocardial infarction. *Am J Epidemiol* 1990;131:1009–16.
18. Thorogood M, Mann J, Murphy M, Vessey M. Is oral contraceptive use still associated with an increased risk of fatal myocardial infarction? Report of a case–control study. *Br J Obstet Gynaecol* 1991;98:1245–53.
19. Petitti DB, Sidney S, Quesenberry CP. Oral contraceptive use and myocardial infarction. *Contraception* 1998;57:143–55.
20. Sidney S, Siscovick DS, Petitti DB, Schwartz SM, Quesenberry CP, Psaty BM, *et al.* Myocardial

infarction and use of low-dose oral contraceptives: a pooled analysis of 2 US studies. *Circulation* 1998;98:1058–63.

21. World Health Organization Collaborative Study of Cardiovascular Disease and Steroid Hormone Contraception. Acute myocardial infarction and combined oral contraceptives: results of an international multicentre case–control study. *Lancet* 1997;349:1202–9.

22. Rosenberg L, Palmer JR, Rao RS, Shapiro S. Low-dose oral contraceptive use and the risk of myocardial infarction. *Arch Intern Med* 2001;161:1065–70.

23. Stampfer MJ, Willett WC, Colditz GA, Speizer FE, Hennekens CH. A prospective study of past use of oral contraceptive agents and risk of cardiovascular diseases. *N Engl J Med* 1988;319:1313–17.

24. Dunn N, Thorogood M, Faragher B, de Caestecker L, MacDonald TM, McCollum C, *et al.* Oral contraceptives and myocardial infarction: results of the MICA case–control study. *BMJ* 1999;318:1579–83.

25. Tanis BC, van den Bosch MA, Kemmeren JM, Cats VM, Helmerhorst FM, Algra A, *et al.* Oral contraceptives and the risk of myocardial infarction. *N Engl J Med* 2001;345:1787–93.

26. Sidney S, Petitti DB, Quesenberry CP, Jr., Klatsky AL, Ziel HK, Wolf S. Myocardial infarction in users of low-dose oral contraceptives. *Obstet Gynecol* 1996;88:939–44.

27. Lewis MA, Heinemann LA, Spitzer WO, MacRae KD, Bruppacher R. The use of oral contraceptives and the occurrence of acute myocardial infarction in young women. Results from the Transnational Study on Oral Contraceptives and the Health of Young Women. *Contraception* 1997;56:129–40.

28. La Vecchia C, Franceschi S, Decarli A, Pampallona S, Tognoni G. Risk factors for myocardial infarction in young women. *Am J Epidemiol* 1987;125:832–43.

29. Dunn NR, Faragher B, Thorogood M, de Caestecker L, MacDonald TM, McCollum C, *et al.* Risk of myocardial infarction in young female smokers. *Heart* 1999;82:581–3.

30. Rosenberg L, Kaufman DW, Helmrich SP, Miller DR, Stolley PD, Shapiro S. Myocardial infarction and cigarette smoking in women younger than 50 years of age. *JAMA* 1985;253:2965–9.

31. Mant J, Painter R, Vessey M. Risk of myocardial infarction, angina and stroke in users of oral contraceptives: an updated analysis of a cohort study. *Br J Obstet Gynaecol* 1998;105:890–6.

32. D'Avanzo B, La Vecchia C, Negri E, Parazzini F, Franceschi S. Oral contraceptive use and risk of myocardial infarction: an Italian case-control study. *J Epidemiol Community Health* 1994;48:324–5.

33. Mann JI, Doll R, Thorogood M, Vessey MP, Waters WE. Risk factors for myocardial infarction in young women. *Br J Prev Soc Med* 1976;30:94–100.

34. Krueger DE, Ellenberg SS, Bloom S, Calkins BM, Maliza C, Nolan DC, *et al.* Fatal myocardial infarction and the role of oral contraceptives. *Am J Epidemiol* 1980;111:655–74.

35. Speroff L, DeCherney A. Evaluation of a new generation of oral contraceptives. The Advisory Board for the New Progestins. *Obstet Gynecol* 1993;81:1034–47.

36. Fotherby K, Caldwell AD. New progestogens in oral contraception. *Contraception* 1994;49:1–32.

37. Chasan-Taber L, Stampfer MJ. Epidemiology of oral contraceptives and cardiovascular disease. *Ann Intern Med* 1998;128:467–77.

38. Spitzer WO, Faith JM, MacRae KD. Myocardial infarction and third generation oral contraceptives: aggregation of recent studies. *Hum Reprod* 2002;17:2307–14.

39. Chan WS, Ray J, Wai EK, Ginsburg S, Hannah ME, Corey PN, *et al.* Risk of stroke in women exposed to low-dose oral contraceptives: a critical evaluation of the evidence. *Arch Intern Med* 2004;164:741–7.

40. Gillum LA, Mamidipudi SK, Johnston SC. Ischemic stroke risk with oral contraceptives: A meta-analysis. *JAMA* 2000;284:72–8.

41. Kemmeren JM, Tanis BC, van den Bosch MA, Bollen EL, Helmerhorst FM, van der Graff, *et al.* Risk of Arterial Thrombosis in Relation to Oral Contraceptives (RATIO) study: oral contraceptives and the risk of ischemic stroke. *Stroke* 2002;33:1202–8.

42. Siritho S, Thrift AG, McNeil JJ, You RX, Davis SM, Donnan GA *et al.* Risk of ischemic stroke among users of the oral contraceptive pill: The Melbourne Risk Factor Study (MERFS) Group. *Stroke* 2003;34:1575–80.

43. Inman WH, Vessey MP. Investigation of deaths from pulmonary, coronary, and cerebral thrombosis and embolism in women of child-bearing age. *BMJ* 1968;2:193–9.

44. Sartwell PE, Stolley PD, Tonascia JA, Tockman MS, Rutledge AH, Wertheimer D. Pulmonary embolism mortality in relation to oral contraceptive use. *Prev Med* 1976;5:15–9.

45. Collaborative Group for the Study of Stroke in Young Women. Oral contraceptives and stroke in young women: associated risk factors. *JAMA* 1975;231:718–22.

46. Jick H, Dinan B, Rothman KJ. Oral contraceptives and nonfatal myocardial infarction. *JAMA* 1978;239:1403–6.

47. WHO Collaborative Study of Cardiovascular Disease and Steroid Hormone Contraception.

Ischaemic stroke and combined oral contraceptives: results of an international, multicentre, case-control study. *Lancet* 1996;348:498–505.

48. Schwartz SM, Petitti DB, Siscovick DS, Longstreth WT, Jr., Sidney S, Raghunathan TE *et al.* Stroke and use of low-dose oral contraceptives in young women: a pooled analysis of two US studies. *Stroke* 1998;29:2277–84.

49. Heinemann LA, Lewis MA, Spitzer WO, Thorogood M, Guggenmoos-Holzmann I, Bruppacher R. Thromboembolic stroke in young women. A European case–control study on oral contraceptives. Transnational Research Group on Oral Contraceptives and the Health of Young Women. *Contraception* 1998;57:29–37.

50. Lidegaard O, Kreiner S. Contraceptives and cerebral thrombosis: a five-year national case-control study. *Contraception* 2002;65:197–205.

51. Hannaford PC, Croft PR, Kay CR. Oral contraception and stroke. Evidence from the Royal College of General Practitioners' Oral Contraception Study. *Stroke* 1994;25:935–42.

52. Lidegaard O. Thrombotic diseases in young women and the influence of oral contraceptives. *Am J Obstet Gynecol* 1998;179:S62–S67.

53. Poulter NR, Chang CL, Farley TM, Marmot MG, Meirik O. Effect on stroke of different progestagens in low oestrogen dose oral contraceptives. WHO Collaborative Study of Cardiovascular Disease and Steroid Hormone Contraception. *Lancet* 1999;354:301–2.

54. Vasilakis C, Jick SS, Jick H. The risk of venous thromboembolism in users of postcoital contraceptive pills. *Contraception* 1999;59:79–83.

55. Heinemann LA, Heinemann LA. Is the stroke risk in OC users higher in Europe than in North America? *Contraception* 1999;60:253–4.

56. Lidegaard O. Oral contraceptives, pregnancy and the risk of cerebral thromboembolism: the influence of diabetes, hypertension, migraine and previous thrombotic disease. *Br J Obstet Gynaecol* 1995;102:153–9.

57. Etminan M, Takkouche B, Isorna FC, Samii A. Risk of ischaemic stroke in people with migraine: systematic review and meta-analysis of observational studies. *BMJ* 2005;330:63–6.

58. Tzourio C, Tehindrazanarivelo A, Iglesias S, Alperovitch A, Chedru F, d'Anglejan-Chatillon J, *et al.* Case-control study of migraine and risk of ischaemic stroke in young women. *BMJ* 1995;310:830–3.

59. Chang CL, Donaghy M, Poulter N. Migraine and stroke in young women: case-control study. The World Health Organisation Collaborative Study of Cardiovascular Disease and Steroid Hormone Contraception. *BMJ* 1999;318:13–18.

60. Lidegaard O. Oral contraception and risk of a cerebral thromboembolic attack: results of a case-control study. *BMJ* 1993;306:956–63.

61. Lidegaard O. Oral contraceptives, pregnancy, and the risk of cerebral thromboembolism: the influence of diabetes, hypertension, migraine and previous thrombotic disease. *Br J Obstet Gynaecol* 1995;102:153–59.

62. MacGregor EA, Guillebaud J. Combined oral contraceptives, migraine and ischaemic stroke. Clinical and Scientific Committee of the Faculty of Family Planning and Reproductive Health Care and the Family Planning Association. *Br J Fam Plann* 1998;24:55–60.

63. WHO Collaborative Study of Cardiovascular Disease and Steroid Hormone Contraception. Haemorrhagic stroke, overall stroke risk, and combined oral contraceptives: results of an international, multicentre, case–control study. *Lancet* 1996;348:505–10.

64. Thorogood M, Mann J, Murphy M, Vessey M. Fatal stroke and use of oral contraceptives: findings from a case-control study. *Am J Epidemiol* 1992;136:35–45.

65. WHO Collaborative Study of Cardiovascular Disease and Steroid Hormone Contraception. Cardiovascular disease and use of oral contraceptives. WHO Collaborative Study. *Bull World Health Organ* 1989;67:417–23.

66. Jick H, Kaye JA, Vasilakis-Scaramozza C, Jick SS. Risk of venous thromboembolism among users of third generation oral contraceptives compared with users of oral contraceptives with levonorgestrel before and after 2000: 1995 cohort and case–control analysis. *BMJ* 321:1190–5.

67. Lewis MA, Spitzer WO, Heinemann LA, MacRae KD, Bruppacher R, Thorogood M. Third generation oral contraceptives and risk of myocardial infarction: an international case-control study. Transnational Research Group on Oral Contraceptives and the Health of Young Women. *BMJ* 1996;312:88–90.

68. Realini JP, Encarnacion CE, Chintapalli KN, Rees CR. Oral contraceptives and venous thromboembolism: a case-control study designed to minimize detection bias. *J Am Board Fam Pract* 1997;10:315–21.

69. Bloemenkamp KW, Rosendaal FR, Buller HR, Helmerhorst FM, Colly LP, Vandenbroucke JP. Risk of venous thrombosis with use of current low-dose oral contraceptives is not explained by

diagnostic suspicion and referral bias. *Arch Intern Med* 1999;159:65–70.

70. Lidegaard O,Edstrom B, Kreiner S. Oral contraceptives and venous thromboembolism: a five-year national case-control study. *Contraception* 2002;65:187–96.

71. Sidney S, Petitti DB, Soff GA, Cundiff DL, Tolan KK, Quesenberry CP, Jr. Venous thromboembolic disease in users of low-estrogen combined estrogen-progestin oral contraceptives. *Contraception* 2004;70:3–10.

72. Vandenbroucke JP, Koster T, Briet E, Reitsma PH, Bertina RM, Rosendaal FR. Increased risk of venous thrombosis in oral-contraceptive users who are carriers of factor V Leiden mutation. *Lancet* 1994;344:1453–7.

73. Andersen BS, Olsen J. Oral contraception and factor V Leiden mutation in relation to localization of deep vein thrombosis. *Thromb Res* 1998;90:191–4.

74. Legnani C, Palareti G, Guazzaloca G, Cosmi B, Lunghi B, Bernardi F *et al*. Venous thromboembolism in young women; role of thrombophilic mutations and oral contraceptive use. *Eur Heart J* 2002;23:984–90.

75. Martinelli I, Taioli E, Bucciarelli P, Akhavan S, Mannucci PM. Interaction between the G20210A mutation of the prothrombin gene and oral contraceptive use in deep vein thrombosis. *Arterioscler Thromb* 1999;19:700–3.

76. Santamaria A, Mateo J, Oliver A, Menendez B, Souto JC, Borrell M, *et al*. Risk of thrombosis associated with oral contraceptives of women from 97 families with inherited thrombophilia: high risk of thrombosis in carriers of the G20210A mutation of the prothrombin gene. *Haematologica* 2001;86:965–71.

77. Spannagl M, Heinemann LA, Schramm W. Are factor V Leiden carriers who use oral contraceptives at extreme risk for venous thromboembolism? *Eur J Contracept Reprod Health Care* 2000;5:105–12.

78. Martinelli I, Battaglioli T, Bucciarelli P, Passamonti SM, Mannucci PM. Risk factors and recurrence rate of primary deep vein thrombosis of the upper extremities. *Circulation* 2004;110:566–70.

79. Emmerich J, Rosendaal FR, Cattaneo M, Margaglione M, De S, V, Cumming T, *et al*. Combined effect of factor V Leiden and prothrombin 20210A on the risk of venous thromboembolism–pooled analysis of 8 case-control studies including 2310 cases and 3204 controls. Study Group for Pooled-Analysis in Venous Thromboembolism. *Thromb Haemost* 2001;86:809–16 [erratum *Thromb Haemost* 2001;86:1598].

80. Vaya A, Mira Y, Mateo J, Falco C, Villa P, Estelles A, *et al*. Prothrombin G20210A mutation and oral contraceptive use increase upper-extremity deep vein thrombotic risk. *Thromb Haemost* 2003;89:452–7.

81. Bloemenkamp KW, Rosendaal FR, Helmerhorst FM, Vandenbroucke JP. Higher risk of venous thrombosis during early use of oral contraceptives in women with inherited clotting defects. *Arch Intern Med* 2000;160:49–52.

82. Creinin MD, Lisman R, Strickler RC. Screening for factor V Leiden mutation before prescribing combination oral contraceptives. *Fertil Steril* 1999;72:646–51.

83. Vandenbroucke JP, van der Meer FJ, Helmerhorst FM, Rosendaal FR. Factor V Leiden: should we screen oral contraceptive users and pregnant women? *BMJ* 1996;313:1127–30.

84. Hennessy S, Berlin JA, Kinman JL, Margolis DJ, Marcus SM, Strom BL. Risk of venous thromboembolism from oral contraceptives containing gestodene and desogestrel versus levonorgestrel: a meta-analysis and formal sensitivity analysis. *Contraception* 2001;64:125–33.

85. Kemmeren JM, Algra A, Grobbee DE. Third generation oral contraceptives and risk of venous thrombosis: meta-analysis. *BMJ* 2001;323:131–4.

86. Heinemann LA, Dinger J. Safety of a new oral contraceptive containing drospirenone. *Drug Saf* 2004;27:1001–18.

87. Spitzer WO. Cyproterone acetate with ethinylestradiol as a risk factor for venous thromboembolism: an epidemiological evaluation. *J Obstet Gynaecol Can* 2003;25:1011–18.

88. World Health Organization Collaborative Study of Cardiovascular Disease and Steroid Hormone Contraception. Venous thromboembolic disease and combined oral contraceptives: results of international multicentre case-control study. *Lancet* 1995;346:1575–82.

89. Nightingale AL, Lawrenson RA, Simpson EL, Williams TJ, MacRae KD, Farmer RD. The effects of age, body mass index, smoking and general health on the risk of venous thromboembolism in users of combined oral contraceptives. *Eur J Contracept Reprod Health Care* 2000;5:265–74.

90. Martinelli I, Taioli E, Battaglioli T, Podda GM, Passamonti SM, Pedotti P, *et al*. Risk of venous thromboembolism after air travel: interaction with thrombophilia and oral contraceptives. *Arch Intern Med* 2003;163:2771–4.

91. van den Bosch MA, Kemmeren JM, Tanis BC, Mali WP, Helmerhorst FM, Rosendaal FR *et al*. The RATIO study: oral contraceptives and the risk of peripheral arterial disease in young women. *J Thromb Haemost* 2003;1:439–44.

92. Martinelli I, Sacchi E, Landi G, Taioli E, Duca F, Mannucci PM. High risk of cerebral-vein thrombosis in carriers of a prothrombin-gene mutation and in users of oral contraceptives. *N Engl J Med* 1998;338:1793–7.

93. de Bruijn SF, Stam J, Koopman MM, Vandenbroucke JP. Case-control study of risk of cerebral sinus thrombosis in oral contraceptive users and in [correction of who are] carriers of hereditary prothrombotic conditions. The Cerebral Venous Sinus Thrombosis Study Group. BMJ 1998;316:589-92 [erratum *BMJ* 1998;316:822].

94. Crook D, Godsland I. Safety evaluation of modern oral contraceptives. Effects on lipoprotein and carbohydrate metabolism. *Contraception* 1998;57:189–201.

95. Dong W, Colhoun HM, Poulter NR. Blood pressure in women using oral contraceptives: results from the Health Survey for England 1994. *J Hypertens* 1997;15:1063–8.

96. Cardoso F, Polonia J, Santos A, Silva-Carvalho J, Ferreira-de-Almeida J. Low-dose oral contraceptives and 24-hour ambulatory blood pressure. *Int J Gynaecol Obstet* 1997;59:237–43.

97. Chasan-Taber L, Willett WC, Manson JE, Spiegelman D, Hunter DJ, Curhan G, *et al.* Prospective study of oral contraceptives and hypertension among women in the United States. *Circulation* 1996;94:483–9.

98. Winkler UH. Blood coagulation and oral contraceptives. A critical review. *Contraception* 1998;57:203–9.

99. Danesh J, Collins R, Peto R. Lipoprotein(a) and coronary heart disease. Meta-analysis of prospective studies. *Circulation* 2000;102:1082–5.

100. Dreon DM, Slavin JL, Phinney SD. Oral contraceptive use and increased plasma concentration of C-reactive protein. *Life Sci* 2003;73:1245–52.

101. Williams MJ, Williams SM, Milne BJ, Hancox RJ, Poulton R. Association between C-reactive protein, metabolic cardiovascular risk factors, obesity and oral contraceptive use in young adults. *Int J Obes Relat Metab Disord* 2004;28:998–1003.

102. Doring A, Frohlich M, Lowel H, Koenig W. Third generation oral contraceptive use and cardiovascular risk factors. *Atherosclerosis* 2004;172:281–6.

103. Rothman KJ. *Epidemiology: An Introduction.* New York: Oxford University Press; 2002.

104. Kesseru E, Albornoz H, Diaz M, Socolsky R. Serum lipid variations in women on copper intrauterine devices, triphasic oral contraceptives and monthly injectable contraceptives. *Contraception* 1991;44:235–44.

105. Haiba NA, el Habashy MA, Said SA, Darwish EA, Abdel-Sayed WS, Nayel SE. Clinical evaluation of two monthly injectable contraceptives and their effects on some metabolic parameters. *Contraception* 1989;39:619–32.

106. Meng YX, Jiang HY, Chen AJ, Lu FY, Yang H, Zhang MY, *et al.* Hemostatic changes in women using a monthly injectable contraceptive for one year. *Contraception* 1990;42:455–66.

107. Kaunitz AM. Lunelle monthly injectable contraceptive. An effective, safe, and convenient new birth control option. *Arch Gynecol Obstet* 2001;265:119–23.

108. Cromie MA, Maile MH, Wajszczuk CP. Comparative effects of Lunelle monthly contraceptive injection (medroxyprogesterone acetate and estradiol cypionate injectable suspension) and ortho-Novum 7/7/7 oral contraceptive (norethindrone/ethinyl estradiol triphasic) on lipid profiles. Investigators from the Lunelle Study Group. *Contraception* 2000;61:51–9.

109. Gallo MF, Grimes DA, Schulz KF. Skin patch and vaginal ring versus combined oral contraceptives for contraception. *Cochrane Database Syst Rev* 2003;CD003552.

110. Bjarnadottir RI, Tuppurainen M, Killick SR. Comparison of cycle control with a combined contraceptive vaginal ring and oral levonorgestrel/ethinyl estradiol. *Am J Obstet Gynecol* 2002;186:389–95.

111. Creasy GW, Fisher AC, Hall N, Shangold GA. Transdermal contraceptive patch delivering norelgestromin and ethinyl estradiol. Effects on the lipid profile. *J Reprod Med* 2003;48:179–86.

112. World Health Organization Collaborative Study of Cardiovascular Disease and Steroid Hormone Contraception. Cardiovascular disease and use of oral and injectable progestogen-only contraceptives and combined injectable contraceptives. Results of an international, multicenter, case-control study. *Contraception* 1998;57:315–24.

113. World Health Organization. Medical Eligibility Criteria for Contraceptive Use. Geneva: WHO; 2004 [www.who.int/reproductive-health/publications/RHR_00_2_medical_eligibility_criteria_3rd/index. htm].

114. McCann MF, Potter LS. Progestin-only oral contraception: a comprehensive review. *Contraception* 1994;50:S1–S195.

115. Hussain SF. Progestogen-only pills and high blood pressure: is there an association? A literature review. *Contraception* 2004;69:89–97.

116. Dorflinger LJ. Metabolic effects of implantable steroid contraceptives for women. *Contraception*

2002;65:47–62.

117. Westhoff C. Depot medroxyprogesterone acetate contraception. Metabolic parameters and mood changes. *J Reprod Med* 1996;41:401–6.

118. Sorensen MB, Collins P, Ong PJ, Webb CM, Hayward CS, Asbury EA, *et al*. Long-term use of contraceptive depot medroxyprogesterone acetate in young women impairs arterial endothelial function assessed by cardiovascular magnetic resonance. *Circulation* 2002;106:1646–51.

119. Heinemann LA, Assmann A, DoMinh T, Garbe E. Oral progestogen-only contraceptives and cardiovascular risk: results from the Transnational Study on Oral Contraceptives and the Health of Young Women. *Eur J Contracept Reprod Health Care* 1999;4:67–73.

120. Wysowski DK, Green L. Serious adverse events in Norplant users reported to the Food and Drug Administration's MedWatch Spontaneous Reporting System. *Obstet Gynecol* 1995;85:538–42.

121. Petitti DB, Siscovick DS, Sidney S, Schwartz SM, Quesenberry CP, Psaty BM, *et al*. Norplant implants and cardiovascular disease. *Contraception* 1998;57:361–2.

122. Gu SJ, Du MK, Zhang LD, Liu YL, Wang SH, Sivin I. A 5-year evaluation of NORPLANT contraceptive implants in China. *Obstet Gynecol* 1994;83:673–8.

123. Meirik O, Farley TM, Sivin I. Safety and efficacy of levonorgestrel implant, intrauterine device, and sterilization. *Obstet Gynecol* 2001;97:539–47.

124. Faculty of Family Planning and Reproductive Health Care CEU. FFPRHC Guidance (October 2003): First prescription of combined oral contraception. *J Fam Plann Reprod Health Care* 2003;29:209–22 [erratum *J Fam Plann Reprod Health Care* 2004;30:63].

125. ACOG. The use of hormonal contraception in women with coexisting medical conditions. ACOG Practice Bulletin Number 18, July 2000. *Int J Gynaecol Obstet* 2001;75:93–106.

126. Mann JI, Vessey MP, Thorogood M, Doll SR. Myocardial infarction in young women with special reference to oral contraceptive practice. *BMJ* 1975;2:241–5.

127. Petitti DB, Wingerd J, Pellegrin F, Ramcharan S. Oral contraceptives, smoking, and other factors in relation to risk of venous thromboembolic disease. *Am J Epidemiol* 1978;108:480–5.

128. Ramcharan S, Pellegrin FA, Ray RM, Hsu JP. The Walnut Creek Contraceptive Drug Study. A prospective study of the side effects of oral contraceptives. Volume III, an interim report: A comparison of disease occurrence leading to hospitalization or death in users and non-users of oral contraceptives. *J Reprod Med* 1980;25:345–72.

129. Adam SA, Thorogood M, Mann JI. Oral contraception and myocardial infarction revisited: the effects of new preparations and prescribing patterns. *Br J Obstet Gynaecol* 1981;88:838–45.

130. Salonen JT. Oral contraceptives, smoking and risk of myocardial infarction in young women. A longitudinal population study in eastern Finland. *Acta Med Scand* 1982;212:141–4.

131. Vessey MP, Lawless M, Yeates D. Oral contraceptives and stroke: findings in a large prospective study. *BMJ* 1984;289:530–1.

132. Vessey M, Painter R, Yeates D. Mortality in relation to oral contraceptive use and cigarette smoking. *Lancet* 2003;362:185–91.

133. Ananijevic-Pandey J, Vlajinac H. Myocardial infarction in young women with reference to oral contraceptive use. *Int J Epidemiol* 1989;18:585–8.

134. Thorogood M, Mann J, Murphy M, Vessey M. Risk factors for fatal venous thromboembolism in young women: a case-control study. *Intl J Epidemiol* 1992;21:48–52.

135. Lewis MA. The Transnational Study on Oral Contraceptives and the Health of Young Women. Methods, results, new analyses and the healthy user effect. *Hum Reprod Update* 1999;5:707–20.

136. Dunn NR, Arscott A, Thorogood M. The relationship between use of oral contraceptives and myocardial infarction in young women with fatal outcome, compared to those who survive: results from the MICA case-control study. *Contraception* 2001;63:65–9.

137. Lidegaard O. Oral contraceptives and myocardial infarction: reassuring new findings. *BMJ* 1999;318:1583–4.

138. Lidegaard O. Smoking and use of oral contraceptives: impact on thrombotic diseases. *Am J Obstet Gynecol* 1999;180:S357–S363.

139. Anon. . Consensus conference on combination oral contraceptives and cardiovascular disease. *Fertil Steril* 1999;71:1S-6S.

Chapter 14
Contraception for young people

Anna Graham

Introduction

Young people under 25 years of age represent the most sexually active age group in the UK, encompassing those with the highest rates of sexually transmitted infections and highest numbers of unplanned pregnancies leading to an abortion. This chapter starts by describing what is known about the sexual behaviour of this age group, behaviour which explains much of the sexual ill health experienced by the under 25s in the UK. Comparative data on conceptions in Western European countries among the under 20s are presented, followed by a summary of the 2003 UK data on common sexually transmitted infections.

Patterns of use of different services for contraceptive advice are described, as well as results from surveys on use of different methods of contraception. Particular issues relating to contraception and young people are then discussed including competence to consent; confidentiality, safety of methods, compliance and service provision. Lastly, training opportunities in sexual health for those working in the community are described.

Sexual behaviour

There are a number of reasons why young people are more likely to conceive and to have a sexually transmitted infection than older people. These include frequency of intercourse, number of sexual partners, concurrent partnerships, increased fertility and relationship factors that may reduce the likelihood of preventing adverse outcomes.

Frequency of intercourse

Young people have more frequent sexual intercourse. This was investigated as part of the first National Survey of Sexual Attitudes and Lifestyles (NATSAL), undertaken in the early 1990s. Wellings et al.[1] reported that the median frequency of sexual intercourse rose to a maximum of five times per month for women aged 20–29 years and for men aged 25–34 years. Women aged 16–24 years reported higher frequencies than men of the same age. The age differences between the genders are likely to be explained by social mixing patterns.

Table 14.1. Heterosexual partners by gender and age group (data collected between 1999 and 2001)[2]

Age group (years)	Partners	
	Mean	**SD**
Men:		
16–24	5.3	10.7
25–34	4.2	8.6
35–44	2.2	3.8
All	3.8	8.2
Women:		
16–24	3.8	6.7
25–34	2.2	3.1
35–44	1.5	3.9
All	2.4	4.6

Number of sexual partners

Young people are more likely to have more sexual partners. Reporting from the second National Survey of Sexual attitudes and Lifestyles (NATSAL 2000), undertaken in 2000–2001, Johnson *et al.*[2] stated that for both men and women the mean number of heterosexual partners in the past 5 years consistently declined with increasing age (Table 14.1).

Table 14.2. Concurrent partners in past year by gender and age group (data collected between 1999 and 2001)[2]

Age group (years)	Partners	
	Percentage	**95% CI**
Men:		
16–24	20.8	17.8–24.3
25–34	15.3	13.3–17.5
35–44	9.8	8.3–11.7
All	14.6	13.4–16.0
Women:		
16–24	15.2	12.7–18.1
25–34	7.6	6.4–8.9
35–44	6.7	5.6–8.0
All	9.0	8.2–10.0

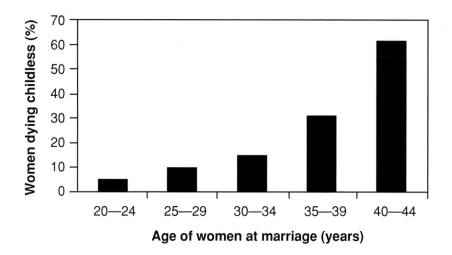

Figure 14.1. Risk of childlessness for women related to age at marriage[3]

Concurrent partnerships

The risks of acquiring a sexually transmitted infection increase with sexual partner-ships that are concurrent (where individuals are engaged in more than one sexual partnership during the same time period). In NATSAL 2000, the authors estimated that 14.6 % of men and 9.0 % of women had concurrent partnerships in the previous year. This decreased with increasing age (Table 14.2).

Fertility

The likelihood of being able to conceive reduces with increasing age. The older a woman is at marriage, the less likely she is to have a child. One-third of women marrying over the age of 35 years will remain childless compared with less than 5 % of those marrying between 20 and 24 years (Figure 14.1).[3]

Relationship issues

It is well known that adverse consequences of sexual activity are more likely if you are a young person living in the UK than if you live in other Western European countries. Researchers explored these differences in the 1990s. Influences on sexual development include both individual and wider contexts. Individual factors have been elucidated from surveys and questionnaire based studies, wider contexts through qualitative interviews. A theory of 'interactional competence' was initially developed by Rademakers, a Dutch researcher in 1992, who described her theory as follows: "a preventative behaviour can never be the result of an individual weighing and deciding but always the consequence of an interaction, in which the wishes and intentions of one partner are being confronted with those of another".[4]

A group of researchers formed a protocol for interviews, focus groups and analysis, for use in 13 European countries. There were three key research aims:

1. To identify explanations of risk related behaviours and the processes through which decisions are reached regarding the adoption of safer sex practices.
2. To identify the personal, social and physical contexts in which sexual activity among young adults takes place.
3. To explore the sources and ranges of meanings of sexual activity, and their relation to the adoption of safer sex techniques.

Results from a comparison of interviews from the UK and the Netherlands, conducted with 16- to 30-year-olds who had had two or more sexual partners in the previous year, were presented at a conference in Italy in 1998.[5] The following findings summarise the events leading up to first sexual intercourse when comparing the two countries:

- similar age of pre-intercourse activities, such as deep kissing
- age at first intercourse higher in the Netherlands
- more likely to have thought about, and discussed with a partner, the issue of contraception prior to intercourse in the Netherlands
- more likely to have used condom at first intercourse in the Netherlands
- 'love' more likely to be reason for first intercourse in the Netherlands
- expressed regret at first intercourse in the UK more likely.

The author suggests that young adults in the Netherlands are more 'competent' than in the UK. This competence could be regarded as a 'cultural feature'. Ingham also described 'associates' of cultural competence, which he suggests could not be called determinants in view of the methodology used:

- Timing of education, extent and nature of discussion regarding sex and sexuality – in the Netherlands this starts earlier (at primary school) and is more realistic, with more discussion at home, including with fathers.
- Role modelling by parents – in the Netherlands parents more likely to have 'weak' gender stereotypes and to display physical intimacy; they are more available to their children and to use physical forms of punishment less.
- Patterns of friendship during early teenage years – in the Netherlands out of school activities are more likely to be in mixed sex groupings and young people are more likely to discuss personal matters with friends of both sexes.

Teenage pregnancy in the UK

It is well known that the UK has the highest rate of teenage pregnancy in Western Europe.[6] Figure 14.2 illustrates this for the latest year for which comparative data are available. The rates in other countries have declined over the last 25 years whereas in the UK they have remained relatively stable. While this fact is of some concern, it needs to be viewed with the background of increased sexual activity at a younger age. It has been suggested by some that the small amount of fluctuation in teenage fertility in the UK can in part be explained by changes in the political culture and other external events such as health concerns related to the pill.[7]

Live births to teenage women   ª **EU comparison, 2001**   ᵇ

Live births per 1,000 women

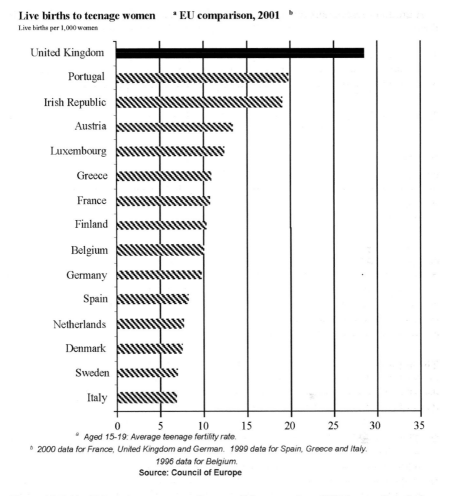

ª Aged 15-19: Average teenage fertility rate.
ᵇ 2000 data for France, United Kingdom and German. 1999 data for Spain, Greece and Italy.
1996 data for Belgium.
Source: Council of Europe

Figure 14.2. Live births to teenage women: European Union comparison, 2001 (source: Council of Europe)

Sexually transmitted infections in young people in the UK

Data on sexually transmitted infections are collected routinely from genitourinary medicine clinics. This is a reliable source of information but obviously excludes testing performed elsewhere in the community. There is some evidence that much testing is undertaken elsewhere. The Avon Surveillance System for Sexually Transmitted Infections (ASSIST) collects data on positive and negative tests for laboratory diagnosed infections taken in any clinical setting from the Health Protection Agency and NHS trust laboratories. In 2001, 50% of chlamydia tests and 44% of positive results came from general practice, family planning or Brook clinics. Nearly two-thirds (62%) of those tested in general practice were over 25 years of age, in whom the positivity rate was 4% compared with 11% for under 25 year olds.[8]

Genital chlamydia infection

Genital chlamydia infection was the most commonly diagnosed bacterial sexually transmitted infection in genitourinary medicine clinics in 2003. *Chlamydia trachomatis* is asymptomatic in up to 70% of cases in women and 50% of cases in men. Undiagnosed infection can develop into serious sequelae, such as pelvic inflammatory disease and infertility in women.

In 2003, the highest rates of diagnosis were among women aged 16–19 years and men aged 20–24 years, at 1334/100 000 and 961/100 000, respectively.[9] The rate of diagnosis declines markedly in those over 25 years because of changes in sexual behaviour and mixing patterns. The rise in diagnoses is, in part, attributable to increased testing following increased awareness of the infection among the general public, as well as health professionals. Additionally, increasing use of more sensitive laboratory testing methods may have an impact on the rising number of diagnoses.

Diagnoses of genital chlamydial infection vary widely throughout the UK but are markedly higher in London, Yorkshire and Humberside and the North West.

Gonorrhoea

The highest rates of uncomplicated gonorrhoea infection in 2003 were seen among women aged 16–19 years (216/100 000) and men aged 20–24 years (291/100 000). Of women diagnosed with gonorrhoea, 40% were under 20 years. Gonorrhoea infection tends to be more highly concentrated in urban and deprived areas.[9]

Genital herpes

During 2003, in England, Wales and Northern Ireland, the highest rates of genital herpes simplex virus (HSV) infection in men were seen in the 20–24 years age group (88/100 000). In women, the highest diagnostic rates were seen in those aged 20–24 years (191/100 000), with only a slightly lower rate in the 16–19 years age group. For both men and women, the overall rate of diagnoses of genital HSV infection was highest in the London region in 2003. Other than in London, there was little variation in the overall diagnostic rate between regions.

Genital warts

Anogenital warts are the most commonly diagnosed sexually transmitted infection in genitourinary medicine clinics and high rates are uniformly distributed across the UK. Highest rates of first episode genital warts in 2003 were among 16- to 19-year-old females and 20- to 24-year-old males (713/100 000 and 785/100 000 respectively).[9]

Abortion

Reducing the length of time to a maximum of 3 weeks from first point of contact with a health professional and a termination being undertaken by 2005 was one of few targets set out in the National Strategy for Sexual Health and HIV in 2001.[10] The abortion rate was highest in women aged 20–24 (Table 14.3).[11]

The reasons for women requesting an abortion are wide ranging. In the past, the need for abortion was thought to be principally due to inappropriate use of contraception. It is likely, however, that the issues are far more complex and more likely to

Table 14.3. Abortion rates in England and Wales in 2002[11]

Age group (years)	Rate/1000 women
< 16	3.5
16–19	25.3
20–24	30.3
25–34	17.5
35 and over	6.7

be highly culturally determined. This is discussed in depth in Chapter 5. There is some evidence that younger women are more likely to request an abortion later than older women. However, the proportion of abortions performed after 20 weeks of gestation is extremely small at any age.

The abortion rate in the under 20s in the UK over the last 30 years of the 20th century has been increasing. This is in contrast to other Western European countries, some of whom have always had low rates, such as France, Germany and the Netherlands, as well as Greece and Italy. The abortion ratio, that is the number of abortions per 1000 live births to under 20s, shows a slightly different picture. In Scandinavian countries, this ratio is greatest, with far more abortions than live births compared with the UK, where there are more live births than abortions. This probably reflects lower acceptance of abortion as a means of contraception or the social acceptance of early childbearing.[6]

Use of services

Over the last quarter of the 20th century, there was an overall decrease in the use of family planning clinics, with increases in attendance at these services seen only in the under 20s.[12] Between 1975 and 1998–99, the proportion of young women under 16 years visiting family planning clinics increased from 1% to 8%. For women aged 16–19 years the proportion increased from a minimum of 12% in 1988–89 to 22% in 1998–99.

Research by Clements *et al.*[13] attempted to determine the spatial variation in teenage conception rates within a region of the UK (Wessex) from data collected between 1991 and 1994. The results showed that the variation in teenage conception rates was principally determined by the age of the teenager and deprivation level. No association was found with distance to a family planning clinic. However, those teenagers living more than 4 km away from the nearest youth-orientated clinic, compared with those under 4 km, had 1.26 times the odds of a maternity rather than a termination, after accounting for other factors.

The majority of contraceptive advice given to the over 20s is through the general practitioner. The challenge is to provide a quality service within the restrictions of a traditionally short consultation. Patients may access practice nurses, many of whom have appropriate qualifications in contraception services.[14] The management of sexually transmitted infections in general practice is less well catered for at the present time. It is possible, however, that, in a climate where integration of sexual health services and chlamydia screening in particular is encouraged,[15] general practice, with its generalist perspective, will find this easier than some specialist settings.

Use of contraception

Data on the provision of contraception are routinely collected from community family planning clinics in England. This does not include returns from general practice, the main source of contraception provision in the UK. The National Statistics Omnibus Survey is one of two main sources of information about contraceptive use and sexual health, the other being the General Household Survey. The latter has been collecting data about contraceptive use since 1983. When the 1997 Survey was suspended, the contraception module carried on the Omnibus Survey was extended to collect information previously gathered by the General Household Survey.

The National Statistics Omnibus Survey is a multipurpose survey based on a representative sample of adults in the UK. The Omnibus Survey interviewed 7258 adults during the 4 months that the contraception module was carried, between June 2003 and March 2004.[16]

The most popular method of contraception in the under 25s was the pill, followed by the male condom. Women responding to the survey used other methods a lot less frequently. The proportion of women aged under 25 years using each method of contraception is shown in Table 14.4.

Table 14.4. Percentage of current use of contraception, by age group (years)[16]

Type of contraception	16–17-year-olds (%)	18–19-year-olds (%)	20–24-year-olds (%)
Non-surgical:			
Pill[a]	26	58	49
Mini pill	1	14	9
Combined pill	20	29	31
Male condom	33	36	37
Withdrawal	3	–	1
Intrauterine device	2	–	1
Injection/implant	3	2	6
Safe period	–	–	1
Cap/diaphragm	–	1	–
Foams/gels	–	–	–
Hormonal IUS	–	–	–
Female condom	–	–	–
Emergency contraception	5	4	2
Total at least one nonsurgical method	50	70	75
Surgical:			
Sterilised	–	1	2
Partner sterilised	–	–	1
Total at least one method	50	71	78

[a] Includes those who did not know type of pill used

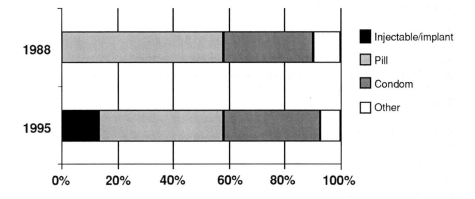

Figure 14.3. Percentage of women age 15–19 years using a contraceptive method[17]

Fourteen percent of women aged 16–49 years were not currently in a heterosexual relationship. Women aged less than 20 years were those most likely *not* to currently be in a heterosexual relationship: 45% of women aged 16–17 years and 25% of those aged 18–19 years were also not in a heterosexual relationship. This proportion fell to around 10% of women aged 25 years or over. The tendency for young people to have periods of time not in relationships requiring contraception makes their contraceptive needs somewhat different to those in longer-term sexual relationships.

Darroch and Singh[17] have suggested that one mechanism for the decline in teenage pregnancy rates in the USA has been a switch to non-user-dependent methods of contraception (specifically, in the US, Depo Provera®). The authors based their analyses on information from the 1988 and 1995 cycles of the National Survey of Family Growth. Long-acting hormonal methods (the injectable and the implant) that have the lowest failure rates of all reversible methods became available in the early 1990s. By 1995, 13% of current contraceptive use was accounted for by these methods, 10% relying on the injectable and 3% the implant. The oral contraceptive pill and condoms were less used compared with 1988. This is illustrated in Figure 14.3.

Particular issues concerning contraceptive methods and young people

Competence to consent to treatment

The Faculty of Family Planning and Reproductive Health Care (FFPRHC) of the RCOG produced guidance on *Contraceptive Choices for Young People* in October 2004.[18] The issue of a young person's competence to consent to treatment is discussed. The guidance suggests that a clinician should assess this by evaluating the young person's ability to understand information provided, to weigh up the risks and benefits and to express her own wishes. If a young person is assessed competent, this should be documented in the case notes. A clinician can provide advice or treatment to a competent young person (under 16 years) without parental consent or knowledge using the Fraser criteria.

Some specialist family planning clinics for young people have devised checklists to ensure that clinicians address the issue of Fraser competence systematically. The Avon Brook Advisory Centre, for example, uses the checklist shown in Box 14.1.

Box 14.1. Avon Brook Advisory Centre guidelines for young people under 16 years

1. Maturity/demonstrates understanding.
2. Discussed parental awareness/consent.
3. Began/continuing sexual intercourse.
4. Physical/mental health.
5. In best interests.

The Fraser criteria emerged following a court case in the mid-1980s. The mother (Victoria Gillick) of a girl aged under 16 years took her health authority to court after her daughter had been provided with contraception without her consent. Lord Fraser, following the House of Lords ruling against the mother in the mid-1980s, produced guidance for health professionals on confidentiality. The Fraser criteria are shown in Box 14.2.

Box 14.2. Outline of the Fraser criteria (source: *Contraceptive Advice and Treatment for Young People Under 16*. HC(86)1. Department of Health 1986)

The Fraser criteria:
- The young person understands the advice.
- The young person cannot be persuaded to inform her parents or to allow the clinician to inform them.
- It is likely that the young person will continue to have sexual intercourse with or without the use of contraception.
- The young person's physical or mental health may suffer as a result of withholding contraceptive advice or treatment.
- It is in the best interests of the young person for the clinician to provide contraceptive advice, treatment or both without parental consent.

Where there is doubt concerning Fraser competence or where there are issues relating to child protection, clinicians must have identified an individual as the local lead in this area, who can be contacted to discuss the young person further.

For most young people, sexual activity is consensual. However, sexual activity should be a positive choice rather than a passive one. Surveys of young people have suggested that high rates of regret follow first intercourse when age at first intercourse is younger. In a survey of school children in Scotland undertaken in the late 1990s (mean age 14 years) one in five girls described being under pressure to have sex for the first and subsequent times, compared with fewer than one in ten boys.[19] NATSAL 2000 defined sexual competence as first intercourse occurring in the absence of duress and regret, with autonomy of decision and with the use of reliable contraceptive method. Lack of sexual competence increases with decreasing age at first intercourse, with 91% of girls and 67% of boys not sexually competent at first intercourse.[20]

Confidentiality

Young people may be especially concerned about confidentiality. The Department of Health published new guidance in 2004 on the duty of confidentiality, care and good practice in providing advice to young people under the age of 16 years.[21]

The duty of confidentiality owed to a young person is similar to that for an adult. Young people should be made aware of the confidentiality to be expected from all members of the healthcare team. Other professionals, such as teachers and youth workers, may not have the same duty of confidentiality. Young people aged under 16 years should be made aware in advance that, if there are concerns regarding maltreatment, exploitation or coercion, confidentiality may need to be breached. This needs to be achieved with the young person's consent, if possible.

The new guidance states that prominent advertising of confidentiality policies in clinics is desirable and that all staff in clinics should receive training on confidentiality issues. The Royal College of General Practitioners has produced, in collaboration with others, a toolkit on *Confidentiality and Young People*.[22] The materials for a training session in the surgery are provided, as well as a recommendation that all staff, reception and domestic as well as clinical, sign confidentiality agreements. Examples of these are given. The toolkit is a valuable resource for individual practices and for sexual health promotion specialists supporting primary care. The toolkit could also be used in other healthcare settings.

Safety of different contraceptive methods

The World Health Organization Medical Eligibility Criteria for Contraceptive Use (WHOMEC) provides guidance on who can use contraceptive methods safely.[23] Young people may have specific risks relating to pubertal development, risk of sexually transmitted infection or ability to comply with contraception. Young people have a lower risk, compared with older women, of cardiovascular and other age-related diseases. However, young people may have concurrent diseases requiring consideration, such as diabetes, inflammatory bowel disease, cystic fibrosis, renal disease, epilepsy or anorexia nervosa.

The WHOMEC recommends unrestricted use of combined and progestogen-only contraceptive pills and the progestogen-only implant from menarche. The benefits outweigh the risks of using medroxyprogesterone acetate (DMPA) from menarche to the age of 18 years and for women over 18 years use is unrestricted. The WHOMEC recommends that the benefits of use of the intrauterine contraceptive device outweigh the risks for women from menarche to age 20 years.

There remains uncertainty about the risks to bone mineral density and the use of DMPA. However, the guidance from the FFPRHC in 2004 stated that other factors such as nutrition, calcium intake and smoking may well influence bone mineral density as much if not more than the use of contraceptive hormones.[18] Many young women who use DMPA do so for a short time and therefore the effect on bone mineral density is likely to be short-lived.

Evidence for the protective effect of condoms against sexually transmitted infections other than HIV is limited. However, consistent and correct use is advocated as reasonable health promotion advice for young people by the guidance.[18] Condoms alone, however, are associated with high contraceptive failure rates. Ideally, young people need to be encouraged to use a reliable method of contraception as well as condoms.

Compliance

Compliance can be an issue with contraceptive provision for any age group and perhaps especially for young people. In order to improve compliance, all people should be offered the full range of contraceptive options, whatever their age.[18] This should include information about back-up methods in the event that no contraception is used or the method used fails. It may be helpful to explicitly discuss health gains from use of some methods of contraception (aside from contraceptive efficacy). Addressing health concerns may also be appropriate. There are a number of leaflets available some specifically targeted at young people.

The FFPRHC guidance from 2004 on *Contraceptive Choices for Young People* states that this age group is especially concerned about the risks of certain cancers and use of the combined pill.[18] Young women can be advised that this method of contraception reduces the risk of ovarian and endometrial cancer and, with less than 5 years of use, does not increase cervical cancer risk. Any increase in risk of breast cancer associated with hormonal contraception is small and there is no effect with duration of use.[24]

The risk of venous thromboembolism increases with use of the combined pill but remains low compared with the risk when pregnant. With use of levonorgestrel or norethisterone containing combined pills the risk is 15/100 000 woman years compared with 25/100 000 woman years for pills containing the newer progestogens such as desogestrel or gestodene.[25] The risk of experiencing a venous thrombo-embolisim in pregnancy is 60/100 000 woman years.

More 'minor' concerns with use of the combined pill, such as weight gain, acne and mood changes, can be a problem for continuation. It is important that women are encouraged to return to discuss these problems in order for their contraceptive method to remain acceptable. Often, changes in prescribing to another brand or method will lead to an acceptable method being found.

Service provision

It has been suggested that the ideal family planning service for young people should be accessible, comprehensive, multidisciplinary, confidential and provided by non-judgemental staff with good communication and counselling skills.[26] This would seem to be the ideal for any health service for any age. The Faculty guidance recommends that sexual health providers adapt services to meet the needs of young people and provide services for vulnerable young people, delivered within mainstream services as well as outreach services.[18]

Qualitative studies show that young people feel that health professionals generally assume too much existing knowledge and underestimate the desire for more information.[27] However, as with much of clinical medicine, the amount of information to convey far outweighs the time available. The provision of written information following a consultation has been shown to be useful in some formats.[28]

Contraceptive and sexual health services need to make links with education authorities and schools to promote and provide the planning and delivery of sex and relationship education. Evidence from Europe suggests that the UK experience provides many mixed messages to young people from home, school, health services and, perhaps most importantly, the media, about sex and relationships and that this is the crucial difference compared with countries where young people have better sexual health.[6]

Training

Clearly one of the main issues facing those working in this field is the need to provide a sexual health service in its broadest sense. This has training implications. Sexual health often affords little time in the undergraduate curriculum and is not part of core general practice training. Specialist training traditionally has concentrated on one-half of the clinical picture.

Courses have been developed in order to give clinicians providing sexual health care, especially in general practice settings, the skills they need to do so. The two most commonly held qualifications are the DFFP (Diploma in the Faculty of Family Planning) and the Sexually Transmitted Infection Foundation (STIF) Course. The former has been around for many years and is run by the FFPRHC. This qualification has been updated and now includes a module on sexually transmitted infections. Trainees in genitourinary medicine are required to attend the contraceptive components of the DFFP.

The STIF course was devised by the Medical Society for the Study of Venereal Diseases (now renamed British Association for Sexual Health and HIV) in response to the National Strategy for Sexual Health and HIV. The aim of the course is to equip participants with the basic knowledge, skills and attitudes for the effective management of sexually transmitted infections. It is a workshop-based 2-day course, with role-playing activities to rehearse sexual history-taking, using scenarios commonly found in everyday general practice. Genitourinary consultants in most parts of the country run the course.

One-off courses are a start but updating is obviously necessary. In 1999, a survey of nearly 600 GP principals in the then-named Avon Health Authority were sent a questionnaire to complete about emergency contraception. The survey had an 84% response rate. Questions concerning family planning qualifications and training were included. In this sample, 399 (82%) of GPs held a family planning qualification. Female GPs were significantly more likely to do so compared with male GPs (178, 93%, versus 221, 76%; $P < 0.001$). Just under 50% (235, 48%) of GPs had attended a family planning refresher in the last 5 years. Again, female GPs were more likely to have done so than male GPs (125/186, 67%, as against 110/285, 39%; $P < 0.001$).[14]

Since this survey was undertaken, the culture of personal learning plans and their fulfilment by a variety of different methods, not only attendance at courses, has evolved. It is likely that health professionals who have an interest in sexual health will continue to update. The challenge is to make it possible for any young person who sees any health professional (in any setting) to be managed appropriately.

It is unfortunate that there is not a qualification in 'sexual health' that includes all facets of this subject. It is possible, in time, that this will be developed nationally and there are some local initiatives to do so such as the Postgraduate Award for Sexual Health in Primary Care for GPs and practice nurses currently running at Warwick University.[29]

Conclusions

Young people undertake the riskiest sexual behaviour. This leads them to experience the highest incidence of sexual ill health: unplanned pregnancy leading to a termination and sexually transmitted infection. In order to address these health needs, both contraception and sexually transmitted infection management (integrated sexual health) need to be provided by services. In order for the above to be possible, the training needs of those working in services should be addressed. Services, for any age group, and perhaps specifically for young people, need to be accessible, comprehensive, confidential and provided by non-judgemental staff with good communication skills.

References

1. Wellings K, Field J, Johnson A, Wadsworth J. *Sexual Behaviour in Britain*. Harmondsworth: Penguin; 1994.
2. Johnson AM, Mercer CH, Erens B, Copas AJ, McManus S, Wellings K, *et al.* Sexual behaviour in Britain: partnerships, practices, and HIV risk behaviours. *Lancet* 2001;358:1835–1842.
3. Menhen J, Larrsen U. Guide to natural fertility with age. In: Mastroianni L, Paulsen L, editors. *Aging, Reproduction and the Climacteric*. New York: Plenum; 1986.
4. Rademakers J, Luijkx JB, Zessen G, va Ziljlmans W, Sratver C, Van der Rijt G. *AIDS-preventie in heteroseksuele contacten*. [Dutch: AIDS –prevention in heterosexual contacts]. Amsterdam: Swets and Zeitlinger; 1992.
5. Ingham, R. Exploring interactional competence: comparative data from the United Kingdom and the Netherlands on young people's sexual development. Paper presented at 24th meeting of the International Academy of Sex Research, Sirmione, Italy, 3–6 June 1998.
6. Kane R, Wellings, K. *Reducing the Rate of Teenage Conception. An International Review of the Evidence. Data from Europe*. Oxford: HEA; 1999.
7. Wellings K, Kane R. Trends in teenage pregnancy in England and Wales: how can we explain them? *J R Soc Med* 1999;92:277–82.
8. Low N, Slater W. Surveillance of sexually transmitted infections in primary care. *Sex Transm Infect* 2004;80:152.
9. UK Collaborative Group for HIV and STI Surveillance. *Focus on Prevention. HIV and other Sexually Transmitted Infections in the United Kingdom in 2003. Annual Report*. London: Health Protection Agency, Centre for Infections; 2004.
10. Department of Health. *The National Strategy for Sexual Health and HIV*. London: DH; 2001.
11. Office for National Statistics. Abortion Rates by Age. London: ONS; 2004.
12. Botting B, Dunnell K. Trends in fertility and contraception in the last quarter of the twentieth century. *Popul Trends* 2000;100(Summer).
13. Clements S, Stone N, Diamond I, Ingham R. Modelling the spatial distribution of teenage conception rates within Wessex. *Br J Fam Plann* 1998;24:61–71.
14. Graham A, Moore L, Sharp D. Provision of emergency contraception in general practice and confidentiality for the under 16s: results of a postal survey by general practitioners in Avon. *J Fam Plann Reprod Health Care* 2001;27:193–6.
15. Department of Health. *Choosing Health: Making Healthier Choices Easier*. London: DH; 2004.
16. Dawe F, Rainford L. *Contraception and Sexual Health, 2003*. London: Office for National Statistics; 2004.
17. Darroch JE, Singh S. *Why is Teenage Pregnancy Declining? The Roles of Abstinence, Sexual Activity and Contraceptive Use*. New York: Alan Guttmacher Institute; 2004.
18. FFPRHC Guidance (October 2004) Contraceptive choices for young people. *J Fam Plann Reprod Health Care* 2004;30:237–51.
19. Wight D, Henderson M, Raab G. Extent of regretted sexual intercourse among young teenagers in Scotland: a cross sectional survey. *BMJ* 2000;320:1243–4.
20. Wellings K, Nanchahal K, Macdowall W, McManus S, Erens B, Mercer CH, *et al.* Sexual behaviour in Britain: early heterosexual experience. *Lancet* 2001;358:1843–50.
21. Teenage Pregnancy Unit, Department of Health. *Best Practice Guidance for Doctors and other Health Professionals on the Provision of Advice and Treatment to Young People Under 16 on Contraception, Sexual and Reproductive Health*. London: The Stationery Office; 2004.
22. Royal College of General Practitioners and Brook. *Confidentiality and Young People. Improving Teenagers' Uptake of Sexual and Other Health Advice*. London: RCGP, Brook; 2000.
23. World Health Organization. *Medical Eligibility Criteria for Contraceptive Use: Improving Access to Quality Care in Family Planning*. Geneva: WHO; 2004.
24. Collaborative Group on Hormonal Factors in Breast Cancer. Breast cancer and hormonal contraceptives: collaborative reanalysis of individual data on 53,297 women with breast cancer and 100,239 women without breast cancer from 54 epidemiological studies. *Lancet* 1996;347:1713–27.
25. Committee on Safety of Medicines. Combined oral contraceptives containing desogestrel or

gestodene and the risk of venous thromboembolism. *Current Problems in Pharmacovigilance* 1999;25:1–2.

26. Cromer BA, McCarthy M. Family planning services in adolescent pregnancy prevention: the views of key informants in four countries. *Fam Plann Perspect* 1999;31:287–93.

27. Kane R, Macdowall W, Wellings K. Providing information for young people in sexual health clinics: getting it right. *J Fam Plann Reprod Health Care* 2003;29:141–5.

28. Little P, Griffin S, Kelly J, Dickson N, Sadler C. Effect of educational leaflets and questions on knowledge of contraception in women taking the combined contraceptive pill: randomised controlled trial. *BMJ* 1998;316:1948–52.

29. Postgraduate award in sexual health in primary care. 2005 [www2.warwick.ac.uk/fac/med/healthcom/primary_care/courses_intro/courses/sexhealth].

Chapter 15
Contraception for older women

Ailsa E Gebbie

Introduction

In the Western World, patterns of contraceptive use vary significantly with age. Women in their later reproductive years may have anxieties about using particular methods at that stage of their life and many abandon contraception altogether before they achieve natural sterility at time of menopause. Although fertility is lower in women over the age of 40 years, it is not zero. A late unplanned pregnancy can have devastating consequences for an individual woman. There is no method of contraception that is contraindicated by age alone and all methods become increasingly effective with age. As a consequence of declining ovarian function, women generally progress from having regular ovulatory menstrual cycles to a phase of menstrual dysfunction until the onset of menopause. Choice of contraceptive method may impact on both menstrual pattern and menopausal symptomatology. Clinicians need to be able to give clear advice about which methods of contraception are suitable for older women and when contraception can be discontinued.

Fertility and pregnancy in older women

Although menopause marks the end of reproduction for women, studies of healthy populations not using contraception have shown significant declines in fertility with age prior to menopause.[1] For example, French Canadians in the 19th century had their last child at an average age of 41 years and 70% of women ended childbearing within the 37–44 years age span.[2]

Pregnancies in women aged over 50 years are uncommon. The oldest known woman to give birth following a spontaneous conception was 57 years and 129 days.[3] Assisted conception techniques have made pregnancies possible well into the postmenopausal age range but only by using donor eggs.[4] A Romanian woman of 67 years reportedly conceived twins following egg donation.[5]

Physiological ageing of the ovary is undoubtedly the main factor in age-related fertility decline. In the mid-to-late 30s, there is acceleration in spontaneous follicle atresia from the ovaries and oocytes are more susceptible to aneuploidy and mitochondrial mutations.[6]

Older women also have significantly increased rates of miscarriage, principally caused by chromosomal abnormalities. A Danish survey showed that the risk of spontaneous miscarriage was 8.9% in women aged 20–24 years and 74.7% in those aged

45 years or more.[7] The risk of Down syndrome at live birth increases from one in nearly 2000 at a maternal age of 20 years to one in 30 at age 40 years.[8] In the UK, nearly 40% of total conceptions in women aged over 40 years will end in therapeutic abortion.[9]

Older mothers have a higher risk of hypertensive disorders, gestational diabetes and operative delivery. Risk of delivering a low-birthweight or preterm infant increases with advancing maternal age and the risk of stillbirth rises to more than 10/1000 births in women over 40 years: more than double the risk in women aged 20 years.[10] There is an increase in pregnancy-related deaths with age and national US data show figures of 9, 21 and 46 deaths per 100 000 live births among women aged 25–29 years, 35–39 years and over 40 years, respectively.[11] The investigators commented that although the risk of pregnancy-related deaths in women aged 35 years or older has declined over the last 20 years, it is still significantly higher than among younger women.

Sexual activity and older women

In adult women, coital frequency is inversely associated with age. Data from the National Survey of Sexual Attitudes and Lifestyles (NATSAL) in the UK showed that frequency of sexual activity in the last 4 weeks was 7.7 for women aged 16–24 years and 5.7 for women aged 35–44 years.[12] Length of relationship is closely associated with frequency of sexual activity at all ages: the number of episodes of coitus decreasing with longer relationships. However, with the current UK divorce rate of two in five, many individuals will be commencing new relationships at relatively older ages with increased frequency of sexual activity. The prevalence of sexual dysfunction is high in women in their older reproductive years. One survey of perimenopausal women in the community reported one-third of women as having sexual problems. Around 17% had impaired sexual interest, 17% had vaginal dryness and 16% had infrequent orgasm. Despite the high frequency of sexual dysfunction in this study, only 4% of the women stated that they would seek help for a sexual problem.[13] Some women report improvement in their sexuality as a result of children leaving home, greater leisure time and lack of menstruation.

Methods of contraception

In the Western World, where contraceptive choice is available, striking changes are seen in patterns of contraceptive use with age (Table 15.1). The risks of the various contraceptive methods will vary with age and some methods may be associated with important noncontraceptive benefits that are particularly relevant to the older woman.

Combined oral contraception

The combined oral contraceptive (COC) is a popular method of reversible contraception worldwide and is of high efficacy in women of all ages. In the UK, it is used by around 6% of women aged 40–44 years and 2% of women aged 45–49 years.[14] A significant reduction in both oestrogen and progestogen dosages has occurred over the last four decades. The modern, low dose preparations containing 20–35 micrograms ethinylestradiol are undoubtedly safer. There is no upper age limit for use of COCs by women who are healthy, at low risk and nonsmokers. It is generally acknowledged that, in practice, such women may continue with COCs until the age of around 50 years.[15]

Table 15.1. Current use of contraception by age in the UK in 2003–04 (reproduced with permission, ONS, 2004)

Current use of contraception	Age (years)								All (%)
	16–17 (%)	18–19 (%)	20–24 (%)	25–29 (%)	30–34 (%)	35–39 (%)	40–44 (%)	44–49 (%)	
Combined pill	20	29	31	31	24	10	6	2	17
Progestogen only pill	1	14	9	6	4	4	5	2	5
Male condom	33	36	37	24	24	22	15	14	23
Withdrawal	3	–	1	3	5	5	1	1	3
Injection/implant	3	2	6	5	4	3	1	1	4
Natural family planning	–	–	1	1	2	1	1	0	3
Diaphragm or cap	–	1	0	0	1	1	1	2	1
Spermicides alone	–	–	–	–	–	–	–	1	0
Intrauterine device	2	–	1	3	5	5	5	4	3
Intrauterine system	–	–	0	1	1	1	1	1	1
Female condom	–	–	–	–	0	0	–	–	0
Emergency contraception	5	4	2	0	0	0	–	–	1
Female sterilisation	–	1	2	3	5	17	17	25	11
Male sterilisation	–	–	1	4	9	15	25	20	12
Total using at least one method of contraception	50	71	78	73	77	80	77	73	75

The World Health Organization (WHO) has stated that, for women aged 40 years and over, the advantages of using the oral contraceptive pill generally outweigh any theoretical or proven risks.[16] Long-term follow-up studies on COCs have been published, which give uniformly reassuring data on safety.[17] Cigarette smoking, however, consistently appears to double risk of mortality from all causes.[18] Women who smoke must always be advised to discontinue COCs at the age of 35 years.

Cardiovascular disease

It is useful to differentiate the cardiovascular events associated with COC use into arterial and venous disease, as the risk factors vary accordingly and are particularly relevant to older women. Venous thromboembolism (VTE) is the most common cardiovascular event among users of modern, low dose COCs, although the associated morbidity and mortality is relatively low compared with that associated with arterial diseases.

Arterial disease

The incidence of arterial disease associated with COCs is now extremely small, as low-dose pills are universally prescribed and women with significant risk factors for arterial disease should not be prescribed COCs.

Myocardial infarction is uncommon in women of reproductive age and deaths are even more rare. Smoking and hypertension are both significant risk factors for myocardial infarction. Nonsmokers of any age without specific risk factors, such as hypertension, can be reassured that they have no increased risk of myocardial infarction with low-dose COC use.[19] From a meta-analysis of studies, there is no evidence of increased risk in past COC users and clear evidence of a dose related effect with older pills.[20] Based on several case–control studies which examined excess risk of myocardial infarction after cessation of smoking, the Clinical Effective Unit of the Faculty of Family Planning and Reproductive Health Care in the UK advised that previous smokers over the age of 35 years may consider the use of COC one year after stopping smoking.[21]

As with myocardial infarction, the risk of stroke is low in women of reproductive age but increases with advancing age.[22] The WHO has comprehensively reviewed risk of both ischaemic and haemorrhagic stroke related to use of hormonal contraception.[19] Normotensive nonsmokers have a two-fold increase in the risk of ischaemic stroke with COC use although the absolute risk is small. No significant increase in risk of haemorrhagic stroke with COC use has been shown. Hypertension increases risk of stroke and COC users with hypertension have up to a ten-fold increased risk of haemorrhagic stroke and a small increase in ischaemic stroke compared with normotensive COC users. Smoking is also a major risk factor for stroke and when smokers take COC the risk of ischaemic stroke is increased significantly (OR 7.2 95%, CI 3.23–16.1). In view of this, it is good clinical practice that COC is not prescribed to older women who smoke over the age of 35 years or who are hypertensive.

Venous thromboembolism

It is well established that COC increases the risk of VTE at least three- to six-fold and the risk seems highest in the first year of use.[23] There is a modest effect on risk of VTE with age in COC users, although the same age-related pattern occurs in women in general, independent of COC use.[24] Obesity, recent surgery, presence of malignancy and inherited thrombophilic disorder are independent risk factors for venous thromboembolism. Selection of appropriate COC preparation for an older woman should be based on using the lowest effective oestrogen dose for cycle control in combination with the progestogen of choice.

Cancer

In premenopausal women, the risk of breast cancer rises sharply with age. A woman of 35 years has a 1/500 risk of developing breast cancer which increases to a 1/100 risk by the age of 45 years.[25] A large reanalysis of the worldwide data on COC use and breast cancer found a small increase in risk of breast cancer in current users (RR1.24; 95% CI 1.15–1.33).[26] Among 10 000 women aged 40–44 years who used COCs for 5 years, 262 cases of breast cancer would be expected up to the age of 55 years: 32 more cases than among never users (230 cases/10 000 women). For women aged 20–24 years, there would only be 1.5 extra cases of breast cancer in 10 000 COC users. Within this reanalysis, the added risk of breast cancer among current COC users takes 10 years to return to normal after stopping therapy but was not influenced by duration of use. Within another case–control study, any excess risk did not appear to be influenced by family history (without *BRCA* gene mutations), age at first use, dose or type of hormone.[27]

There is a complex association between COCs and cervical cancer. Data suggest that long duration use of COCs appears to be associated with an increased risk of cervical cancer: 10 year use of COCs gave a relative risk of 2.2 (95% CI 1.9–2.4).[28] One multicentre case–control study identified a four-fold increased risk of cervical cancer in women using COCs in excess of 10 years who were positive for cervical human papillomavirus.[29] It is simply not known whether there is any lasting effect on risk of cervical cancer at older ages after COC use has ceased. Numerous studies confirm a protective effect of COC on ovarian, endometrial and bowel cancer. COC use decreased risk of epithelial ovarian cancer by over 50% and the reduction in risk lasted for at least 15 years after discontinuing COCs.[30] Similarly, COC use reduced risk of endometrial cancer by at least 50% with protection continuing for 15 years after stopping.[31] COCs offer a degree of protection against colorectal cancer and one meta-analysis of the data showed a relative risk of 0.82 (95% CI 0.74–0.92), although the possible mechanism for this benefit is not understood.[32]

COCs reduce the incidence of benign breast disease, particularly development of fibroadenomas and cystic disease.[33] Although older studies show that COCs decrease risk of functional ovarian cysts, this appears to be dose related and it is less clear that modern low-dose preparations offer the same degree of protection.[34]

Menstrual benefits

As women reach their later reproductive years, they frequently experience irregular, heavy or painful menstruation, which often results in inconvenience to lifestyle, days off work and gynaecological consultations. A Cochrane systematic review failed to identify adequate evidence that COCs reduce menstrual blood loss and dysmenorrhoea.[35] Small studies have shown a reduction in measured menstrual blood loss of around 40% and, in clinical practice, it is a useful agent in this respect.[36] COC users have significantly fewer hospital referrals for menstrual problems and are less likely to undergo hysterectomy.[37]

Osteoporosis

Evidence-based analysis suggests that COCs have a favourable effect on bone mineral density.[38] Long-term users seem to reach the menopause with bone density 2–3% higher than nonusers but it is not known whether this effect confers any benefit to prevent lifetime risk of fracture. In one study of women aged 40–60 years, COCs suppressed bone turnover more than standard hormone replacement therapy (HRT) and only COCs significantly increased femoral neck bone mineral density.[39] In terms of actual fracture risk, a population-based case–control study of hip fracture in Swedish postmenopausal women aged 50–81 years found a decreased risk in women who used COCs late in reproductive life.[40] Ever-users of COCs were associated with a 25% reduction in hip fracture risk (OR 0.75; 95% CI 0.59–0.96) and there was a trend of increased protection with higher-dose COCs.

Progestogen-only methods

Progestogen-only methods of contraception offer particular advantages for older women. They can be prescribed for older women with contraindications to COCs: in particular, women aged over 35 years who smoke or have other risk factors for cardiovascular disease. There seems to be no significant increase in the relative risk of stroke, myocardial infarction or venous thromboembolic disease among women using progestogen-only methods, although relatively few studies have assessed this area.[19] They are associated with both menstrual irregularity and amenorrhoea which may cause concern regarding possible underlying gynaecological disease or confusion over onset of menopause.

Progestogen-only pills

The overall failure rate of the progestogen-only pill (POP) is 2–3/100 women-years, which is significantly highly than COCs. However, because of increased inhibition of ovulation at older ages, the failure rate of POP is only 0.3/100 women-years in women over 40 years, which is equivalent to efficacy of COC in young women.[41] The POP is a useful contraceptive for older women who wish to continue with an oral method which avoids the small risks associated with oestrogen containing pills.

Depot medroxyprogesterone acetate

Depot medroxyprogesterone acetate (DMPA) is an extremely effective contraceptive method for women of all ages and is given by intramuscular injection at a dose of 150 mg. It will help dysmenorrhoea and menorrhagia and is a useful strategy to treat premenstrual syndrome and menstrual migraine. It has few adverse effects and most long-term users will become amenorrhoeic.

DMPA has significantly suppressive effects on ovarian production of oestradiol and there are concerns about its prolonged use and potential development of osteoporosis. There is conflicting evidence and it is not possible to give a definitive evidence-based answer. Some data are reassuring and show similar bone density in past users of DMPA and those who have never used it.[42] Other data show bone loss at the hip and spine in DMPA users compared with controls.[43] Any loss of bone mineral density appears to recover when DMPA is stopped.[44] There is no consensus on whether it is of value to check an oestradiol level, perform a 'routine' bone density scan or prescribe exogenous oestrogen to long-term or older DMPA users.

It seems reasonable to recommend women consider discontinuing DMPA at around the age of 45 years, to allow for any spontaneous recovery of bone density prior to the actual menopause. For some women, the menstrual advantages of using DMPA far outweigh any theoretical risk of developing osteoporosis.

Etonorgestrel implant

The etonorgestrel implant is a single polyethylene vinyl acetate rod inserted subdermally into the upper arm. The rod releases the progestogen etonorgestrel at a dose of around 67 mg/day.[45] It is effective for up to 3 years and is generally well tolerated, with 82% of women in clinical trials continuing its use beyond 2 years. Although most studies excluded women aged over 40 years, there is no reason that would contraindicate its use in women purely because of age.

Hormonal emergency contraception

Levonorgestrel-only is the hormonal emergency contraception of choice. It has virtually no contraindications and can be purchased over the counter without prescription in the UK.[46] It can be recommended for a woman of any age if an episode of unprotected intercourse has occurred and she is deemed to be at risk of pregnancy. A single dose (1500 micrograms) is taken within 72 hours of unprotected intercourse.

Intrauterine device

The modern copper intrauterine device (IUD) is a highly effective and cost-effective method of contraception for women of all ages.[47] Older women who use IUDs have a lower incidence of pelvic infection, expulsion and failure, including ectopic pregnancy, compared with younger IUD users.[48] Most IUD users have a modest increase in menstrual blood loss, slightly earlier onset of bleeding in the luteal phase and a degree of increased dysmenorrhoea.[49] Women who become perimenopausal with an IUD in place may well experience bleeding difficulties, although this menstrual disturbance is generally related to the effect of hormonal changes on the endometrium rather than the device itself.

Intrauterine system

The intrauterine system (IUS), which releases levonorgestrel at 20 micrograms/day, offers highly effective contraception and can reduce menstrual blood loss by around 90%.[50] It therefore has particular advantages for older women with menstrual dysfunction who require contraception. Although erratic bleeding is a frequent initial problem, studies have shown rates of amenorrhoea of nearly 50% at 12 months after insertion.[51] Several small studies have demonstrated a decrease in mean uterine volume and size of uterine fibroids in women using an IUS for treatment of menorrhagia.[52]

An older woman using an IUS for contraception plus menstrual dysfunction may have it replaced every 5 years until she becomes menopausal. In addition, the IUS is licensed for use as the progestogen component of HRT in many Western countries. The combination of systemic oestrogen and an IUS has been shown to diminish menopausal symptoms and induce endometrial atrophy.[53] A woman may have an IUS inserted just for this indication or may be a pre-existing user who simply adds the oestrogen of choice. The probability of irregular bleeding and spotting in the first few months after insertion when combined with systemic oestrogen is high, although thereafter amenorrhoea is common.[54] The IUS may also have a role in the reversal of endometrial hyperplasia through its potent endometrial effect, particularly in women unsuitable for surgery.[55]

Anecdotally, some women report improvement in symptoms of premenstrual syndrome, particularly in the early phase of using an IUS. Although one noncomparative study of women using IUS did report a reduction in subjective premenstrual symptoms of nearly 56%, there is insufficient evidence that the IUS alone is effective in this respect.[47]

Barrier methods

In the Western World, condoms are widely used across the age ranges.[22] Older individuals entering into new relationships should be advised to use condoms for personal protection against infection. The diaphragm and cervical cap are of declining popularity in many Western countries. They are low-risk, woman-controlled methods of contraception that older women use more reliably, with significantly lower failure rates, than younger users.[56]

Sterilisation

The sterilisation rates for both men and women in the UK are significantly higher than in many other European countries. Around 45% of women aged 45–49 years in the UK rely on a permanent surgical procedure for contraception.[14] In Europe, more than 50% of sterilised women will have undergone their procedure before the age of 35 years.[57] It seems logical that older women, who are close to natural sterility, should avoid a surgical procedure but individual assessment and choice are important. Women who are sterilised at older ages are much less likely to regret having the procedure performed.[58] Women requesting sterilisation can be reassured that there is no known association between tubal occlusion and increased risk of heavier or longer periods.[59]

Stopping contraception

The standard advice is that women should continue contraception for 1 year following their last spontaneous menstrual period, if aged over 50 years. Women under the age of 50 years should continue with contraception for 2 further years following their last period to exclude the likelihood of further ovulation. Levels of hormones, such as follicle-stimulating hormone (FSH) and oestradiol, fluctuate widely during the perimenopause and, in general, it is not helpful to base guidance on when contraception can be stopped on isolated hormone analyses.[60]

It is good practice to advise most women to stop the combined pill at the age of 50 years, as the risks of COCs increase with age and around 50% will already be postmenopausal.[61] Women who use COCs for contraception can be advised to change to a POP or a barrier method to allow assessment of menstrual cycle, menopausal status and thereby the requirements for contraception or possibly HRT. There is evidence of a rise in FSH at the end of the pill-free interval in COC users who have reached menopause but insufficient data to be helpful in clinical practice.[62]

Women aged over 45 years who are taking a POP and are amenorrhoeic can have a random serum FSH level checked. If two FSH levels at least 1 month apart are within the menopausal range, then contraception can be discontinued after one further year.[21] It is accepted clinical practice that a copper-containing IUD inserted at or after the age of 40 years can remain in place until the women becomes menopausal.[63]

Hormone replacement therapy

The onset of menopausal symptoms generally predates the final menstrual period. Once a perimenopausal woman has commenced HRT, it becomes impossible to assess accurately when natural sterility has been achieved. Conventional sequential HRT is not a reliable method of contraceptive and women may still ovulate and potentially conceive.[64] High-dose HRT regimens have been shown to suppress ovulation.[65] Barrier methods of contraception, an IUD or the POP can all be continued in conjunction with HRT. In practice, it usually is most convenient to recommend that women who started HRT prior to the menopause should continue contraception to the age of 55 years, when natural sterility can be assumed.

References

1. Eaton JW, Mayer AJ. The social biology of very high fertility among the Hutterites. The demography of a unique population. *Hum Biol* 1953;25:206–64.
2. Desjardins B, Bideau A, Brunet G. Age of mother at last birth in two historical populations. *J BioSoc Sci* 1994;26:509–16.
3. Guinness World Records. *Guinness Book of Records*. London: Bantam Books; 2000.
4. Navot D, Bergh PA, Williams MA, Garrisi GJ, Guzman I, Sandler B, *et al.* Poor oocyte quality rather than implantation failure as a cause of age-related decline in female infertility. *Lancet* 1991;337:1375–7.
5. Woman expecting twins at age of 67 years. *The Scotsman.* Friday 31 December 2004.
6. Faddy MJ, Gosden RD. Mathematical model for follicle dynamics in human ovaries. *Hum Reprod* 1995;10:770–5.
7. Andersen AM, Wohlfahrt J, Christen P, Olsen J, Melbye M. Maternal age and fetal loss: population based register linkage study. *BMJ* 2000;320:1708–12.
8. Hook EB, Cross PK, Schreinemachers DM. Chromosomal abnormality rates at amniocentesis and in live-born infant. *JAMA* 1983;249:2034–8.
9. Office of National Statistics. Conceptions by age of woman at conception, *2002 Health Statistics Quarterly 24*. London: HMSO; 2004.
10. Salihu HM, Shumpert MN, Slay M, Kirby RS, Alexander GR. Childbearing beyond maternal age 50 and fetal outcomes in the United States. *Obstet Gynecol* 2003;102:1006–14.
11. Callaghan WM, Berg CJ. Pregnancy related mortality among women aged 35 years and older, United States. 1991–1997, *Obstet Gynecol* 2003;102:1015–21.
12. Johnson AM, Mercer CH, Erens B, Copas AJ, McManus S, Wellings K, *et al.* Sexual behaviour in Britain: partnerships, practices and HIV risk behaviour. *Lancet* 2001;358:1835–42.
13. Osborn M, Hawton K, Gath D. Sexual dysfunction among middle aged women in the community. *Br Med J (Clin Res Ed)* 1988;296:959–62.
14. Dawe F, Rainford L. *Contraception and Sexual Health, 2003*. London: Office for National Statistics; 2004.
15. Fortney JA. Oral contraceptives for older women. *IPPF Med Bull* 1990;24:3–4.
16. World Health Organization. *Improving Access to Quality Care in Family Planning. Medical Eligibility Criteria for Contraceptive Use*. WHO/FRH/FPP/96.9. Geneva: World Health Organization; 1996.
17. Beral V, Hermon C, Kay C, Hannaford P, Darby S, Reeves G. Mortality associated with oral contraceptive use: 25 year follow up of cohort of 46,000 women from the Royal College of General Practitioners' oral contraception study. *BMJ* 1999;318:96–100.
18. Vessey MP, Painter R, Yeats D. Mortality in relation to oral contraceptive use and cigarette smoking. *Lancet* 2003;362:185–91.
19. World Health Organization. Cardiovascular disease and use of oral and injectable progestogen-only

contraceptive and combined injectable contraceptives. Results of an international multicentre, case-control study. *Contraception* 1998;57:315–24.

20. Khader YS, Rice J, John L, Abueita O. Oral contraceptives use and the risk of myocardial infarction: a meta-analysis. *Contraception* 2003;68:11–17.

21. Faculty of Family Planning and Reproductive Health Care Clinical Effectiveness Unit. Contraception for women over 40 years. *J Fam Plann Reprod Health Care* 2005;31:51–63.

22. Office of National Statistics. *Deaths by Age, Sex and Underlying Causes, 2003 Registrations.* London: HMSO Publications; 2004.

23. Jick H, Kaye JA, Vasilakis-Scaramozza C, Jick S. Risk of venous thromboembolism among users of third generation oral contraceptives compared with users of oral contraceptives with levonorgestrel before and after 1995: cohort and case-control analysis. *BMJ* 2000;321:1190–5.

24. Burkman R, Schlesselman JJ, Zieman M. Safety concerns and health benefits associated with oral contraception. *Am J Obstet Gynecol* 2004;190(4 Suppl):S5–22.

25. Tuckey J. Combined oral contraception and cancer. *Br J Fam Plann* 2000;26:237–40.

26. Collaborative Group on Hormonal Factors in breast Cancer. Breast Cancer and hormonal contraceptives: collaborative reanalysis of individual data on 53,297 women with breast cancer and 100,239 women without breast cancer from 543 epidemiological studies. *Lancet* 1996;347:1713–27.

27. Marchbanks PA, McDonald JA, Wilson HG, Folger SG, Mandel MG, Daling JR, *et al.* Oral contraceptives and the risk of breast cancer. *N Engl J Med* 2002;346:2025–32.

28. Smith JS, Green J, Berrington de Gonzalez A, Appleby P, Peto J, Plummer M, *et al.* Cervical cancer and use of hormonal contraception: a systemic review. *Lancet* 2003;361:1159–67.

29. Moreno V, Bosch FX, Munoz N, Meijer CJ, Shah KV, Walboomers JM, *et al.* Effect of oral contraceptives on risk of cervical cancer in women with human papilloma infection: the IARC multicentric case-control study. *Lancet* 2002;359:1085–92.

30. International Agency for Research on Cancer. *Hormonal Contraception and Postmenopausal Hormonal Therapy.* Monographs on the Evaluation of Carcinogenic Risks to Humans. Lyons: IARC; 1999.

31. Weiderpass E, Adami H, Baron JA, Magnusson C, Lindgren A, Persson I. Use of oral contraceptives and endometrial cancer (Sweden). *Cancer Causes Control* 1999;10:277–84.

32. Fernandez E, Vecchia CL, Balducci A, Chatenoud L, Francheschi S, Negri E. Oral contraceptives and colorectal cancer risk: a meta-analysis. *Br J Cancer* 2001;84:722–7.

33. Rohan T, Miller A. A cohort study of oral contraceptive use and benign breast disease. *Int J Cancer* 1999;82:191–6.

34. Chiaffarino F, Parazini F, La Vecchia C, Ricc E, Crosignani PG. Oral contraceptive use and benign gynecologic condition: a review. *Contraception* 1998;57:11–18.

35. Iyer V, Farquhar C, Jepson R. Oral contraceptive pills for heavy menstrual bleeding *Cochrane Database Syst Rev* 2003;(2):1–2.

36. Larsson G, Milson I, Lindstedt G, Rybo G. The influence of low-dose combined oral contraception on menstrual blood loss and iron status. *Contraception* 1992;46:327–34.

37. Vessey M, Painter R, Mant J. Oral contraception and other factors in relation to hospital referral for menstrual problems without known underlying cause: findings in a large cohort study. *Br J Fam Plann* 1996;22:166–9.

38. Kunhong W, Borgatta L, Stubblefield P. Low dose oral contraceptives and bone mineral density: an evidence base analysis. *Contraception* 2000;61:77–82.

39. Taechakraichana N, Limpaphayom K, Ninlagarn T, Panyakhamlerd K, Chaikittisilpa S, Dusitsin N. A randomised trial of oral contraceptive and hormone replacement therapy on bone mineral density and coronayr heart disease risk factors in postmenopausal women. *Obstet Gynecol* 2000;95:87–94.

40. Michaelsson K, Baron J, Farahmand B, Persson I, Ljunghall S. Oral contraceptive use and risk of hip fracture: a case control study. *Lancet* 1999;353:1481–4.

41. Vessey MP, Lawless M, Yeats D, McPherson K. Progestogen only oral contraception. Findings in a large prospective study with special reference to effectiveness. *Br J Fam Plann* 1985;10:117–21.

42. Orr-Walker BJ, Evans MC, Ames RW, Clearwater JM, Cundy T, Reid IR. The effect of past use of the injectable contraceptive depot medroxyprogesterone acetate on bone mineral density in normal postmenopausal women. *Clin Endocrinol* 1998;49:615–18.

43. Banks E, Berrington A, Casabonne D. Overview of the relationship between the use of progestogen only contraceptives and bone mineral density. *BJOG* 2001;108:1214–21.

44. Cundy T, Cornish J, Evans MC, Roberts H, Reid IR. Recovery of bone density in women who stop using medroxyprogesterone acetate. *BMJ* 1994;308:247–8.

45. Drugs and Therapeutic Bulletin. Etonogestrel implant (Implanon) for contraception. *Drug Ther Bull* 2001;39:57–9.

46. Trussell J, Ellertson C, Stewart F, Raymond EG, Shochet T. The role of emergency contraception.

Am J Obstet Gynecol 2004;190 (4 Suppl):S30–8.

47. Barrington JW, Bowen-Simpkins P. The levonorgestrel intrauterine system in the management of idiopathic menorrhagia. *Br J Obstet Gynaecol* 1997;104:614–16.

48. Chi IC. What we have learned from recent IUD studies: a researcher's perspective. *Contraception* 1993;48:81–108.

49. Faundes A, Segal SJ, Adejuwon CA, Brache V, Leon P, Alvarez-Sanchez F. The menstrual cycle in women using an intrauterine device. *Fertil Steril* 1980;34:427–30.

50. Andersson K, Rybo G. Levonorgestrel-releasing intrauterine device in the treatment of menorrhagia. *BJOG* 1990;97:690–4.

51. Hidalgo M, Bahamondes L, Perrotti M, Diaz J, Dantas-Monteiro C, Petta C. Bleeding patterns and clinical performance of the levonorgestrel-releasing intrauterine system up to two year. *Contraception* 2002;65:129–32.

52. Grigorieva V, Chen-Mok M, Tarasova M, Mikhailov A. Use of a levonorgestrel-releasing intrauterine system to treat bleeding related to uterine leiomyomas. *Fertil Steril* 2003;79:1194–8.

53. Riphagen FE. Intrauterine application of progestins in hormone replacement therapy: a review. *Climacteric* 2000;3:199–212.

54. Raudaskoski T, Tapanainen J, Tomas E, Luotola H, Pekonen F, Ronni-Sivula H, *et al.* Intrauterine 10 micrograms and 20 micrograms levonorgestrel systems in postmenopausal women receiving oral oestrogen replacement therapy: clinical, endometrial and metabolic response. *BJOG* 2002;109:136–144.

55. Wildemeersch D, Dhont M. Treatment of non-atypical endometrial hyperplasia with a levonorgestrel-releasing intra-uterine system. *Am J Obstet Gynecol* 2003;188:1297–8.

56. Gallo MF, Grimes DA, Schulz KF. Cervical cap versus diaphragm for contraception. *Cochrane Database Syst Rev* 2002;(4):CD003551.

57. Skouby SO. Contraceptive behaviour in the 21st century: a comprehensive study across five European countries. *Eur J Contracept Reprod Health Care* 2004;9:57–68.

58. Hillis SD, Marchbanks PA, Tylor LR, Peterson HB. Poststerilization regret: findings from the United States review of sterilisation. *Obstet Gynecol* 1999;93:889–95.

59. Royal College of Obstetricians and Gynaecologists. *Male and Female Sterilisation*. Evidence based Clinical Guidelines Number 4. London: RCOG Press; 2004.

60. Bastien LA, Smith CM, Nanda K. Is this woman perimenopausal? *JAMA* 2003;289:895–902.

61. Treloar AE. Menstrual cyclicity and the pre-menopause. *Maturitas* 1981;3:249–64.

62. Creinin MD. Laboratory criteria for menopause in women using oral contraceptive. *Contraception* 1996;66:101–4.

63. Newton J, Tacchi D. Long term use of copper intra-uterine devices. *Lancet* 1990;335:1322–3.

64. Gebbie AE, Glasier A, Sweeting V. Incidence of ovulation in perimenopausal women before and during hormone replacement therapy. *Contraception* 1995;52:221–2.

65. Smith RNJ, Studd JWW, Zamblera D, Holland EFN. A randomised comparison over 8 months of 100 micrograms and 200 micrograms twice weekly dose of trandermal oestradiol in the treatment of severe premenstrual syndrome. *BJOG* 1995;102:475–84.

SECTION 2
MAKING THINGS BETTER

Chapter 16
Potential new targets for female contraception

David T Baird

Introduction

Effective contraception is one of the keystones of reproductive health.[1] Without easy access to a range of contraceptive services, couples are unable to plan the number of children they wish. Women, in particular, are denied the opportunity of developing their full potential by participating in all aspects of society because of 'the burden of excess fertility'.[2] The introduction of the combined oral contraceptive pill in the early 1960s was truly a major breakthrough in methods of contraception.[3] Since the 1960s, the contraceptive pill has been refined by lowering the doses of oestrogen and progestogen. In addition, steroid hormones have been administered by a variety of routes, such as intramuscular injection or subcutaneous implant, allowing choice from a wider range of contraceptive methods.[4] However, all of these methods have involved steroid hormones, which are associated with some common minor adverse effects as well as rare major adverse events. There has been no totally novel method of contraception marketed since the 1960s, in spite of the fact that our knowledge of the female reproductive system has expanded enormously. There is no shortage of potential targets.

Is there a need?

The rate of increase in the world's population is slowing.[5] Contraceptive prevalence has increased worldwide, from around 10% in the 1960s up to over 60% by the year 2000. In most developed countries, where the prevalence is over 70%, the total fertility rate is below replacement level.[6] These figures alone are evidence that, given the will, people can regulate the number of children they have using existing methods of contraception. However, these overall figures disguise certain disadvantages of current methods.

Many of the hormonal methods are associated with minor adverse effects, such as breakthrough bleeding, weight gain and premenstrual symptoms.[7] These minor adverse effects are tolerated but are certainly not welcomed by many women and are a frequent cause for discontinuation of a method. In addition, there are certain rare serious adverse effects, such as thromboembolic events, which are contraindications to use by certain women who are at risk.[8] Thus, although modern methods overall are extremely safe (much safer than the risk of dying during pregnancy), they are not ideal.

Even in developed countries where there is easy access to modern methods of effective contraception, there is evidence that many pregnancies are unplanned and/or unwanted.[9] In many Western European countries and North America about one in four pregnancies are terminated by induced abortion.[10] About one-third of those pregnancies which continue and result in a live birth are unplanned. Combining these two facts, it is apparent that up to 50% of conceptions are unplanned, even in a society where men and women have easy access to modern effective methods of contraception. The reasons for this high incidence of unplanned pregnancies are complex and include ambivalence about the desire to avoid pregnancy, organisation of services, education and other factors.[11] However, a significant proportion of unplanned pregnancies occur because of failure of the method. Most modern methods are highly effective if used perfectly. In practice, their failure rate is determined not only by the intrinsic efficacy of the method but also by how well it is used (effectiveness).[12] Thus, methods such as the progestogen-only pill, which rely on the woman taking a pill at a specific time every day, are much less effective than those which make fewer demands on the user, such as depot injections.[13]

For some methods, there are some concerns about their long-term risks. For example, there is now good evidence that there is a small increased risk of developing breast cancer in women while taking the combined oral contraceptive pill and for up to 10 years after stopping it.[14] In contrast, the long-term risk of developing endometrial and ovarian cancer is decreased.[15] Breast cancer is much more common than either ovarian or endometrial cancer in modern society. There is an increased risk of breast cancer associated with delay in age of first pregnancy, which is probably a product of repeated sterile ovarian cycles. It has been suggested that suppression of ovarian activity with, for example, gonadotrophin-releasing hormone (GnRH) agonists or antagonists could reduce the risk of developing breast cancer.[16] Such a method would be popular with individual women, as well as conveying a huge public health advantage.

In summary, in spite of the declining fertility rates worldwide modern methods of contraception still leave a lot to be desired. In view of its complexity, it is not surprising that the female reproductive system has many potential targets for disruption for contraceptive purposes. It is likely that any new method will be better accepted if it also has health benefits over the 'normal' state of repeated menstrual cycles.

Since the 1970s, there have been a number of reviews attempting to identify new approaches and predict new contraceptive developments.[17–21] In the 1970s and 1980s, as our knowledge about the functioning of the reproductive system was better understood, a number of potential physiological systems were targeted, such as the hypothalamus, ovulation and so on. With the discovery of the molecular mechanisms involved in many of these processes, the structure of specific potential targets, such as the follicle-stimulating hormone (FSH) receptor, have been identified.[21] The fact that no product has yet been developed is not due to lack of scientific knowledge but for other commercial reasons. Compared with many drugs, the product development of a new contraceptive is expensive and relatively high in risk. It has been calculated that the time from discovery to marketing a product is approximately 15 years and costs up to US$800 million.[22] Large numbers of healthy men and women will be exposed to potentially harmful drugs for much of their life. The long-term consequences of such exposure might not become apparent for several decades. For this reason, it is unlikely that the pattern of contraceptive use will change radically in the next 10 years. No one method will be suitable for everyone. Hence, although it is often talked about, we are not looking for the 'ideal contraceptive'.

What is the preferred approach?

The establishment of pregnancy involves growth and development of the follicle, ovulation and fertilisation of a mature oocyte and implantation of the early embryo in the decidua of the uterus. It is often thought that the 'ideal contraceptive' would be one that prevented pregnancy by targeting a process that was unique to the reproductive system and, hence, had no effects elsewhere in the body (Table 16.1).[21] For example, if the maturation of the oocyte were to be disrupted, cyclical ovarian activity would persist but pregnancy would not occur because the oocyte could not be fertilised.

Methods such as this, however, which result in the persistence of recurrent sterile ovarian and menstrual cycles, are by no means 'natural'. Most female mammals have long periods of natural infertility when ovarian cycles cease.[23] Women are no exception. The amenorrhoea which occurs during pregnancy and lactation is a sign of inhibition of ovulation. These natural periods of infertility provide a clue to novel ways of interfering with reproductive function for contraception.[24] Recurrent menstrual cycles are a relatively recent occurrence and a product of the marked decline in fertility rate in many societies in the 20th century. The occurrence of monthly menstrual bleeding in association with the combined oral contraceptive pill is a consequence of the 21-day regimen of administration of the pills.[25] At the time of the introduction of the contraceptive pill, it was thought that it would be better accepted by women and providers if cyclical bleeding persisted. However, this view is now being challenged, particularly because of the inconvenience and morbidity associated with menstruation.[26-28] Thus perhaps we should reconsider whether the profile of the 'ideal contraceptive' should change from one which perpetuates repeated menstrual cycles to one which involves simulating periods of natural infertility.

It is assumed that any new contraceptive should be highly effective, safe, easy to use and acceptable to women. Current hormonal methods meet many of these criteria and will be difficult to beat. It is desirable, therefore, that new methods convey additional health benefits. Continuation rates are higher in women whose dysmenorrhoea is improved while taking oral contraceptives.[29] In the long term, a pill or regimen which reduced rather than increased the risk of breast cancer, would prove popular. These factors are of importance when deciding which of the hundreds of potential targets are worth pursuing as new contraceptives.

Targets

Each component of the hypothalamic–pituitary–ovarian axis, as well as the uterus, is a potential target for contraception.[24] The combined oral contraceptive pill works principally by inhibiting the release of gonadotrophins from the anterior pituitary by suppressing the function of the hypothalamus. Because receptors for estradiol and progesterone are distributed in many tissues, these compounds have generalised effects (some favourable and some undesirable) throughout the body. Any compound which affects hypothalamic function will alter the ovarian and menstrual cycles through alteration in the pattern of secretion of gonadotrophins.

Hypothalamus

By 1976, the structure of GnRH had already been identified and several analogues synthesised, providing the opportunity to disrupt the secretion of gonadotrophins by selectively targeting the hypothalamus.[30] Agonists of GnRH have an established place in the treatment of a range of clinical disorders including cancer, fibroids and prior to stimulation of the ovary with FSH in assisted conception. By downregulating the GnRH receptor in the anterior pituitary, the secretion of FSH and luteinising hormone (LH) is inhibited. More recently, a number of GnRH antagonists have been developed which rapidly induce a profound hypogonadotrophic state.[31]

Proof of concept studies using GnRH agonists as contraceptives were published over 20 years ago in the 1980s.[32] There has been no further development of this approach for contraception, however. Initially, the analogues were expensive to make and required frequent administration by injection or nasal spray.[33] Long-acting implants lasting up to 3 months are now available which would make their use more practical. Because of the suppression of gonadotrophins and inhibition of follicular development, oestrogen secretion in these women is suppressed to very low levels. It is necessary, therefore, to supply replacement oestrogen. However, the dose of oestrogen necessary to maintain bone mineral density is less than that required to suppress ovulation. It has been suggested that a regimen could be used which induced amenorrhoea, reduced adverse effects and was protective against bone loss and breast cancer.[16,34] There is also convincing evidence that even the low doses of oestrogen and progestogen which are used for replacement treatment are associated with an increased risk of breast cancer and cardiovascular disease at least in postmenopausal women.[35]

Although the concept of suppressing gonadotrophins with analogues of GnRH is feasible, there are great difficulties in adjusting the dose to one which suppresses ovulation but maintains some follicular development while avoiding one which requires oestrogen replacement because of profound suppression of ovarian function.

Ovary

There have been spectacular advances in the identifying molecules involved with development of the follicle and the oocyte.[36] Folliculogenesis in women takes about 4–6 months from recruitment of primordial follicles through to the development of an ovulatory follicle.[37] This process involves a series of maturational events controlled by a number of key factors. Only the terminal few weeks of follicle development are directly controlled by pituitary gonadotrophins. Interference with any of these steps allows potential ways of developing new contraceptives. Much information has been obtained from mice with selective mutations of key molecules.[36] For example, animals homogeneous for GDF9K/O are infertile because primary follicles fail to develop normally after recruitment of primordial follicles.[38] Although these experimental studies have provided much information about the fundamental process of folliculogenesis, it seems unlikely that this approach, involving inhibition of follicle development at such an early stage, could be used to develop new contraceptive. In the absence of antral follicles, the women would be oestrogen deficient and would require replacement therapy with all the problems mentioned in the previous section. An intriguing possibility would be to inhibit recruitment from the pool of primordial follicles, thus preventing the progressive depletion of follicles in the ovary which eventually leads to ovarian failure at the menopause.[39] However, it is unlikely that the total inhibition of recruitment that would be necessary for contraception would be easy to achieve pharmacologically.

A more realistic approach would be the inhibition of follicle rupture.[40] The mid-cycle LH surge leads to a sequence of events involving progesterone and its receptor, prostaglandins and the cyclo-oxygenase enzymes, which results in rupture of the follicle wall.[41] Administration of inhibitors of progesterone and prostaglandin synthesis, as well as progesterone antagonists, results in failure of ovulation, with the oocyte trapped within the luteinized unruptured follicle.[41–43] The granulosa cells luteinise and secrete progesterone so that regular menstrual cycles are maintained. Specific inhibitors of cyclo-oxygenase-2 are now widely used in clinical medicine but their use for contraception remains largely unexploited.[44] Reports of an increased risk of myocardial infarction in long-term users of rofecoxib will not encourage further studies for contraception.[45]

As mentioned in the previous section, inhibition of the final maturation of the oocyte has many theoretical advantages. During folliculogenesis, the oocyte grows in size as the cytoplasm and nucleus matures.[46] The nucleus is arrest in the dictyate phase of the first meiotic division until a few hours before ovulation when, in response to the LH surge, meiosis recommences.[47] It is only after this has taken place that the oocyte achieves full developmental competence.

A number of molecular events are involved in the arrest of meiosis, including cyclic adenosine monophosphate (cAMP).[47] Inhibition of phosphodiesterase3, an enzyme responsible for the break down of cAMP in the ovary, results in failure of oocyte maturation in the mouse and infertility.[48] This is an example of an approach involving disruption of the terminal stages of maturation of the gamete without interfering with the endocrine function of the ovary.

The corpus luteum is an obvious target for contraception.[49] An attractive concept would be to develop a 'once-a-month' pill that worked by causing regression of the corpus luteum.[49] The secretion of progesterone by the corpus luteum is necessary to prepare the endometrium for implantation and to maintain the pregnancy for a few weeks afterwards.[50] The cause of luteal regression in women remains a mystery, in spite of extensive research. We do know that secretion of human chorionic gonadotrophin (hCG) by the early embryo is necessary for maintenance of the corpus luteum of pregnancy.[51] Administration of antisera to hCG in monkeys results in regression and termination of pregnancy.[52] Phase II trials in women have demonstrated the contraceptive potential of active vaccination against the beta subunit of hCG, although the titre of antibodies is variable.[53] With the molecular structure of LH/hCG receptor now known, the synthesis of antagonists which would block the luteotrophic action of LH and hCG is a real possibility.[54]

Uterus

The uterus must be exposed to a sequence of oestrogen followed by progesterone if it is to be receptive to an early embryo.[55] The process of implantation involves scores of genes many of which are induced by progesterone secreted by the corpus luteum.[56] Antagonists of progesterone, such as mifepristone, are contraceptive by preventing the formation of a secretory endometrium[57] or if given in the luteal phase by inducing menstrual bleeding. In two pilot studies, 200 mg mifepristone was given in the early luteal phase of the cycle to 53 women.[58,59] Only three pregnancies occurred in over 300 cycles of treatment. However, it is likely that the use of this approach as the basis of a once-a-month pill will need to wait until there are easier more accurate methods of detecting ovulation. Even in these volunteers, many women failed to take the pill at the correct time at midcycle because they omitted to test their urine for LH at a critical stage of the cycle.[60]

It has been suggested that mifepristone given at the end of the luteal phase could be used as a once-a-month pill.[61] However, mifepristone with or without misoprostol prevented pregnancy in only 85% of women and, hence, this combination is too inefficient to be used as a menstrual inducer.[62]

In the future, it may be possible to develop a new contraceptive method based on antagonising a key molecule involved in implantation, such as leukemia inhibitory factor (LIF). Transgenic mice, in which the gene for LIF has been mutated, are infertile because of the failure of implantation.[63] There is a range of other molecules which are necessary for successful implantation, including those involved with angiogenesis.[64] Antagonists of angiogenesis are contraceptive by preventing vascularisation of the follicle and corpus luteum as well as the implantation site. Although these antagonists are not selective for reproductive for the ovary and/or uterus, there is relatively little requirement for the formation of new blood vessels in tissues of healthy women outside the reproductive system.[65] Thus, short-term administration of an inhibitor of angiogenesis for a day or so once a month is unlikely to impair the function of other organs in the body.

Those approaches which mainly target the uterus, leaving the secretion of ovarian hormones, will retain repeated menstrual cycles. If follicular development and ovulation is disrupted, the endometrium may be exposed to oestrogen unopposed by progesterone. In these circumstances, there may be a risk of developing cystic hyperplasia of the endometrium and, eventually, cancer.[66] It will be necessary to protect the endometrium by cyclical administration of progestogen or continuous antigestogen.

Sperm transport and fertilisation

After deposition of the ejaculate in the vagina at coitus, sperm rapidly ascend the female reproductive tract to reach the site of fertilisation in the ampulla of the fallopian tube.[67] Although the motility necessary for the successful completion of this journey is an intrinsic property of the sperm, the environment of the cervix, uterus and tube are all important. The sperm can only pass through the cervical mucus when it is under the oestrogen domination at midcycle. Under the influence of progesterone, cervical mucus is converted to a sticky consistency and is resistant to the passage of sperm; this is basis of the contraceptive action of the progestogen-only pill. Chemokines associated with follicular fluid guide the passage of sperm through the uterus and tubes.[68] As the sperm ascend the tract, they undergo a process of capacitation, which must occur before fertilisation. When the sperm reaches the oocyte, it must first traverse the surrounding cumulus cells before binding to the specific surface proteins on the cell surface.[69]

All these processes are potential contraceptive targets. For example, it was shown many years ago that marmoset monkeys were rendered sterile when they were immunised against one of the proteins in the zona pellucida involved in sperm–egg interaction: ZP3.[70] This approach was dropped when it was found that the antibodies were cytotoxic and the monkeys underwent ovarian failure because of irreversible loss of primordial follicles. It should be noted that it is possible to target the sperm while it is resident in the female reproductive tract. For example, sperm motility is critically dependent upon a specific calcium channel involved in the hypermotility of sperm which is necessary to traverse the cumulus.[71] Blockage of this CATsper calcium channel should result in infertility due to failure of fertilisation. Such an antagonist could be given to either the man or the woman.

New contraceptives in the next 5 years

Presented with this comprehensive list of potential targets, the optimist might be tempted to list a large number of new contraceptives which will be developed in the next 5 years. It would be more realistic to predict that it is unlikely that any totally new contraceptive for women will be developed in the near future unless it has considerable advantages over the existing methods. Current methods are potentially good at preventing pregnancy but their effectiveness is constrained in practice by noncompliance and discontinuation. Thus, as argued above, any new method will need to be easy to use as well as highly effective. Ideally, it will have several short-term benefits, such as the relief of menstrual symptoms, which will improve acceptability and compliance and hence effectiveness. There should be the prospect that, in the long term, it will do no harm: ideally it would reduce the risk of developing one of the diseases which are a cause of morbidity and mortality.

Owing to the long and expensive lead time from discovery to product, any new product is likely to be a compound that is already in clinical trials and been shown to be relatively safe. In 1999, Anna Glasier and I reviewed contraceptive developments which were likely to occur in our life time (Table 16.2).[4] The new delivery systems such as are the basis of Implanon® (Organon) were easy to predict because they were already in phase-3 development. In spite of huge investment in microbicides, we still have no contraceptive which is protective against sexually transmitted disease such as chlamydia or HIV.[72] In fact, research has shown that one of the marketed microbicidal gels (nonoxinol-9) may actually increase the susceptibility to infection in certain populations.

Table 16.1. Defining the key criteria for novel contraceptive target development: IOM 2004[21]

Criterion	Example of desirable characteristics
Expression	Uniquely or selectively expressed in reproductive tract tissue or organs involved in reproduction
Function	Inhibiting functions specifically and completely disrupts or alters a process unique to reproduction
Timing of action	Close to time of fertilisation (e.g. post-meiotic events in gametogenesis)
Potential for reversible modulation by a drug	Druggable protein classes, e.g. enzymes, membrane proteins, receptors and ion channels and transporter proteins
Potential route of administration	Amenable to simple delivery systems, ensuring ease of use and high rates of compliance
Potential for product manufacture	Inexpensive and easy to produce
Potential for noncontraceptive benefits	Dual protection against sexually transmitted infections and conception; protection against cancer and other diseases

Table 16.2. New contraceptives: predicted developments[4]

Timing of predicted development	Development
Within 5 years	New delivery systems of conventional contraceptives, such as vaginal rings, transdermal patches and gels
	Contraceptives that also protect against sexually transmitted diseases
Short term (< 10 years)	Once-a-month pill that inhibits implantation
	Oestrogen-free daily pill for women (antioestrogens)
	Hormonal male contraception
	Orally active, nonpeptide antagonists of GnRH for men and women
Long term (> 10 years)	Antagonists of FSH receptor
	Arrest of spermatogenesis or sperm maturation
	Arrest of final maturation of oocyte
	Inhibitors of follicle rupture, such as with phosphodiesterase inhibitors

A major advance has been the development of vaccines against papillomavirus which are now in phase-3 trials.[73] The ability to prevent carcinoma of the cervix should have a huge impact on alleviating disease in women worldwide.

In our paper in 1999, we predicted that, by 2009, the most likely new female contraceptive would be a daily pill based on an antigestagen.[4] Phase-2 studies with mifepristone since then have confirmed the safety and efficacy of this approach.[74] The increasing wish for amenorrhoea should make this an attractive approach for many women.[75] Only time will tell as to whether the theoretical long-term benefits, such as the reduction in the risk of breast, ovarian and uterine cancer, are realised.[76] A number of pharmaceutical companies have shown interest in the therapeutic potential of this class of compounds for the management of benign and malignant reproductive disease as well as contraception.

While it is possible that an antigestagen may be available as a new daily pill by 2009, it is less likely that there will be commercial interest in the other contraceptive uses of this class of compounds. Mifepristone is highly effective as an emergency contraceptive pill and is licensed in China at a dose of 10 mg and 25 mg for this purpose.[77] It has fewer adverse effects than levonorgestrel or the Yuzpe regimen (ethinyloestradiol 100 micrograms plus levonorgestrel 0.5 mg: two doses 12 hours apart) and is probably more effective because it inhibits implantation as well as ovulation.[78] As mentioned above, pilot studies have demonstrated that it could form the basis of a once-a-month pill. However, in spite of the obvious attraction of this approach to many women, it is unlikely to be developed commercially for this purpose. Many pharmaceutical companies are cautious about incurring the displeasure of the so called 'pro-life' anti-abortion lobby. Also, the legal situation of abortifacient pills, which induce menses at the time of implantation, is doubtful in many countries. An agent which selectively induced luteal regression (such as an LH/hCG receptor antagonist) might be ethically and legally more acceptable.

Conclusions

Modern methods of contraception are extremely effective if used as instructed. Their effectiveness is limited in practice by the fact that some are inconvenient to use and are associated with a number of minor adverse effects. If we are to reduce the number of unplanned pregnancies, we must try and develop new methods which are easy to use and which are associated with health benefit.[79] Compliance and continuation rates are likely to be higher if women felt better while taking contraception. A reduction in serious life-threatening diseases should be the aim in the long term.[80]

References

1. Diczfalusy E. Reproductive health: a rendezvous with human dignity. *Contraception* 1995;52:1–12.
2. Baird D. A fifth freedom. *BMJ* 1965;(ii):1141–8.
3. Diczfalusy E. Contraception and society. *Eur J Contracept Reprod Health Care* 2002;7:199–209.
4. Baird DT, Glasier AF. Contraception. *BMJ* 1999;319:969–72.
5. United Nations. *World Population Prospects: The 2002 Revision Highlights*. ESA/P/WP180. New York: UN; 2003.
6. Population Reference Bureau. World Population Data Sheet 2004 [http://www.prb.org].
7. Guillebaud J. Combined oral contraception. In: Glasier AF, Gebbie A, editors. *Handbook of Family Planning*. 4th ed. Edinburgh: Churchill Livingstone; 2000. p. 29–76.
8. Beral V, Hermon C, Kay C, Hannaford P, Darby S, Reeves G. Mortality associated with oral contraceptive use: 25 year follow up of cohort of 46000 women from Royal College of General Practitioners oral contraceptive study. *BMJ* 1999;318:96–100.
9. World Health Organization. *Unsafe Abortion: Global estimates of the incidence of unsafe abortion and associated mortality in 2000*. Geneva: WHO; 2004.
10. Jones RK, Darroch JE, Henshaw SK. Contraceptive use among US women having abortions in 2000-2001. *Perspect Sex Reprod Health* 2002;34:294–303.
11. Barrett G, Smith SC, Wellings K. Conceptualisation, development, and evaluation of a measure of unplanned pregnancy. *J Epidemiol Community Health* 2004;58:426–33.
12. Trussel J. Contraceptive failure. In: *Contraceptive Technology*. 18th ed. New York: Ardent Media; 2004. p. 77 –846.
13. Fraser IS. Progestagen-only contraception. In: Glasier AF, Gebbie A,eds. *Handbook of Family Planning*. 4th ed. Edinburgh: Churchill Livingstone; 2000. p. 77–103.
14. Collaborative Group on Hormonal Factors in Breast Cancer. Breast cancer and hormonal contraceptives: a collaborative re-analysis of individual data on 53,297 women with breast cancer and 100,239 women without breast cancer from 54 epidemiological studies. *Lancet* 1996;347:1717–27.
15. World Health Organization. Oral contraceptives and neoplasia. *World Health Organ Tech Rep Ser* 1992;817:1–46
16. Pike MC, Spicer DV. Hormonal contraception and chemotherapy of female cancers. *Endocr Relat Cancer* 2000;7:73–83.
17. Royal Society. *Contraceptives of the Future*. London: Royal Society; 1976.
18. Harper MJK, editor. *Birth Control Technologies: Prospect by the Year 2000*. London: William Heinemann Medical Books; 1983.
19. Millar RP, Baird DT, editors. Human reproduction: pharmaceutical and technical advances. *Br Med Bull* 2000;56;577–837.
20. Harrison PF, Rosenfield A, editors. *Contraceptive Research and Development. Looking to the Future*. Washington: National Academy Press; 1996.
21. Nass JN, Strauss III JF, editors. *New Frontiers in Contraceptive Research: A Blueprint for Action*. Institute of Medicine, Washington: National Academies Press; 2001.
22. Van Look PFA. Contraceptives of the future. In: Glasier A, Gebbie A, editors. *Handbook of Family Planning and Reproductive Healthcare*. Edinburgh: Churchill Livingstone; 2000. p. 397–8.
23. Short RV. The evolution of human reproduction. *Proc R Soc Lond B* 1976;195:3–24.
24. Baird DT. Manipulation of the menstrual cycle. *Proc R Soc Lond B* 1965;195:137–48.
25. Pincus G. *The Control of Fertility*. New York: Academic Press; 1965.
26. Den Tonkelaar I, Oddens BJ. Preferred frequency and characteristics of menstrual bleeding in relation to reproductive status and contraceptive use and hormone replacement therapy use. *Contraception* 1999;59;357–62.

27. Kaunitz AM. Menstruation: choosing whether…and when. *Contraception* 2000;62:277–84.
28. Thomas SL, Ellertson C. Nuisance or natural and healthy: should monthly menstruation be optional for women? *Lancet* 2000;355:922–924.
29. Robinson JC, Plichta S, Weisman CS, Nathanson CA, Ensminger M. Dysmenorrhoea and use of oral contraceptives in adolescent women attending a family planning clinic. *Am J Obstet Gynecol* 1992;166:578–83.
30. Coy DH, Labrie F, Savary M, Coy EJ, Schally AV. Antagonistic activity of analogs of luteinizing hormone-releasing hormone (LH-RH) *in vitro*. *Mol Cell Endocrinol* 1976;5:201–8.
31. Huirne JAF, Lambalk CB. Gonadotrophin-releasing hormone: receptor antagonists. *Lancet* 2001;358:1793–803.
32. Nillius SJ, Bergquist C, Wide L. Inhibition of ovulation in women by chronic treatment with a stimulatory LRH analogue – A new approach to birth control? *Contraception* 1978;17:537–45.
33. Fraser HM. GnRH analogues for contraception. *Br Med Bull* 1993;49:62–72.
34. Medina D, Sivaraman L, Hilsenbeck SG, Conneely O, Ginger M, Rosen J, *et al*. Mechanisms of hormonal prevention of breast cancer. *Ann N Y Acad Sci* 2001;952:23–35.
35. Beral V, Banks E, Reeves G. Evidence from randomised trials on the long-term effects of hormone replacement therapy. *Lancet* 2002;360:942–4.
36. Matzuk MM, Lamb DJ. (2002) Genetic dissection of mammalian fertility pathways. *Nat Cell Biol* 2002;4 Suppl:41–9.
37. Gougeon A. Regulation of ovarian follicular development in primates: facts and hypotheses. *Endocr Rev* 1996;17:121–55.
38. Dong J, Albertini DF, Nishimori K, Kumar TR, Lu N, Matzuk MM. Growth differentiation factor-9 is required during early ovarian folliculogenesis. *Nature* 1996;10:531–5.
39. Gruijters MJ, Visser JA, Durlinger AL, Themmen AP. Anti-Mullerian hormone and its role in ovarian function. *Mol Cell Endocrinol* 2003;15:85–90.
40. Priddy AR, Killick SR. (1993) Eicosanoids and ovulation. *Prostaglandins Leukot Essent Fatty Acids* 1993;49:827–31.
41. Richards JS, Russell DL, Ochsner S, Espey LL. Ovulation: new dimensions and new regulators of the inflammatory-like response. *Annu Rev Physiol* 2002;64:69–92.
42. Killick S, Elstein M. Pharmacologic production of luteinized unruptured follicles by prostaglandin synthetase inhibitors. *Fertil Steril* 1987;47:773–7.
43. Duffy DM, Stouffer RL. Follicular administration of a cyclooxygenase inhibitor can prevent oocyte release without alteration of normal luteal function in rhesus monkeys. *Hum Reprod* 2002;17:2825–31.
44. Anon. Taking stock of coxibs. *Drug Ther Bull* 2005;43:1–6.
45. Mayor S. Rofecoxib caused heart disease. *BMJ* 2005;330:212.
46. Hardy K, Wright CS, Franks S, Winston RM. *In vitro* maturation of oocytes. *Br Med Bull* 2000;56:588–602.
47. Picton H, Briggs D, Gosden R. The molecular basis of oocyte growth and development. *Mol Cell Endocrinol* 1998;145:27–37.
48. Jensen JT, Zelinski-Wooten MB, Schwinof KM, Vance JE, Stouffer RL. The phosphodiesterase 3 inhibitor ORG 9935 inhibits oocyte maturation during gonadotropin-stimulated ovarian cycles in rhesus macaques. *Contraception* 2005;71:68–73.
49. Croxatto H, Harper M, McDonnell D, Vale W. (1996) Female methods. In: Harrison PF, Rosenfield A, editors. *Contraceptive Research and Development*. Washington DC: National Academy Press; 1996. p. 351–80.
50. Stouffer RL, Chandrasekher YA, Slayden OD, Zelinski-Wooten MB. Gonadotrophic and local control of the developing corpus luteum in rhesus monkeys. *Hum Reprod* 1993;8 Suppl 2:107–11.
51. Csapo AI, Pulkkinen M. Indispensability of the human corpus luteum in the maintenance of early pregnancy: Luteectomy evidence. *Obstet Gynecol Surv* 1978;33:69–81.
52. Hearn JP. Immunization against pregnancy. *Proc R Soc Lond B* 1976;195:149–60.
53. Talwar GP, Singh O, Pal R, Chatterjee N, Sahai P, Dhall K, *et al*. A vaccine that prevents pregnancy in women. *Proc Natl Acad Sci U S A* 1994;91:8532–6.
54. Ascoli M, Fanelli F, Segaloff DL. The lutropin/choriogonadotropin receptor, a 20002 perspective. *Endocr Rev* 2002;23:141–7.
55. Martin J, Dominguez F, Avila S, Castrillo JL, Remohi J, Pellicer A, Simon C. Human endometrial receptivity: gene regulation. *J Reprod Immunol* 2002;55:131–9.
56. Giudice LC. Microarray expression profiling reveals candidate genes for human uterine receptivity. *Am J Pharmacogenomics* 2004;4:299–312.
57. Bygdeman M, Swahn ML, Gemzell-Danielsson K, Svalander P. Mode of action of RU 486. *Ann Med* 1993;25:61–4.

58. Gemzell-Danielsson, KSwahn ML, Svalander P, Bygdeman M. Early luteal phase treatment with mifepristone (RU 486) for fertility regulation. *Hum Reprod* 1993;8:870–873.

59. Hapangama DK, Brown A, Glasier AF, Baird DT. Feasibility of administering mifepristone as a once a month contraceptive pill. *Hum Reprod* 2001;16:1145–50.

60. Hapangama DK, Glasier AF, Baird DT. Noncompliance among a group of women using a novel method of contraception. *Fertil Steril* 2001;76:1196–201.

61. Bygdeman M. The possibility of using mifepristone for menstrual induction. *Contraception* 2003;68:495–8.

62. Xiao B, von Hertzen H, Zhao H, Piaggio G. Menstrual induction with mifepristone and misoprostol. *Contraception* 2003;68:489–94.

63. Cheng JG, Rodriguez CI, Stewart CL. Control of uterine receptivity and embryo implantation by steroid hormone regulation of LIF production and LIF receptor activity: towards a molecular understanding of "the window of implantation". *Rev Endocr Metab Disord* 2002;3:119–26.

64. Fraser HM, Lunn SF. Angiogenesis and its control in the female reproductive system. *Br Med Bull* 2000;56:787–97.

65. Wulff C, Weigand M, Kreienberg R, Fraser HM. Angiogenesis during primate placentation in health and disease. *Reproduction* 2003;126:569–77.

66. Baird DT. Antigestogens: the holy grail of contraception. *Reprod Fertil Dev* 2001;13:723–8.

67. Croxatto HB. Gamete transport. In: Rock JA, Rosenwalks Z, editors. *Reproductive Endocrinology, Surgery and Technology , Volume I*. Philadelphia, PA: Lippincott-Raven; 1996. p. 386–402.

68. Spehr M, Gisselmann G, Poplawski A, Riffell JA, Wetzel CH, Zimmer RK, et al. Identification of a testicular odorant receptor mediating human sperm chemotaxis. *Science* 2003;299:2054–8.

69. Wassarman PM, Jovine L, Litscher ES, Qi H, Williams Z. Egg-sperm interactions at fertilization in mammals. *Eur J Obstet Gynecol Reprod Biol* 2004;115 Suppl 1:S57–60.

70. Aitken RJ. Immunocontraceptive vaccines for human use. *J Reprod Immunol* 2002;57:273-87.

71. Ren D, Navarro B, Perez G, Jackson AC, Hsu S, Shi Q, et al. A sperm ion channel required for sperm motility and male fertility. *Nature* 2001;413:603–9.

72. McCormack S, Hayes R, Lacey CJN, Johnson AM. Microbicides in HIV prevention. *BMJ* 2001;322:410–413.

73. Tomson TT, Roden RB, Wu TC. Human papillomavirus vaccines for the prevention and treatment of cervical cancer. *Curr Opin Investig Drugs* 2001;5:1247–61.

74. Baird DT, Brown A, Chneg L, Critchley HOD, Lin S, Narvekar N, Williams ARW. Mifepristone: a novel estrogen-free daily pill. *Steroids* 2003;68:10–13.

75. Glasier AF, Smith KB, van der Spuy ZM, Ho PC, Cheng L, Dada K, et al. Amenorrhoea associated with contraception – an international study of acceptability. *Contraception* 2003;67:1–8.

76. Spitz IM. Progesterone antagonists and progesterone receptor modulators: an overview. *Steroids* 2003;68:891–994.

77. Xiao B, Zhao H, Piaggio G, von Hertzen H. Expanded clinical trial of emergency contraception with 10 mg mifepristone. *Contraception;* 2003;68:431–7.

78. Croxatto HB, Devoto L, Durand M, Ezcurra E, Larrea F, Nagle C, et al. Mechanism of action of hormonal preparations of emergency contraception: a review of the literature. *Contraception* 2001;63:111–21.

79. Baird DT. Overview of advances in contraception. *Br Med Bull* 2000;56:704–16.

80. ESHRE Capri Workshop. Non-Contraceptive Health Benefits of Contraception. *Hum Reprod Update* 2005 (in press).

Chapter 17
Improving male contraceptive methods

Fred CW Wu

Introduction

That one-third of couples worldwide (and 41% in the UK in 2001) chooses a male contraceptive method is a testament to substantial male participation in family planning. Yet only two options are currently available to men: a reversible method (the condom) that is not reliable and the only reliable method (vasectomy) that is generally not reversible. While younger men without a regular partner are best served by the dual protection against sexually transmitted infections and unintended pregnancy offered by condoms, there is a real and substantial unmet need for men in stable relationships eager to share the responsibility for family planning. In this respect, a new reversible male method as reliable as modern female products would significantly expand the currently limited choice and encourage increased contraceptive uptake and continuation in men.

In principle, the series of unique cell types and biologically processes that underlie the physiological functions of the testis (spermatogenesis, spermiogenesis, spermiation) epididymis (sperm volume regulation, surface membrane protein interaction and acquisition of motility) and the maturing and ejaculated spermatozoa in the female genital tract (acrosome reaction, egg recognition/binding/fusion) should provide numerous potential opportunities for contraceptive targeting. Indeed, an increasing range of key molecules has been identified from knockout animal models of infertility, which could provide theoretical candidates for potential contraceptive development. However, the enormous economic investment required in developing preventive medications in the current drug regulatory climate, excessive liability risks and relative lack of public funding all conspire to make it unlikely that completely novel contraceptive products will emerge from basic science leads in the foreseeable future. In contrast, hormone contraception for men relies mainly on off-the-shelf (and often forgotten) compounds and formulations, some of which have good safety profiles from many years of clinical use in androgen replacement and in female contraception. This relatively 'low-technology' approach, bypassing or expediting some of the obstacles inherent to the development of completely new agents, offers realistic prospects of marketing a new reversible and effective contraceptive product within a reasonable time span. Such a method would instantly broaden the contraceptive options for men who seek alternatives to female methods used for many years by their partners, who may have developed adverse effects, medical contraindications or simply wish a break; men whose partners are lactating in the postpartum period and for those who are undecided or wish to defer vasectomy.[1]

Mechanism of action

The aim of male hormonal contraception is to suppress or arrest spermatogenesis reversibly and to induce temporary infertility while preserving other androgen-dependent physiological functions without unwanted metabolic effects. Sperm-atogenesis is regulated by the pituitary gonadotrophins, luteinising hormone (LH) and follicle-stimulating hormone (FSH). FSH is required specifically for the Sertoli cells' support of the mitotic and meiotic germ cells, while testosterone synthesis by the Leydig cells is stimulated by LH. Both FSH and high concentrations of intra-testicular testosterone (as a proxy for LH action) are critical to the quantitative maintenance of spermatogenesis in the adult testis, the actions of both being to some extent interchangeable when either one of the two signals is abrogated. It follows that, for the purpose of hormonal contraception, both FSH as well as LH have to be suppressed concurrently in order to turn off spermatogenesis. It is fortuitous and fortunate that virtually all known therapeutic anti-gonadotrophic agents (such as androgens, oestrogens, progestins and gonadotrophin-releasing hormone, GnRH, analogues) suppress both FSH and LH simultaneously. Thus, hormonal male contra-ception will create a state of iatrogenic hypogonadotrophic hypogonadism, which dictates the use of exogenous androgens (5–7 mg daily) to maintain extra-testicular androgen-dependent physiological functions, somewhat analogous to the use of oestrogens (50–200 micrograms daily) to provide and regulate menstrual cyclicity in the female combined oral contraceptive pill.

Many phase-1 and -2 dose-finding and proof of principle studies have investigated the efficacy of spermatogenesis suppression and, to a lesser extent, contraceptive efficacy.[1,2] These have included androgen-only regimens and androgen combinations with other agents such as progestins and GnRH analogues.

Contraceptive regimens

Androgen alone

Most early studies have used testosterone alone because of the expedient that gonadotrophin suppression and androgen replacement can be achieved with a single agent. However, oral bioavailability of unmodified testosterone is poor because of hepatic first-pass metabolism and orally active 17 alpha-alkylated testosterone ana-logues are hepatotoxic. The daily physiological requirement for milligram amounts of testosterone in men can only be achieved with depot preparations of injectable testosterone esters or implantable testosterone pellets.

Testosterone enanthate

Intramuscular preparations of esterified testosterone, such as testosterone enanthate, are the most commonly used preparations for physiological androgen replacement therapy in adult hypogonadal men at a dose of 200 mg every 2 weeks (transdermal and other newer preparations have only become available in the last few years). Early studies in the 1970s have shown that, for suppression of gonadotrophins and spermatogenesis in eugonadal men, doses of testosterone enanthate higher than needed for physiological replacement are required. Two landmark multinational studies sponsored by the World Health Organization Special Programme of Research, Development, and Research Training in Human Reproduction[3] were conducted between 1986 and 1995, using weekly intramuscular injections of 200 mg of testosterone enanthate as a prototype male contraceptive to determine the contraceptive efficacy of hormone-induced azoo- and oligozoopermia. These studies confirmed that supraphysiological doses of testosterone induced azoospermia in 60% of Caucasian but in 91% of oriental subjects, the remainder becoming severely oligozoospermic, with mean sperm concentrations of around 3 million/ml.[4] During the 403.7 person-years of exposure accumulated from 655 subjects in 15 centres distributed in ten countries, a relationship between sperm concentration (the extent of spermatogenesis suppression) and pregnancy rate (contraceptive failure) was demonstrated for the first time. The pregnancy rate for azoospermia was 0.8 (95% CI 0.02–4.5) per 100 person years in the first study. In the second study, the pregnancy rate was 0 (95% CI 0.0–1.6) for azoospermia and 8.1 (95% CI 2.2–20.7) per 100 person-years for oligozoospermia (0.1–3.0 million/ml). The combined failure rate for men with sperm concentrations in the range of 0–3 million/ml was 1.4 (95% CI 0.4–3.7) pregnancies per 100 person years,[5] which is comparable to the female oral contraceptive pill and better than the typical first year failure rate of condoms (12%). These important proof-of-principle studies demonstrated that hormonal suppression of spermatogenesis could provide effective and reversible contraception for men with few adverse events. They also suggested that targets of suppression to ensure effective contraceptive protection were either azoospermia or severe oligozoospermia (less than 1 million/ml).

The prototype regimen of weekly intramuscular injections of testosterone enanthate highlighted major drawbacks in the androgen-only approach. Unsatisfactory pharmacokinetics of injectable testosterone esters, available at that time, resulted in widely fluctuating levels of testosterone with frequent supraphysiological peaks. Frequent injections were required to prevent troughs falling to levels that allow breakthrough of suppression.[3] Relatively high doses of testosterone required to induce and maintain adequate suppression of spermatogenesis were the likely cause of androgen-dependent adverse effects including acne, weight gain, behavioural change, decreased high density lipoprotein-cholesterol (HDL-C) and increased haemopoiesis. For these reasons longer acting testosterone preparations with improved pharmacokinetics and alternative strategies using combinations with other anti-gonadotrophic agents were sought.

Testosterone implants

Pellets of crystalline testosterone (one 200 mg pellet releasing 1.3 mg/day) inserted surgically into the subcutaneous tissue of the lower abdominal wall under local anaesthetic have been used for androgen replacement since the 1950s. The quasi-zero-order pharmacokinetics of testosterone implants, maintaining stable testosterone levels for many weeks without supraphysiological peaks, can be exploited to confer dose-sparing advantages in achieving hormonal suppression of spermatogenesis. Thus, a single implantation of 1200 mg (six pellets) has been shown to induce and maintain azoospermia and oligozoospermia for 16 weeks with similar efficacy to testosterone enanthate alone (200 mg weekly), while physiological testosterone levels prevented most androgen-related metabolic adverse effects.[6] This demonstrated the critical importance of pharmacokinetic properties of androgen formulations in male contraceptive development.

Testosterone undecanoate

Testosterone undecanoate is an unsaturated ester of testosterone with a long hydrophobic aliphatic fatty acid side chain which renders it highly fat-soluble. Formulation of testosterone undecanoate in teaseed oil (125 mg/ml in China) and castor oil (Nebido™ 250 mg/ml, Jenapharm/Schering, Germany) yielded long-acting depot preparations for intramuscular use. testosterone undecanoate (in castor oil) has a long half-life of 70 days, with more stable pharmacokinetics when administered at 4–8 weekly intervals. Testosterone undecanoate (in teaseed oil) 500 mg monthly, given intramuscularly, can induce azoospermia or oligozoospermia (less than 3 million/ml) in 97% of Chinese subjects with high contraceptive efficacy (one pregnancy in 143 person-years' exposure, a failure rate of 2.3 (95% CI 0.5–4.2) per 100 couple-years.[7] These encouraging results are being followed-up by phase-3 studies involving more than 1000 men in ten centres in China, where a new and more concentrated formulation of testosterone undecanoate in soybean oil (250 mg/ml) is also under investigation.

Transdermal testosterone preparations

Several novel transdermal delivery systems (patches and gels) of testosterone have become available. While self-administration and maintenance of physiological testosterone blood levels offer obvious convenience and advantages in androgen replacement for hypogonadism, the requirement for daily application and higher levels of variability in skin absorption raises an important issue of compliance, not to mention the high incidence of skin irritation with the reservoir patch. Unsurprisingly, transdermal testosterone on its own has not been investigated as a potential contraceptive formulation.

7α-methyl-19-nortestosterone

MENT (7α-methyl-19-nortestosterone) is a highly potent synthetic androgen that is resistant to 5α-reductase but sensitive to aromatase. This metabolic idiosyncrasy underlies the tissue selectivity that confers a prostate-sparing profile. In a preliminary dose-finding study, four subdermal MENT acetate implants (each delivering 400 micrograms/day) have been shown to suppress gonadotrophins and induce azoospermia in 64% of men, with a suggestion of reduction in prostate volume by 10–17% after 6 months.[8]

Summary

The androgen-only approach to male hormonal contraception is attractive conceptually and proof-of-principle studies have confirmed the feasibility of this approach, especially in oriental men. The efficacy, however, is significantly lower in White men. While newer testosterone formulations may avoid the relatively high dose of older testosterone esters required to suppress spermatogenesis, the spectre of long-term androgen-related adverse effects remains a significant disincentive to product development unless synthetic androgens with desirable tissue selectivity can be seriously explored.

Progestin/androgen combinations

Exogenous progestins can inhibit gonadotrophin secretion in men and suppress spermatogenesis. Combining a progestin with androgens for male contraception exploits the synergistic actions of the two steroids so that they can be used at lower doses, thus minimising the potential for adverse effects. The plethora of available synthetic progestin preparations, including oral, injectable and implants, also serves to broaden the choice of potential regimens. Some of the more interesting progestogen/androgen combinations studied to date are summarised here.

Depot medroxyprogesterone acetate

Depot medroxyprogesterone acetate (DMPA) has been combined with 19-nortestosterone, testosterone enanthate and testosterone implants. Studies with 19-nortestosterone and testosterone enanthate in combination with DMPA in Indonesian men documented azoospermia rates of 98%. In White men, the combination of DMPA with T implants achieved lower azoospermia rates similar to testosterone enanthate alone.[9] The main limitation of DMPA is the prolonged period (more than 6 months) necessary for spermatogenesis recovery following cessation of treatment.

Cyproterone acetate

Cyproterone acetate (CPA) combines anti-gonadotrophic and anti-androgenic properties, which may be particularly favourable for suppression of spermatogenesis. Oral CPA at doses of 25–100 mg combined with testosterone enanthate induces rapid suppression of spermatogenesis, with the time taken to achieve azoospermia being significantly shorter compared with that with testosterone enanthate alone (49 days as against 98 days).[10] While this is encouraging, a dose-dependent decrease in haemoglobin and body weight related to the anti-androgen action of CPA and the potential for hepatic dysfunction limit the prospects of this combination.

Levonorgestrel

Levonorgestrel has been extensively studied in combination with a variety of androgens. Initially a dose of 500 micrograms daily with testosterone enanthate 100 g weekly confirmed greater sperm suppression than with testosterone enanthate alone (azoospermia 67% versus 33%).[11] Further study with lower doses of levonorgestrel (250 micrograms and 125 micrograms) did not compromise suppression rates.[12] Metabolic effects were dose dependent and included lowered HDL-C and weight gain. Oral levonorgestrel 250 micrograms daily and intramuscular testosterone undecanoate 1000 mg 6-weekly in combination has been compared with testosterone undecanoate 1000 mg 6-weekly alone. There was no difference in suppression to azoospermia (50–57%),[13] suggesting that the addition of levonorgestrel did not confer any advantage. Testosterone patches have been combined with oral levonorgestrel (125 micrograms daily) and long-acting levonorgestrel implants (four rods Norplant® II).[14] Relatively poor sperm suppression (severe oligozoospermia in less than 60%) probably relates to the unreliable administration or absorption of testosterone, so that circulating levels in the low normal range only can be achieved. This highlights the critical role of testosterone as a necessary suppressor of gonadotrophins in combination contraceptive regimens in addition to its role in androgen replacement.

Desogestrel and etonogestrel

Desogestrel is an oral third-generation synthetic progestin with potent progestational activity but lower androgenicity. These potentially favourable properties led to the study of desogestrel in combination with testosterone enanthate. Oral desogestrel 300 micrograms in combination with various testosterone enanthate doses produced a high rate of azoospermia.[15] A lowering of HDL-C of 20–25% was observed. A cross-national study confirmed that desogestrel (150 micrograms daily) in combination with 400 mg testosterone implants (every 12 weeks) can induce azoospermia in virtually all men in the 300-microgram group, with a significant decline in HDL-C in White men only.[16] Etonogestrel is the active metabolite converted by the liver from desogestrel with dose-equivalent biopotency. Etonogestrel has been formulated as a subdermal nonbiodegradable implant for female contraception (Implanon®, NV Organon). Three etonogestrel rods (68 mg etonogestrel/rod) in combination with testosterone implants (400 mg every 12 weeks).[17] All nine men became azoospermic, although the time to achieve this varied from 8 weeks to 28 weeks and one man showed partial recovery after 40 weeks. Treatment did not result in weight gain, change in body composition or decline in HDL-C. Further study of this promising progestin implant in combination with testosterone undecanoate injections is in progress. This effort not only represents the beginnings of public/private collaboration but also indicates for the first time a willingness of industry to invest in hormone contraceptive products for men.

Norethisterone enanthate

Norethisterone (NET) is an androgenic progestin which can be delivered as NET enanthate (NETE), an intramuscular aqueous depot preparation available in Europe for female contraception. NETE 400 mg and testosterone undecanoate 1000 mg have been administered at 6-weekly intervals[18] and have induced azoospermia in 92% of men. Moderate increases in haemoglobin (within the normal range) and decreases in HDL-C were observed. The dosing interval of the two steroids can be prolonged to 8-weekly without losing efficacy.[19] This promising regimen consisting of two long-acting depot injectable preparations is being further investigated in planned multi-centre studies.

Summary

There is a perception that progestin and androgen combinations are more effective than testosterone alone,[20] possibly related to an additional action of the progestins in the testis, and therefore more suited to White men, who are less responsive to steroid suppression. However, the small numbers of subjects and relatively short duration of treatment make valid comparisons between regimens difficult, thus limiting the ability to generalise from these studies. The potential of progestin-related adverse effects (short- and long-term) merits greater attention. Current research efforts sponsored by industry are directed towards developing a combination of long-acting depot testosterone injections and progestin implants or injections as the first contraceptive product to be marketed.

GnRH antagonists

GnRH antagonists are competitive blockers of GnRH receptor binding and suppress gonadotrophins within 24 hours. Studies have shown rapid spermatogenic suppression with a high rate of azoospermia. While these complex synthetic peptides clearly have contraceptive potential (their main advantage being faster suppression than sex steroids), the disadvantages are their high cost, short half-life and the need for frequent subcutaneous injection. Adverse effects encountered have included local skin reactions at the site of injection. When the GnRH antagonist Nal-Glu and testosterone enanthate were used to initiate spermatogenic suppression, this could then be maintained with testosterone enanthate alone.[21] New long-acting depot preparations of potent GnRH antagonists may therefore have a place in male contraception where rapid induction of spermatogenic suppression can subsequently be maintained by testosterone with or without progestins.

Ethnic differences

There are clear ethnic differences in the response to sex steroid suppression of spermatogenesis between Asian (more responsive) compared with White men (less responsive), independent of anthropometry and circulating hormone levels. In studies using androgens alone (testosterone enanthate and testosterone undecanoate) azoospermia was achieved in more than 90% of Asian men as against fewer than 60% of European or American men. The potential explanations for these differences may include genetic[22] and dietary/environmental factors[23,24] that are not yet fully understood. Intra-ethnic variation is also seen within White populations. Only 40–60% of men usually suppress azoospermia while others remain oligozoospermic in response to sex steroids. Gonadotrophin-dependent and -independent factors have been suggested[25,26] but the exact mechanism(s) evades current understanding.

Conclusions

There is evidence to support couple dissatisfaction with currently available contraceptive methods and choice. A cross-cultural survey also found that women felt the contraceptive burden too frequently falls to them and they welcomed the availability of a reversible male contraceptive which they trust their partners to take.[27] An important aspect of the male hormonal method is the variable and relatively long time lag (8–10 weeks) after commencing treatment until sperm suppression is sufficient for effective contraceptive. However, a similar lag time also applies to vasectomy (irreversible) and a lag of 1 month applies to the female oral contraceptive pill. Another potential drawback is the need for semen analysis to signal sufficient suppression of sperm count, although this can be simplified in future with self-administered dipstick methods or even dispensed with altogether with more clinical experience in the field.

Publicly funded research has reached a stage where realisation of male hormonal contraception is within our reach and the pharmaceutical industry is beginning to embark on the necessary steps leading to product development. A progestogen/androgen combination is most likely to be the first product to be marketed. Further development of long-acting depot formulations or oral and nonsteroidal compounds will provide a variety of contraceptive formulations that will allow men to have a widened choice, improve acceptability and encourage continued usage.

References

1.   Anderson RA, Baird DT. Male Contraception. *Endocr Rev* 2002;23:735–62.
2.   Kamischke A, Nieschlag E. Progress towards hormonal male contraception. *Trends Pharmacol Sci* 2004;25:49–57.
3.   Waites GM. Development of methods of male contraception: impact of the World Health Organization Task Force. *Fertil Steril* 2003;80:1–15.

4.   World Health Organization Task Force on Methods for the Regulation of Male Fertility. Contraceptive efficacy of testosterone-induced azoospermia in normal men. *Lancet* 1990;336:955–9.
5.   Contraceptive efficacy of testosterone-induced azoospermia and oligozoospermia in normal men. *Fertil Steril* 1996;65:821–9.
6.   Handelsman DJ, Conway AJ, Boylan LM. Suppression of human spermatogenesis by testosterone implants. *J Clin Endocrinol Metab* 1992;75:1326–32.
7.   Gu Y-Q, Wang X-H, Xu D, Peng L, Cheng L-F, Huang M-K, et al. A multicenter contraceptive efficacy study of injectable testosterone undecanoate in healthy chinese men. *J Clin Endocrinol Metab* 2003;88:562–8.
8.   von Eckardstein S, Noe G, Brache V, Nieschlag E, Croxatto H, Alvarez F, et al. A clinical trial of 7 alpha-methyl-19-nortestosterone implants for possible use as a long-acting contraceptive for men. *J Clin Endocrinol Metab* 2003;88:5232–9.
9.   Handelsman DJ, Conway AJ, Howe CJ, Turner L, Mackey MA. Establishing the minimum effective dose and additive effects of depot progestin in suppression of human spermatogenesis by a testosterone depot. *J Clin Endocrinol Metab* 1996;81:4113–21.
10. Meriggiola MC, Farley TM, Mbizvo MT. A review of androgen-progestin regimens for male contraception. *J Androl* 2003;24:466–83.
11. Bebb RA, Anawalt BD, Christensen RB, Paulsen CA, Bremner WJ, Matsumoto AM. Combined administration of levonorgestrel and testosterone induces more rapid and effective suppression of spermatogenesis than testosterone alone: a promising male contraceptive approach. *J Clin Endocrinol Metab* 1996;81:757–62.
12. Anawalt BD, Bebb RA, Bremner WJ, Matsumoto AM. A lower dosage levonorgestrel and testosterone combination effectively suppresses spermatogenesis and circulating gonadotropin levels with fewer metabolic effects than higher dosage combinations. *J Androl* 1999;20:407–14.
13. Kamischke A, Ploger D, Venherm S, von Eckardstein A, von Eckardstein S, Nieschlag E. Intramuscular testosterone undecanoate with or without oral levonorgestrel: a randomized placebo-controlled feasibility study for male contraception. *Clin Endocrinol (Oxf)* 2000;53:43–52.
14. Gonzalo IT, Swerdloff RS, Nelson AL, Clevenger B, Garcia R, Berman N, et al. Levonorgestrel implants (Norplant II) for male contraception clinical trials: combination with transdermal and injectable testosterone. *J Clin Endocrinol Metab* 2002;87:3562–72.
15. Wu FC, Balasubramanian R, Mulders TM, Coelingh-Bennink HJ. Oral progestogen combined with testosterone as a potential male contraceptive: additive effects between desogestrel and testosterone enanthate in suppression of spermatogenesis, pituitary-testicular axis, and lipid metabolism. *J Clin Endocrinol Metab* 1999;84:112–22.
16. Kinniburgh D, Zhu H, Cheng L, Kicman AT, Baird DT, Anderson RA. Oral desogestrel with testosterone pellets induces consistent suppression of spermatogenesis to azoospermia in both Caucasian and Chinese men. *Hum Reprod* 2002;17:1490–501.
17. Brady BM, Walton M, Hollow N, Kicman AT, Baird DT, Anderson RA. Depot testosterone with etonogestrel implants result in induction of azoospermia in all men for long-term contraception. *Hum Reprod* 2004;19:2658–67.
18. Kamischke A, Heuermann T, Kruger K, von Eckardstein S, Schellschmidt I, Rubig A, et al. An effective hormonal male contraceptive using testosterone undecanoate with oral or injectable norethisterone preparations. *J Clin Endocrinol Metab* 2002;87:530–9.
19. Meriggiola (in press 2005) [published yet?]
20. Nieschlag E, Zitzmann M, Kamischke A. Use of progestins in male contraception. *Steroids* 2003;68:965–72.
21. Swerdloff RS, Bagatell CJ, Wang C, Anawalt BD, Berman N, Steiner B, et al. Suppression of spermatogenesis in man induced by Nal-Glu gonadotropin releasing hormone antagonist and testosterone enanthate (TE) is maintained by TE alone. *J Clin Endocrinol Metab* 1998;83:3527–33.
22. Wang C, Berman NG, Veldhuis JD, Der T, McDonald V, Steiner B, et al. Graded testosterone infusions distinguish gonadotropin negative-feedback responsiveness in Asian and white men: a Clinical Research Center study. *J Clin Endocrinol Metab* 1998;83:870–6.
23. Santner SJ, Albertson B, Zhang GY, Zhang GH, Santulli M, Wang C, et al. Comparative rates of androgen production and metabolism in Caucasian and Chinese subjects. *J Clin Endocrinol Metab* 1998;83:2104–9.
24. Wang C, Catlin DH, Starcevic B, Heber D, Ambler C, Berman N, et al. Low fat high fiber diet decreased serum and urine androgens in men. *J Clin Endocrinol Metab* 2005;90:3550–9.
24. Handelsman DJ, Farley TM, Peregoudov A, Waites GM. Factors in nonuniform induction of azoospermia by testosterone enanthate in normal men. World Health Organization Task Force on Methods for the Regulation of Male Fertility. *Fertil Steril* 1995;63:125–33.

25. McLachlan RI, Robertson DM, Pruysers E, Ugoni A, Matsumoto AM, Anawalt BD, *et al.* Relationship between serum gonadotropins and spermatogenic suppression in men undergoing steroidal contraceptive treatment. *J Clin Endocrinol Metab* 2004;89:142–9.

26. Martin CW, Anderson RA, Cheng L, Ho PC, van der SZ, Smith KB, *et al.* Potential impact of hormonal male contraception: cross-cultural implications for development of novel preparations. *Hum Reprod* 2000;15:637–45.

27. Glasier AF, Anakwe R, Everington D, Martin CW, van der SZ, Cheng L, *et al.* Would women trust their partners to use a male pill? *Hum Reprod* 2000;15:646–9.

Chapter 18
Strategies to reduce unintended pregnancy among young people

Catherine Dennison and Cathy Hamlyn

Introduction

The past few years have seen major developments in policy and practice concerning young people and their reproductive and sexual health. The impetus for these has come from a number of sources, most notably the high rates of unintended pregnancy among young women and evidence surrounding the increased risk of negative outcomes for teenage parents and their children. This chapter provides an outline of government strategy surrounding prevention of pregnancy among young women, progress being made towards strategy objectives and direction for the future.

The Teenage Pregnancy Strategy for England

In 1999, the Government's Social Exclusion Unit launched a Teenage Pregnancy Strategy for England.[1] The strategy was a reaction to worrying trends in relation to young people's sexual activity:

- sex before the age of 16 years is common but associated with low levels of contraceptive use and high levels of regret
- high levels of unplanned teenage pregnancies, many of which are terminated by abortion
- high levels of sexually transmitted infections among young people
- links between teenage parenthood and poverty, unemployment, health problems and other negative outcomes.

The Prime Minister had specifically charged the Social Exclusion Unit with this task. Reflecting on the UK's high rates of teenage pregnancy in comparison with other European countries, in 1999 he stated: "Britain has the worst record on teenage pregnancies in Europe. It is not a record in which we can take any pride. As a country, we can't afford to continue to ignore this shameful record. Few societies find it easy to talk honestly about teenagers, sex and parenthood. It can seem easier to sweep such uncomfortable issues under the carpet. But the consequences of doing this can be seen all round us in shattered lives and blighted futures".

The resulting 10-year Teenage Pregnancy Strategy for England has two main goals: to reduce the rate of conceptions in under 18s by 50% by 2010 and set a firmly established downward trend in conceptions in the under-16-years age group and to increase to 60% the proportion of teenage mothers in education, training or employment in order to reduce their risk of long-term social exclusion. A 30-point action plan was set out for the first phases of the strategy. The plan covered a wide range of issues under four broad headings:

- joined-up action
- a national media campaign to reach young people and parents
- better prevention
- better support for teenage parents.

Following successful implementation of the original action plan, new work programmes have been developed under the same four themes in subsequent years. The following section details what has been achieved so far and how the strategy is being taken forward.

'Joined-up' action

A comprehensive structure has been put in place to ensure that the strategy is implemented across all areas of England. The emphasis is on groups of professionals working together so that action is coordinated and strengthened and clear messages about sex, pregnancy and sexually transmitted infections are sent to young people.

In order to coordinate activities related to the strategy, a national Teenage Pregnancy Unit was established. Initially based in the Department of Health, the unit is now located in the Children, Young People and Families Directorate, Department for Education and Skills (DfES). The unit continues to work closely with staff in several other government departments to ensure implementation of the action plan. The prevention goal is now a shared commitment, a public service agreement, between the DfES and the Department of Health. Crucially, it is also incorporated in a number of key planning frameworks, delivery plans and indicator sets for national and local level; for example, the National Health Service Plan, as a Best Value Indicator for Excellent Council status, primary care trust local delivery plan and data monitoring lines, local authority performance within the 'Change for Children' programme and the *Choosing Health* White Paper delivery plan.

To ensure effective implementation at local level, the unit interfaces with a network of teenage pregnancy coordinators based within local authorities. Each local authority has constituted a Teenage Pregnancy Partnership Board, membership of which is drawn from partner organisations. Together, boards and coordinators have developed and are implementing a 10-year strategy for their area that reflects the national strategy. Each local authority has agreed conception rate reduction targets for both 2004 and 2010. Coordinators are responsible for the instigation of activities aimed at making progress towards these targets, ensuring that these activities match the needs of the area and making sure that relevant partners, such as education, social services and housing authorities, are involved. Funds are available to every local area, in proportion to their conception rate, to facilitate this. Local teenage pregnancy coordinators are supported by nine regional teenage pregnancy coordinators, one in each government office of the regions.

A national independent advisory group, with a wide-ranging membership of experts from outside of government, advises on the direction of the strategy and the work of the Teenage Pregnancy Unit. Individual group members also act as advocates for the strategy among their own professional groups.

A number of policy developments have reinforced the aim of reducing the rate of conceptions in the under 18s as being a priority and the role of joined-up working in achieving this. In 2003, the Government published *Every Child Matters*,[2] its vision for children and young people based around five outcomes: being healthy, staying safe, enjoying and achieving, making a positive contribution and enjoying economic wellbeing. The Teenage Pregnancy Strategy is expected to be key in contributing to these outcomes. The Children Act 2004 places a duty on local authorities and their partners to cooperate towards meeting the five outcomes through joint planning and commissioning via pooled budgets. New performance management and inspection arrangements are being introduced to ensure progress towards these outcomes is made.

Both the National Service Framework for Children, Young People and Maternity Services[3] and the *Choosing Health*[4] public health White Paper have included teenage pregnancy. As part of its wider agenda to improve the health and wellbeing of all children, young people and their families, the National Service Framework highlights the importance of young-people-centred services in the prevention of teenage pregnancies and sexually transmitted infections and in the support for teenage parents. *Choosing Health* sets down the Government's commitment to building on the work of the Teenage Pregnancy Strategy. The new Green Paper, *Youth Matters*, led by the DfES, provides further endorsement of strategy goals and the need for joined up working and funding streams at local level.[5]

National media campaign

In an attempt to counteract media messages that promote sexual activity in young people and to inform them about the risks of unprotected sex, a national media campaign aimed at young people was launched in 2000. It addresses the themes of dealing with peer pressure, negotiating the use of contraception, encouraging condom use and informing young people about the consequences of unprotected sex. The campaign materials, developed in consultation with young people, use humour and straight talking to get their message across. Advertisements are featured on commercial radio stations, in teenage magazines and on washroom doors in shopping centres.

The campaign is supported by the Sexwise help line. Although operating nationally, it provides young people with advice and signposting to confidential services in their area. Sexwise advisers answer an average of 10 284 calls per day. The website, www.ruthinking.co.uk, provides comprehensive information and a database of local confidential services online. From March 2004 to February 2005, an average of 73 093 visits were made to the site each month. Public relations work in the teenage media and partnerships with youth brands reinforce campaign messages and further publicise the helpline and website.

To complement campaign activity aimed at young people, the 'Time to Talk' initiative, a partnership with the parenting support organisation, Parentline Plus, has been initiated to encourage parents to communicate with their children around sex and relationships. The need to facilitate improved parent–child communication has been shown by research which, as well as finding links between communication and delayed age of first intercourse and use of contraception, shows that many young people report receiving little or no information on sex and relationships from their parents.

Better prevention

A wide range of activities is being undertaken to tackle the causes of teenage pregnancy. These include improving the sex and relationship education that young people receive and enabling better access to confidential sources of advice about, and methods of, contraception. The international evidence base supports taking a multifaceted approach to prevention of pregnancy.[6] Analysis of countries with lower rates concludes that they are characterised by provision of quality sex education, improving access to contraception and building incentives to avoid early parenthood.[6,7] Reviews of 'what works' show support for school-based sex education, linked to contraceptive services and community based education and services.[8] Research has shown a positive association between total number of school sex education lessons received and not becoming pregnant.[9]

Ensuring that all young people receive good quality sex and relationships education is a central part of the prevention component. In 2000, the DfES issued guidance to schools on how sex and relationships education, within the context of personal, social and health education, should be delivered, with the expectation that schools would use this to develop and review their own policies.[10] The Office for Standards in Education (Ofsted) subsequently issued a review of current provision and set clear learning outcomes.[11] Ofsted now includes personal, social and health education within their full inspection of schools. To ensure that teachers are equipped to deliver sex and relationships education effectively, a programme of professional development in personal, social and health education was introduced. Community nurses can also access a linked programme in recognition of the contribution that they can make.

The National Healthy Schools Programme has been a key mechanism for improving delivery of sex and relationships education, within the context of personal, social and health education. Participating schools have received support to improve their policy and practice. The programme has already reached over 16 000 schools: encompassing primary, secondary, independent and special schools. Healthy Schools was relaunched in September 2005 and delivery of good quality personal, social and health education is now a core requirement of achieving the new Healthy School Standard. The DfES 5-Year Strategy and the *Choosing Health* White Paper set a goal for all schools to become 'Healthy Schools' by 2009. In September 2005, the QCA published assessment guidance for schools on the skills and knowledge young people should gain through personal, social and health education at each key stage. This should help schools to evaluate their delivery of personal, social and health education, an area that the 2005 Ofsted report cited as weak.[12]

The needs of young people who are likely to be outside of school but who are known to be at increased likelihood of becoming teenage parents are also being addressed. For example, in recognition that at least 25% of young males in prison custody are already fathers, all young offender institutions must now offer sex education and parenting courses.

Sex and relationships education, wherever and however it is delivered, needs to provide young people with details of where and how they can access local contraceptive services. However, unless such services are confidential and 'young-people friendly' young people will not use them. The Teenage Pregnancy Unit issued guidance on what good services should look like.[13] The Teenage Pregnancy Unit and the Department of Health are working in partnership to support development of quality standards for provision of services. The resource *Getting it right for young people*

'*You're Welcome: Quality Standards*' will be issued in Autumn 2005, to assist services in making improvements and sustaining the quality of the services they provide to young people.

An emphasis has also been placed on taking services to where young people are, resulting in sexual health advice being given in leisure centres, mobile units, Connexions centres and schools. Increasingly schools are interested in providing on-site health services to improve young people's access to advice on a range of health and emotional issues, including sexual health. Provision of a young people's sexual health drop-in service is one of the options schools may consider as part of the Extended Schools Programme.

Reaching groups at higher risk of pregnancy, as well as the mainstream, has been a key element of the Strategy. National and local links have been made with groups experienced in working with vulnerable young people to develop materials and interventions tailored to the needs of Black and minority ethnic young people, asylum seekers and refugees, those looked after in the public care system and care leavers, those with special educational needs, and young offenders. Specific guidance has been issued to those working with young people in the public care system and to youth support workers[14]. National and local links between Strategy and regeneration initiatives have also been developed to reach young people in the highest rate areas.

Better support

An equivalent level of energy is being directed towards improving the level of support given to those who do become pregnant and those who go on to become parents. An essential part of this is to improve the support given to young women when they find they are pregnant, to inform the choices they make and to assist them in accessing the help they need. This includes support to prevent subsequent unplanned pregnancies. It is estimated that 20% of births conceived to under 18s are second pregnancies. New guidance on commissioning maternity services for teenage parents is one illustration of how the strategy is attempting to improve the care young women receive if they continue with their pregnancy.[15] For those who become young parents, support tailored to match need should now be available to them in their local area. Support should be available to them to address housing need; help with negotiating the benefit system; access education and training, including funding for childcare to enable them to attend; and provision of emotional support, through peers or professionals. Sure Start Plus has been a pilot programme in 35 local authorities to deliver packages of coordinated support to pregnant teenagers and teenage parents.

The Sexual Health Strategy

The launch of the National Strategy for Sexual Health and HIV in 2001 extended government commitments in relation to sexual health.[16] Rather than being restricted to teenagers, this new strategy relates to the population as a whole. Alongside goals relating to reducing prevalence and transmission of HIV and sexually transmitted infections improving the health and social care for people living with HIV reductions and reducing the stigma associated with HIV and sexually transmitted infections, the strategy aims to reduce unintended pregnancy.

Much of what is in the Sexual Health Strategy complements the Teenage Pregnancy Strategy. A focus is being placed on improving contraceptive, as well as broader sexual health, service provision. Additional funding has been made available to modernise sexual health services, to increase access and to extend the locations where advice and treatment are available. A national audit of contraceptive services is planned, in order to identify gaps in local services where investment should be focused.

The need to improve access to information on sexual health is also a theme of the Sexual Health Strategy. A national media campaign has been instigated to reach an older age group than the teenage pregnancy one. Following *Choosing Health*, a new, larger-scale, national campaign will be launched. It will be aimed at younger men and women to ensure that they understand the real risk of unprotected sex and convince them of the benefits of using condoms to avoid sexually transmitted infections and unintended pregnancy.

Evidence of effectiveness

Current trends

The rate of under-18s conceptions is the main marker of progress on the prevention goal of the Teenage Pregnancy Strategy. The most recent data available are for 2003, which show a reduction of 9.8% since 1998, the baseline year for the strategy. The rate of under-16s conception has decreased by 9.9%. Eight of nine government regions have seen a decline in their rates of between 8% and 16% since 1998. Four of five local authorities have reduced their rates between 1998 and 2003. As Figure 18.1 illustrates, although this trend is in the right direction, meeting the 2010 target remains extremely challenging.

Explaining trends

To help build an understanding of how the Teenage Pregnancy Strategy is having impact and what are the most effective elements, a 4-year independent evaluation was commissioned in 2000. A multidisciplinary team from the London School of Hygiene

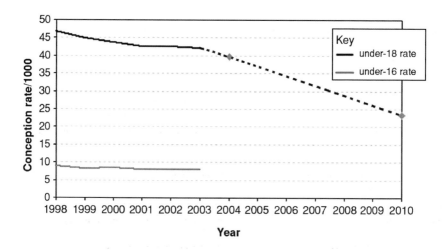

Figure 18.1. Progress in reducing conception rates

and Tropical Medicine, University College London, and the British Market Research Bureau undertook the project. They used a range of methodologies to identify factors that have enhanced or hindered implementation over the first 4 years and provided feedback on what appears to be contributing to conception rate reductions.[9]

The evaluation team confirmed perceptions that implementation is working well:

- joint working has progressed
- substantial proportions of young people recognise the media campaign
- more young people agree that sex and relationships education meets their needs
- young people have increased their use of school-based services, help lines and websites to access contraceptive advice.

The evaluation highlighted that the rate of decline has been steeper in areas of high deprivation and low educational attainment and in areas that received most funding to implement the strategy. This has been taken as confirmation that the strategy has been well targeted at areas of greatest need but that future efforts need to be focused on tackling the underlying socioeconomic determinants of teenage pregnancy.

In-depth qualitative analysis in a small number of areas tried to identify characteristics of areas with increasing and decreasing rates. The methodology used must have caveats placed around it, most notably that it relied upon retrospective interpretation, where informants were aware of local trends in looking to single out contributing elements. However, the factors in Table 18.1 tended to characterise decreasing and increasing areas.

To extend our knowledge of 'what works', the team looked to other European countries to identify what factors could be seen as contributing to their current patterns. Birth rates in Denmark, France, Germany, the Netherlands and Switzerland are all considerably lower than the UK, but their most recent trends differ. The team concluded that: "countries in which teenage pregnancy rates have remained low appear to be characterised by ample educational and career opportunities, and a high

Table 18.1. Characteristics of areas with increasing and decreasing rates

Increasing rates	Decreasing rates
Base line statistics unfavourable	Base rate favourable to interpretation
Population instability	Small population size
Multiple deprivation indices	Increasing affluence in area
Socioeconomic heterogeneity	Access to young people's sexual health services
Social norms favouring early motherhood	Strong, senior coordination
History of effective preventative work predating strategy	Effective partnerships
Delay in start of strategy	Prompt start to strategy
Junior coordinator	Support from local education authority
Local opposition to strategy	Local support for the strategy
Organisational change unhelpful	Organisational change helpful

value placed on the achievement of young women; by the widespread provision of sex education, unaccompanied by controversy and political resistance; by an absence of conflicting and confusing media representations of sexuality, particularly among the young; and by good access to sexual health services".

The future

Informed by the national evaluation and other sources of analysis, the next phase of the strategy will see an increased focus on reaching those young people most at risk. With 50% of conceptions in the under-18s occurring in 20% of areas with the highest rates, there will be an emphasis on intensifying delivery of all-strands of the strategy to high-rate neighbourhoods and vulnerable groups.

Although all young people need to continue to 'receive' key elements of the strategy, such as improved sex and relationships education and enhanced services, it is recognised that some young people require greater levels of support. We need to reach those young people who take most risks, who are reckless with their own health and their own bodies. In order to steer this work, we need to understand better why such girls and young women have sex; why they don't use contraception effectively and what would motivate them to avoid early pregnancy. We also need to increase our understanding of how to influence those young men who do not treat girls and young women with respect; who will not use contraception; and who seem indifferent to sexually transmitted infections and pregnancy risks. Again, understanding what would make a difference to these young men is essential.

International comparisons offer warning against reticence in efforts to prevent unintended teenage conceptions. The Netherlands, where pregnancy rates have been just a fraction of those in the UK, has seen an increase coinciding with reduced investment in sexual health services, sex and relationship education and removal of universal entitlement to free contraception. Each new wave of young people needs to receive messages about resisting peer pressure and how to protect themselves. They need to know how to access advice and that advice needs to be kept relevant and they need access to, and confidence to participate in, a range of opportunities so that postponing pregnancy becomes desirable. Local and national political will, as indicated in policy statements such as the *Choosing Health* White Paper, offers long-term support for these objectives. Politicians, policy makers, practitioners and researchers need to work together to ensure that they are realised.

References

1. Social Exclusion Unit. *Teenage Pregnancy*. London: TSO; 1999.
2. Department for Education and Skills. *Every Child Matters*. CM5860. London: DfES; 2003 [www.everychildmatters.gov.uk].
3. Department of Health. *The National Service Framework for Children, Young People and Maternity Services*. London: DH; 2004.
4. Department of Health. *Choosing Health. Making Healthier Choices Easier*. London: DH; 2004.
5. Department for Education and Skills. *Youth Matters*. Cm 6629. London: TSO; 2005 [www.dfes.gov.uk/publications/youth].
6. Darroch J, Singh S. *Why is Teenage Pregnancy Declining? The roles of abstinence, sexual activity and contraceptive use*. Occasional Report No. 1. New York: Alan Guttmacher Institute; 1999.
7. UNICEF. *A League Table of Teenage Births in Rich Nations*. Innocenti Report Card No. 3. Florence: UNICEF; 2001.
8. Swann C, Bowe K, McCormick G, Kosmin M. *Teenage Pregnancy and Parenthood: a review of reviews*. Evidence briefing. London: Health Development Agency; 2003.

9   Wellings K, Wilkinson P, Grundy C, Kane R, Lachowycz K, Jacklin P, *et al. Teenage Pregnancy Strategy: Evaluation Final Report Synthesis.* Report RW38. London: Department for Education and Skills; 2005.

10.   Department for Education and Skills. *Sex and Relationship Education Guidance. Guidance: Curriculum and Standards. Head Teachers, Teachers and School Governors.* London: DfES; 2000.

11.   Office for Standards in Education. *Sex and Relationships Education in Schools.* London: OFSTED; 2002.

12.   Office for Standards in Education. *Personal, Social and Health Education in Secondary Schools.* London: OFSTED; 2005.

13.   Teenage Pregnancy Unit. *Best Practice Guidance on the Provision of Effective Contraception and Advice Services.* London: TPU; 2000.

14.   Teenage Pregnancy Unit. *Enabling Young People to Access Contraceptive and Sexual Health Information and Advice: Legal and Policy Framework for Residential Social Workers, Foster Carers and other Social Care Practitioners.* London: TPU; 2004.

15.   Teenage Pregnancy Unit, Royal College of Midwives. *Teenage Parents: Who Cares? A Guide to Commissioning and Delivering Maternity Services for Young Parents.* London: Department of Health; 2004.

16.   Department of Health. *The National Strategy for Sexual Health and HIV.* London: DH; 2001.

Chapter 19
Fertility control: improving prescribing

Gillian Penney

Background

Primary clinical research continually generates new findings that can contribute to effective and efficient patient care. Secondary research, in the form of systematic review and meta-analysis, and guideline development or consensus exercises, such as this Study Group, endeavour to collate and synthesise the evidence on discrete clinical topics. However, all this evidence and effort cannot change patient outcomes unless healthcare professionals adopt new recommendations in practice.

For more than 15 years, the UK National Health Service (NHS) has dedicated substantial funding to a series of 'quality' initiatives aimed at 'getting evidence into practice'. The evolution of this NHS quality agenda has encompassed medical and clinical audit,[1,2] clinical guidelines,[3] clinical effectiveness[4] and clinical governance.[5] Despite this long-term investment, there is continuing acknowledgement of a gap between evidence and practice. This gap was highlighted by Archie Cochrane as long ago as 1972.[6] It was the topic of a major review by the NHS Centre for Reviews and Dissemination in 1999[7] and is the theme of the evidence-based medicine approach advocated by the Canadian group led by David Sackett.[8]

The UK health quality organisation, the National Institute for Clinical Excellence, recognises that changes to improve patient care may need to be implemented at any or all of three levels: the **individual** practitioner, the healthcare **team** and the local or national **service**.[9] The focus of this chapter is on one specific component of healthcare: prescribing. Interventions aimed at improving prescribing are appropriately targeted at the individual, rather than the team or service. Thus, this chapter examines strategies for improving professional behaviour in general but focuses specifically on strategies aimed at individual practitioners for improving prescribing behaviour.

Method of review

This chapter is based on a structured review of published literature. Initially, the Cochrane Effective Practice and Organisation of Care Group section within the Cochrane Library was searched for systematic reviews on changing professional behaviour. Sixty reviews and protocols were identified. In view of this substantial body of 'level 1a' evidence[10] from systematic reviews, individual studies relating to changing professional behaviour in general were not systematically sought. The Ovid

Table 19.2. Specific types of intervention for changing professionals' behaviour (adapted from Cochrane Library, Effective Practice and Organisation of Care Group)

Type of intervention	Current Cochrane Reviews and (Protocols) (*n*)	Cochrane Reviews summarised in this chapter
Continuing education and quality assurance:		
Distribution of educational materials (including guidelines)	0 (2)	
Educational meetings (including lectures and workshops)	1 (0)	Yes
Local consensus processes	0 (1)	No
Educational outreach visits	1 (0)	Yes
Local opinion leaders	1 (0)	Yes
Patient-mediated interventions	0 (0)	No
Audit and feedback	1 (0)	Yes
Reminders (computerised and paper-based)	0 (3)	No
Marketing	0 (1)	No
Mass media	1 (0)	Yes
Other (interprofessional education/continuous quality improvement)	1 (1)	Yes
Financial interventions:		
Provider oriented	2 (0)	Yes
Patient oriented	0 (1)	No
Organisational interventions:		
Provider oriented	21[a]	No
Patient oriented		
Structural interventions		
Regulatory interventions	0 (0)	No

[a] Reviews and protocols not separated

structured case records, and promotion of a patient information leaflet. Despite delivery of the implementation package by an energetic researcher under the auspices of a respected national organisation, there was no significant impact on compliance with key guideline recommendations.

Thus, although substantial national investment in the development of clinical guidelines continues, there is little, if any, objective evidence that they are effective in changing professional behaviour, even when supported by carefully designed implementation strategies.

Educational meetings

A current Cochrane Review addresses 'Continuing education meetings and workshops: effects on professional practice and healthcare outcomes'.[16] Thirty-two studies were included, involving a total of 2995 professionals. Ten comparisons assessed the effects of interactive workshops; seven showed significant effects (mostly moderately large effects) and three showed nonsignificant, small but positive effects. Nineteen comparisons assessed the effects of workshops in combination with didactic lectures; 12 showed significant effects (mostly moderately large effects) and seven showed nonsignificant but positive effects. In contrast, seven comparisons assessing didactic presentations alone showed no significant effects (with the single exception of one of four outcomes measured in one study). Thus, the Cochrane reviewers concluded 'Interactive workshops can result in moderately large changes in professional practice. Didactic sessions alone are unlikely to change professional practice'.

Educational outreach visits

An educational outreach visit has been defined as 'a personal visit by a trained person to a healthcare provider in his own setting'[17] and is also known as 'university-based academic detailing', 'public interest detailing' and 'academic detailing'. Clearly, this approach closely resembles the strategy used by pharmaceutical companies in sending their representatives to visit individual doctors. Outreach visits have been identified as an intervention that may improve professionals' practice – particularly prescribing. A current Cochrane Review addresses 'Educational outreach visits: effects on professional practice and healthcare outcomes'.[17]

Eighteen studies were included, involving a total of 1896 doctors. All of the outreach interventions comprised multiple components: including written materials, conferences, reminders and audit and feedback. Thirteen studies specifically related to prescribing behaviour. Positive effects on practice were observed in all 18 studies; only one study measured a patient outcome. Thus, the Cochrane reviewers concluded, 'Educational outreach visits appear to be a promising approach to modifying health professional behaviour, especially prescribing'.

Local opinion leaders

The theoretical models of behaviour and behaviour change outlined above suggest that using local opinion leaders to transmit norms and model appropriate behaviour may improve health professionals' practice. A local opinion leader has been defined as 'a health professional nominated by his colleagues as being educationally influential'.[18] A current Cochrane Review addresses 'Local opinion leaders: effects on professional practice and healthcare outcomes'.[18] Eight studies were included involving a total of 296 professionals. Only two trials showed a statistically significant and clinically important effect. Nevertheless, almost all trials demonstrated some improvement for at least one of the outcomes measured. Thus, the Cochrane reviewers concluded, 'Using local opinion leaders has mixed effects on professional practice'.

Audit and feedback

Audit and feedback (defined by the Cochrane Collaboration as 'any summary of clinical performance over a specified period of time'[19]) is widely used as a strategy to improve professional practice. Intuitively, one would expect that professionals would be prompted to modify their practice if given feedback that their practice was inconsistent with that of their peers or accepted guidelines. A current Cochrane Review addresses 'Audit and feedback: effects on professional practice and healthcare outcomes'.[19]

Eighty-five studies were included. Of these, 47 (with over 3500 professionals) directly compared audit and feedback to no intervention. Overall, the median adjusted risk difference of noncompliance with desired practice was 0.07 (representing a 7% absolute decrease in noncompliance). However, some studies showed adjusted risk differences of up to 0.71 (representing a 71% decrease in noncompliance). The overall conclusion of the Cochrane reviewers was that 'Audit and feedback can be effective in improving professional practice. When it is effective, the effects are generally small to moderate'. This conclusion is in line with our own experience. By means of before-and-after surveys, we assessed the impact of a national audit of gynaecological topics on clinicians' practice.[20] Significant changes in reported practice, in line with project recommendations, were found for seven of 12 specific elements of care examined.

Mass media

The mass media frequently cover health-related topics. They are the leading source of information about important health issues and are targeted by those who aim to influence the behaviour of health professionals and patients.[21] A current Cochrane Review addresses 'Mass media interventions: effects on health services use'.[21] Twenty interrupted time series were included; generally, methodological quality was poor. Despite the limitations of the studies, the Cochrane reviewers concluded that 'mass media may have an important role in influencing use of healthcare interventions'. However, these findings relate to behaviour of patients, rather than professionals. We have no information on the extent to which the mass media influence clinicians' practice.

Interprofessional education

A current Cochrane Review addressed the specific topic of 'Interprofessional education: effects on professional practice and healthcare outcomes'.[22] Despite identifying 1042 studies, none was deemed to meet the inclusion criteria for a Cochrane Review and no conclusions could be drawn about the effects of interprofessional education.

Provider-oriented financial interventions

It is widely believed that the method of payment of doctors may affect their clinical behaviour. However, little is known about the effects of different payment systems on policy objectives such as cost-containment or quality of care. Two current Cochrane Reviews address forms of provider oriented financial interventions.[23,24]

The first review assesses the impact of target payments (a payment system which remunerates professionals only if they provide a minimum level of care).[23] Only two studies (involving 149 practices) were included. Target payments increased immunisation rates (significantly in only one study). The Cochrane reviewers concluded that the available evidence was of insufficient quality and power to provide an answer as to the impact of target payments.

The second review sought to assess the impact of various payment systems (capitation, fee-for-service and mixed) on primary-care physicians' behaviour.[24] Four studies (involving 640 doctors and 6400 patients) were included. Findings were complicated: with fee-for-service systems resulting in more patient visits, greater continuity of care and higher compliance with recommended number of visits but in lower patient satisfaction with access to their doctors. The reviewers could only conclude that there is some evidence that payment systems affect clinicians' behaviour but that the ability to generalise from the findings is unknown.

Other types of intervention

Table 19.2 includes other types of intervention which, theoretically, might serve to change clinicians' behaviour. Some have not been discussed here because of the lack of published systematic reviews: local consensus processes, patient-mediated interventions, reminders, marketing and patient-oriented financial interventions. Others have not been discussed because they relate to organisational or regulatory interventions. Issues related to improving services are addressed elsewhere in this volume.

Interventions to improve prescribing

Within the Cochrane Library, interventions to change professional behaviour are categorised according to the type of intervention (as discussed above) and also according to the type of behaviour to be changed. One review and two protocols relate to changing prescribing behaviour. The one full review addresses 'Computerised advice on drug dosage to improve prescribing practice'.[25] Fifteen trials involving 1229 patients were included. However, none of the studies related to contraceptive prescribing. The findings supported the use of computer assistance in determining drug dosage. The findings are unlikely to be generalisable to contraceptive practice, where dosage schedules are uncomplicated and seldom individualised according to patient weight or other characteristics.

Studies relating to contraceptive practice

The Medline search (1996–2004) for studies specifically relating to 'practice patterns' and 'contraception/fertility control' identified only 11 broadly relevant abstracts. Of these, only three related to interventions designed to change prescribing by professionals.[26–28] The others related to interventions designed to change patients' knowledge or behaviour (which may, in turn, affect clinicians' behaviour) or to the effects of service redesign.

One study from the USA assessed changes in the prescribing practices of healthcare providers after an educational programme about emergency contraception.[26] The educational programme, or demonstration project, had four main components, including written materials and training sessions. Before-and-after questionnaires were completed by 102 doctors and 'mid-level professionals'. After the educational programme, the number of professionals who reported prescribing emergency contraception at least once a year increased by almost 20%.

A study from Thailand assessed changes in practice relating to emergency contraception among pharmacy personnel after an educational intervention.[28] Sixty pharmacies participated; 50% being allocated to receive the educational programme. Knowledge and practice in dispensing emergency contraception was assessed by 'well-trained secret shoppers'. Sellers in the intervention group improved significantly in choice of drug, advice provided and knowledge of the time limit for initiating emergency contraception but those in the control group did not.

A third study, from the Netherlands, assessed the quality of data recording (rather than actual prescribing) after introduction of a new electronic medical record.[27] For the contraceptive pill, the percentage of cases where information on indications was missing fell from 34% to 1%. While not directly relevant to quality of prescribing or of immediate patient care, accurate data recording is, of course, an important element of health care.

Improving prescribing: a pragmatic approach

This brief overview of models of professional behaviour and of the available evidence about interventions to change behaviour indicates that the research base is currently incomplete. What is clear is that it is relatively easy to improve the knowledge of professionals (through written materials, didactic lectures or other means) but more difficult to improve behaviour, including prescribing practice.

Cochrane Reviews indicate that approaches to changing professional behaviour that are consistently effective (albeit to a modest extent) include interactive workshops and educational outreach visits. Audit and feedback is widely used and is often a component of educational outreach but there is less consistent evidence of its effectiveness. There is even less robust evidence to support the other types of intervention that have been proposed (such as financial incentives; use of opinion leaders and patient-mediated interventions).

Despite these difficulties, health policy makers, heads of services and individual clinicians must strive to continually improve practice (including prescribing) in order to meet the goals of the clinical effectiveness[4] and clinical governance[5] initiatives. In 1999, the *Effective Health Care Bulletin* on 'Getting evidence into practice'[7] outlined a systematic, stepwise approach to achieving change in practice involving a 'diagnostic analysis' to inform the development of an appropriate action plan. Such an approach remains relevant today and is summarised in Table 19.3.

Recommendations

On a regular basis, each and every health policy maker, head of service and individual clinician should identify recently published guidelines, consensus statements (such as these Study Group proceedings) and policy documents which are relevant to his own area of practice. Policy makers, heads of services and individual clinicians should compare their own practice (or practice within the service for which they are responsible) with the recommendations in these identified documents. If necessary, local audits should be undertaken to assess the extent to which practice measures up to recommendations. For each aspect of practice for which a need for change is identified, a systematic diagnostic analysis should be undertaken, leading to a three-point action plan for change:

- **What** are we going to do?
- **Who** is going to make it happen?
- **When** will it be done?

Table 19.3. A systematic approach to changing professional practice (adapted from *Effective Health Care Bulletin*)[7]

Stage no.	Stage	Components and activities
1	Identify area of practice requiring change	Clinical audit may identify areas where local practice is inconsistent with colleagues or relevant guidelines. Critical incidents or patient/carer complaints may also highlight areas requiring change
2	Identify all groups ('stakeholders') involved	For action planning and change to be successful, all groups affected by a change must be involved in the process
3	Assess characteristics of the proposed change	The extent to which an aspect of practice is evidence-based, requires new skills, fits with patient expectations, etc. and can influence ease of achieving change[29]
4	Assess 'preparedness' of target clinicians to change	Interactive discussions with all those affected
5	Identify barriers to change	Categorising barriers can assist action planning. There are published frameworks[30] but a simple classification is: invalid standard; knowledge; skills; attitudes; resources
6	Identify enabling factors, or facilitators, of change	The diagnostic analysis should aim to identify positive factors, as well as negative
7	Agree a three-point action plan	On completion of the 'diagnostic analysis', for each area of practice requiring change, the stakeholder group should agree an action plan: **What** are we going to do? **Who** is going to make it happen? **When** will it be done?

References

1. Department of Health. *Working for Patients.* London: HMSO; 1989.
2. Department of Health, NHS Management Executive. *Clinical Audit: Meeting and Improving Standards in Healthcare.* London: DH; 1993.
3. Mann, T. *Clinical Guidelines: Using Clinical Guidelines to Improve Patient Care Within the NHS.* London: NHS Executive; 1996.
4. NHS Executive. *Promoting Clinical Effectiveness: A Framework for Action in and through the NHS.* London: NHS Executive 1996.
5. Department of Health. *A First Class Service: Quality in the New NHS.* London: DH; 1998.
6. Cochrane AL. *Effectiveness and Efficiency. Random Reflections on Health Services.* London: Nuffield Provincial Hospitals Trust; 1972.
7. University of York. NHS Centre for Reviews and Dissemination, Getting evidence into practice. *Effective Health Care* 1999;5:16.
8. Sackett DL, Straus SE, Richardson WS, Rosenberg W, Haynes RB. *Evidence-based Medicine: How to*

Practise and Teach EBM. 2nd ed. London: Churchill-Livingstone; 2000.

9. National Institute for Clinical Excellence. *Principles for Best Practice in Clinical Audit*. Oxford: Radcliffe Medical Press; 2002.

10. US Department of Health and Human Services Agency for Health Care Policy and Research. *Acute Pain Management: Operative or Medical Procedures and Trauma*. Clinical Practice Guideline No. 1. Publication No. AHCPR 92-0032. Rockville, MD: Agency for Health Care Policy and Research; 1992.

11. Lomas J. Retailing research: increasing the role of evidence in clinical services for child birth. *Milbank Quarterly* 1993;71:439–75.

12. Foy R, Ramsay CR, Grimshaw JM, Penney GC, Vale L, Thomson A, *et al*. The impact of guidelines on mild hypertension in pregnancy: time series analysis. *BJOG* 2004;111:765–70.

13. Scottish Obstetric Guidelines and Audit Project. *The Management of Mild, Non-proteinuric Hypertension in Pregnancy*. Aberdeen: Scottish Programme for Clinical Effectiveness in Reproductive Health; 1997.

14. Foy R, Penney GC, Grimshaw JM, Ramsay CR, Walker AE, MacLennan G, *et al*. A randomised controlled trial of a tailored multifaceted strategy to promote implementation of a clinical guideline on induced abortion care. *BJOG* 2004;111:726–33.

15. Royal College of Obstetricians and Gynaecologists Clinical Effectiveness Support Unit. *The Care of Women Requesting Induced Abortion*. Evidence-based Guideline No 7. London: RCOG Press; 2004.

16. Thomson O'Brien MA, Freemantle N, Oxman AD, Wolf F, Davis DA, Herrin J. Continuing education meetings and workshops: effects on professional practice and health care outcomes. *Cochrane Database Syst Rev* 2001; CD003030. DOI:10.1002/14651858.CD003030.

17. Thomson O'Brien MA, Oxman AD, Davis DA, Haynes RB, Freemantle N, Harvey EL. Educational outreach visits: effects on professional practice and health care outcomes. *Cochrane Database Syst Rev* 1997;(4).

18. Thomson O'Brien MA, Oxman AD, Haynes RB, Davis DA, Freemantle N, Harvey EL. Local opinion leaders: effects on professional practice and health care outcomes. *Cochrane Database Syst Rev* 1999;(1).

19. Jamtvedt G, Young JM, Kristoffersen DT, Thomson O'Brien MA, Oxman AD. Audit and feedback: effects on professional practice and health care outcomes. *Cochrane Database Syst Rev* 2003;(3).

20. Penney GC, Templeton A. Impact of a national audit project on gynaecologists in Scotland. *Qual Health Care* 1995;4(1):37–9.

21. Grilli R, Ramsay C, Minozzi S. Mass media interventions: effects on health services utilisation. *Cochrane Database Syst Rev* 2002;(1).

22. Zwarenstein M, Reeves S, Barr H, Hammick M, Koppel I, Atkins J. Interprofessional education: effects on professional practice and health care outcomes. *Cochrane Database Syst Rev* 2000;(3).

23. Giuffrida A, Gosden T, Forland F, Kristiansen IS, Sergison M, Leese B, *et al*. Target payments in primary care: effects on professional practice and health care outcomes. *Cochrane Database Syst Rev* 1999;(4).

24. Gosden T, Forland F, Kristiansen IS, Sutton M, Leese B, Giuffrida A, *et al*. Capitation, fee-for-service and mixed systems of payment: effects on the behaviour of primary care physicians. *Cochrane Database Syst Rev* 2000;(3).

25. Walton RT, Harvey E, Dovey S, Freemantle N. Computerised advice on drug dosage to improve prescribing practice. *Cochrane Database Syst Rev* 2000;(1).

26. Beckman LJ, Harvey SM, Sherman CA, Petitti DB. Changes in providers' views and practices about emergency contraception with education. *Obstet Gynecol* 2001;97:942–6.

27. Hiddema-Van de Wal A, Smith R, van der Werf G, Meyboom-De Jong B. Towards improvement of the accuracy and completeness of medication registration with the use of an electronic medical record (EMR). *Fam Pract* 2001;18:288–91.

28. Ratanajamit C, Chongsuvivatwong V, Geater AF. A randomized controlled educational intervention on emergency contraception among drugstore personnel in southern Thailand. *J Am Med Womens Assoc* 2002;57:196–9.

29. Foy R, MacLennan G, Grimshaw J, Penney G, Campbell M, Grol R. Attributes of clinical recommendations that influence change in practice following audit and feedback. *J Clin Epidemiol* 2002;55:717–22.

30. Foy R, Walker A, Penney GC. Barriers to clinical guidelines: the need for concerted action. *British Journal of Clinical Governance* 2001;6:166–74.

Chapter 20

Improving services: increasing options and encouraging use

Anna Glasier

Introduction

Contraceptive prevalence in the UK in the early 21st century is high. According to the Office for National Statistics Omnibus Survey,[1] only 2% of sexually active, potentially fertile women not wishing to conceive reported not using a method of contraception in 2003/04. This reassuring statistic hides the fact that the majority of women at risk of pregnancy are using methods associated with relatively high failure rates when used typically. Among women using a reversible method, just under 50% are using oral contraception with typical use failure rates of 8%. Well over 50% are using a barrier method, periodic abstinence (natural family planning) or withdrawal, with typical-use failure rates of between 15% (male condom) and 32% (cap).[2]

There are few good data on patterns of contraceptive use with time and most come from the USA or Sweden. It is probably reasonable to extrapolate these data to the UK and assume that incorrect or inconsistent use of condoms[3] and oral contraception[4] is common. It is also likely that discontinuation rates are high,[5] method switching frequent and that when they do switch, women or couples often change to a less effective method of contraception, despite wishing to avoid pregnancy.[5,6]

Most data suggest that somewhere between 33% and 50% of women in the UK[7,8] having an abortion used no method of contraception at the time they conceived. Most of the others were using a method inconsistently or incorrectly. Fewer than 10% of unintended pregnancies result from a true method failure. Given these statistics, and in the knowledge that unintended pregnancy is related to a multitude of social factors, it is worth considering what services can do to improve patterns of contraceptive uptake, use and continuation in the UK.

It is difficult to improve on a contraceptive prevalence of 98%. Health professionals should concentrate their efforts on increasing uptake of the most effective methods and ensuring correct and consistent use of all contraceptives. Initiatives that may improve the pattern of contraceptive use include:

- expanding service provision
- improving accessibility of services
- increasing the range of methods available at services
- improving education/information about correct and consistent use

- involving men in service use
- improving the accessibility of the methods.

Expanding services

Services can be expanded either by increasing the number of 'outlets' for contraceptive methods and/or by increasing the range of providers.

Increasing the number of outlets

Contraception is available in the UK free of charge to women and men attending their general practitioner (and the vast majority of UK residents are registered with a GP) and from National Health Service (NHS) family planning clinics. It is also available free from some other NHS services, such as genitourinary medicine clinics, accident and emergency departments (usually only emergency contraception), and from charitable organisations such as Brook clinics (usually limited to young people). Condoms and emergency contraception can be purchased without prescription from pharmacies and condoms are sold in other retail outlets.

Most women in the UK obtain contraception from their GP surgery (81% in the 2003/04 Omnibus Survey). A significant proportion (32%), however, choose to attend a family planning clinic. Over time, many women will visit both. The number of people attending family planning clinics increased by 2% in 2003/04. Young people are particularly likely to attend family planning clinics: 23% of all 16 to 17-year-olds and almost 40% of 16 to 19-year-olds using a service had attended a family planning clinic.[1] Unpublished data from surveys in a large family planning clinic in Edinburgh (and almost certainly echoed in other clinics) reveal a number of reasons why people choose to attend a family planning clinic in preference to the GP. Those most commonly cited include perceived expertise; a guarantee of seeing a female doctor; better opening times, including evening sessions; and ease of obtaining appointments. Young people appreciate the anonymity and confidentiality they perceive in services provided outside their GP surgery.[9] These same factors are echoed in findings from studies in other areas. Data from Wessex have suggested that close geographical proximity to a dedicated young peoples' service is associated with lower rates of teenage pregnancy.[10]

Eight percent of women completing the 2003/04 Omnibus Survey had used a pharmacist for family planning services. Most men use pharmacists and other retail outlets for purchasing condoms (at present, the only reversible method available to them). In urban areas, pharmacies are to be found in most main streets and are open on Saturdays and sometimes on Sundays. The availability of emergency contraception from pharmacies has demonstrably resulted in women experiencing fewer problems obtaining it. In the 2003/04 Omnibus Survey only 4% of respondents reported difficulty in obtaining emergency contraception compared with 13% in 2000/01.

A number of non-medical settings have been evaluated as sites for family planning service provision including schools,[11] city-centre pharmacies[12] and 'healthy living centres'. A study of pupils in Baltimore demonstrated increased rates of attendance for family planning advice if health centres were available within schools.[11] Non-medical settings often present practical difficulties, such as the availability of case notes and supplies but may be particularly attractive to vulnerable groups, who appreciate the complete anonymity associated with entering a building which is not obviously a sexual health setting. Not all sites suit all people and costs and practical issues often dictate what premises are available. In general, a setting that is geographically central, well served by public transport, with car parking available and in or near a place visited regularly by the target group while simultaneously offering some anonymity, is likely to be an acceptable setting.

Increasing the range of contraceptive providers

Expanding the role of a variety of nonmedical health professionals in reproductive health services should improve access to contraception. Recent years have seen an expanding role for nurses in sexual health. In a GP setting, much of the routine contraceptive advice and provision is from the practice nurse. Many school nurses provide sex education and some also provide contraception in schools according to patient group directions. For many years, nurses in most community family planning clinics have extended their role beyond that of handmaiden to the doctor. The use of patient group directions and nurse prescribing allows well-trained nurses to practise independently, offering a much better service than in the past and complementing that provided by doctors.[13,14] The nature of general nurse training and the lack of a broad training structure for nurses in sexual and reproductive health inevitably means that they offer a narrower breadth of care and expertise than experienced doctors.[15] In the climate of a cash-strapped NHS, there is a danger that nurses will be regarded as a cheaper substitute for doctors[16] when, for a high quality service, both are needed.

Linking services providing for different reproductive and sexual health needs (such as genitourinary medicine and family planning clinics[17]) or, better still, integrating the two services should facilitate access to advice and supplies. Multi-agency working (recommended for young people[18]) should facilitate access to contraception for a number of vulnerable groups regardless of age. In a US survey designed to explore the acceptability of a number of different sites for contraceptive provision, community centres and even churches were considered acceptable to some women.[19]

Pharmacists also play an increasing role in contraceptive service provision. Many are now trained to provide emergency contraception, offering a convenient service to people prepared to pay in order to avoid the inconvenience of making an appointment to see a doctor. Around the UK, a number of pharmacists working to patient group directions are able to offer emergency contraception free of charge to particular target groups, such as young people and those living in more deprived areas, who may be effectively denied the convenience by virtue of the cost of the treatment.[20]

Improving the accessibility of services

Staff attitudes

What probably matters most in attracting users and encouraging them to attend and return to services is the attitude and approach of the staff providing them.[21] Many people find contraception a sensitive subject and can be embarrassed to ask for supplies. Many doctors find sexual health issues difficult to discuss.[22] A moralistic attitude on the part of providers is counter productive. Many health professionals have negative ideas about the 'sort of women who need to use emergency contraception'.[23] Surveys of pharmacists providing emergency contraception demonstrate that the most frequent concern about it is that it will be 'abused' or 'misused'.[20] Even women themselves regard the need for emergency contraception as being a sign of irresponsible behaviour.[24] None of these views encourages women to use emergency contraception whenever they need it.

Patient–provider interaction

There is some evidence that compliance and continuation rates are influenced by the relationship between the provider and the user.[4] In a US study of the consistency of oral contraceptive use,[25] the less satisfied the user was with her interactions with the provider, the more likely she was to be dissatisfied with her contraceptive pills. A UK survey in primary care suggested that teenage pregnancy rates decreased when young people had access to female doctors or young doctors, or where there was more nurse time available.[26] Female doctors report less difficulty in discussing sexual problems with teenagers.[27] Association between client–provider interaction and contraceptive use is poorly researched and much of what has been published relates to services for adolescents. The authors of a comparison of teenage sexual behaviour in the USA, Sweden, France, Canada and Great Britain[28] concluded that 'easy access to contraceptives and other reproductive health services in the UK (and elsewhere) contributes to better contraceptive use and therefore lower teenage pregnancy rates than in the US'. The report further suggests that integrating contraceptive services into other types of primary care lends support to the notion that contraceptive use is normal and important.

Opening times

Accessibility of services can also be improved by optimising opening hours. Extended opening times (particularly over lunchtime) and drop-in clinics where no appointment time is required have been shown to increase access for young people.[29] For women who work full time or who have responsibility for childcare during the day, evening clinics may be particularly acceptable.

Increasing the range of methods available at family planning services

Cost considerations

The last decade of the 20th century saw an increase in the number of contraceptive methods available in the UK. Although not radically different from the traditional trio of condom, intrauterine device (IUD) or contraceptive pill, more recently available methods do offer a variety of routes of administration and duration of action and some are arguably easier to use. In a randomised controlled trial, for example, compliance was better among women using the contraceptive patch than among oral contraceptive users.[30] New methods are inevitably more expensive, particularly implants and hormone-releasing intrauterine systems which, although extremely cheap if used for their full duration, are expensive to purchase. In the drive to cut the cost of prescribing to the NHS, national and local formulary organisations often limit the availability of new methods because of their high cost relative to the extremely cheap copper IUD (less than £10 per device) or second-generation combined oral contraceptives (less than £1 per packet). In comparison with other drugs, all contraceptives are cheap and all have been shown to be cost-effective.[31] While accepting the need for a limited NHS budget to cover seemingly limitless healthcare needs, purchasers need to recognise the importance of the acceptability of a method in determining its correct and consistent use. The 'expensive' long-acting implants have been demonstrated to reduce pregnancy rates among teenagers,[32,33] while the additional health benefits of the intrauterine system in conferring oligo/amenorrhoea on older women with menstrual dysfunction must represent added value to meeting contraceptive needs. Hospital-based abortion services with limited pharmacy budgets are commonly unable or unwilling to provide the more expensive methods, despite serving a population of women with a one in four chance of a repeat unintended pregnancy.

Technical expertise

While 98% of GP surgeries offer some form of contraception, not all provide the full range of services or provide information about those that do.[9] Implants and IUDs require technical expertise for their insertion and removal. Many GPs (and even some of the smaller community family planning clinics) lack this expertise and the number of women for whom they will provide these methods is insufficient for them to gain and maintain the skills. This argues the need for specialist community family planning clinics or formal arrangements for specialist GPs who can provide a full contraceptive service for a locality.

Improving education and information

More than 50% of couples using a reversible method of contraception in the UK use either condoms or contraceptive pills. Few people are formally taught to use a condom correctly, and correct use of the combined pill with its 'missed pill rules' is complicated. Many couples have preconceived (often erroneous) ideas about particular methods of contraception and will not contemplate even trying them. Long-acting methods – many of which involve no action on the part of the user – are used by fewer than 10% of women.[1] Many women discontinue a method because of adverse effects, most of which will resolve quickly, or because of perceived risks such as cancer or weight gain. In a small interview study of UK women undergoing abortion,[34] the effectiveness of contraceptive counselling was described as disappointing. Women had limited knowledge of contraception and services, misconceptions about methods and about their own fertility and reported cursory or limited counselling. In a similar UK study of women undergoing repeat abortion, only 40% had had a comprehensive discussion of contraceptive options in relation to their individual circumstances.[35] Both studies concluded that more and better-quality information and advice should help to improve patterns of contraceptive use.

Many compliance problems relate to misinformation about contraceptive methods, the importance of their adverse effects and how to use them correctly. In their review of the causes and consequences of oral contraceptive noncompliance, Rosenberg and Waugh list a number of steps to be taken to improve use, many of which depend on good counselling.[5] There is, however, considerable diversity in the needs and preferences of contraceptive users and it can be difficult to get the counselling right. Some find the information they are given too much and too complicated, while others find it insufficient and oversimplified. Health professionals often assume too much knowledge and underestimate people's ability to cope with information. It can be hard to strike a balance, particularly for groups who tend to be rather passive during consultations, such as adolescents. In an interview study of young people using sexual health services, Kane *et al.* concluded that 'effective provision of information has considerable potential to enhance sexual health services', demonstrating that it impacted measurably on 'client satisfaction' encouraging use of the service.[36]

There is evidence that the provision of written information enhances understanding. A US study demonstrated that the distribution of written material about contraception helped women make an informed choice about a postpartum method.[37] A randomised controlled trial in the UK[38] assessed the effectiveness of providing educational leaflets in improving knowledge among women taking the combined pill. Knowledge of contraception was poor in those receiving no information. Written information had a significant effect on knowledge of factors associated with pill failure (OR 3.43, 95% CI 1.45–8.09 if the Family Planning Association leaflet was given and OR 3.03, 95% CI 1.30–7.00 if interactive questions were used). Even after the intervention, however, fewer than one in three women were well informed.

Only a few studies have demonstrated that improved knowledge about contraception can increase uptake, adherence or continuation rates. In a randomised controlled trial carried out in the USA, exposure to a half-hour slide-tape presentation followed by a personal consultation with a specialist provider increased the (self-reported) use of effective contraception among young men.[39] In developing country settings, structured counselling about bleeding disturbances (usually amenorrhoea) associated with the use of Depo-Provera® (Pharmacia) has been shown to reduce discontinuation rates.[40] Other studies have failed to demonstrate any measurable benefit of improved information giving and none has shown any long-term benefit in reducing pregnancy rates. In a systematic review of US data, Moos *et al.* concluded that there was no robust evidence to determine effective counselling approaches for changing knowledge, attitudes or behaviours.[41] Almost no studies address the effects of counselling to prevent unintended pregnancy in clinical settings in the UK.

Telephone helplines are increasingly being used to provide information to individuals seeking advice about contraceptive methods and services. A telephone hotline set up in the USA to inform women about emergency contraception was deemed to be influential in promoting the method.[42]

The print and broadcast media and the internet have been used to promote responsible sexual behaviour and inform the public about contraception. The mass media may be particularly useful for teaching young people about reproductive health because elements of popular culture can be used to articulate messages in young people's terms.[43] The Teenage Pregnancy Unit in England has a package of measures aimed at reducing teenage pregnancy including a national publicity campaign to reinforce key messages.[18] The Scottish Executive has funded a health demonstration project (Healthy Respect) aimed at helping young people develop a positive attitude to sexual health and reducing unplanned teenage pregnancies. The project uses the internet as a means of providing information to young people, their parents and reproductive health providers.[44] A Cochrane review concluded that these channels of communication may have an important role in influencing the use of healthcare interventions.[45]

Involving men

In the UK, men take substantial responsibility for contraception. The male condom is the second most commonly used reversible method and more men then women are sterilised.[1] Condoms are provided free of charge by family planning services but not by

GPs. The number of men attending family planning clinics has been increasing in recent years. Until the mid-1980s, about 20 000 men/year attended family planning clinics for the first time while, in 1995–96, 67 000 first contacts were recorded.[46] Nevertheless, most men are notoriously reluctant to attend health services and this will be a factor to be considered when hormonal methods for men become available necessitating provision and follow up. In most developed countries, efforts have concentrated on involving young men, who have been overlooked in the past. Much has been said about the importance of involving men in family planning, particularly young men,[47] but little has been done to address their needs and even less to evaluate the effect of their involvement on contraceptive use or unintended pregnancy.

Making methods more accessible

Most women of reproductive age are involved full time either in employment or in child care and find it difficult to take time off work to visit a health service for contraceptive supplies. Many young women are simply not sufficiently well organised to make the arrangements to obtain supplies and some are too embarrassed to seek them. Only condoms and emergency contraception are available without a prescription and neither is cheap (nor effective at preventing pregnancy). In an interview study of 305 women undergoing termination of pregnancy in Edinburgh, 10% claimed that they had not used contraception at the time of conception because they had run out of supplies. A further 6% were not expecting to have intercourse when it happened and easier access to supplies may have prevented some of those pregnancies.[48]

Making oral contraceptives (the most commonly used method in the UK) available off prescription has been discussed repeatedly over the years. A prescription drug generally becomes a candidate for off-prescription availability if it is used for a condition that is easy to self-diagnose and has low potential for harm from abuse under conditions of widespread availability.[49] Both conditions can be said to apply to oral contraception. Nevertheless, a number of concerns are expressed in support of keeping oral contraceptives as prescription-only medicines:

- it is feared that more women with contraindications may use them
- women would no longer then be a captive audience for cervical cancer screening and (in other countries) other tests
- oral contraceptives do not protect against sexually transmitted infections
- imperfect use (because of lack of good counselling) would increase.[50]

The World Health Organization recommends that oral contraceptives can be provided by people with limited clinical judgement, except under a few circumstances where pre-existing medical conditions (most of which are rare in women of reproductive age and all of which the user herself knows she has) make their use less safe.[51] The WHO also recommends that no test other than the measurement of blood pressure (which can be done in pharmacies) for combined hormonal contraceptives (but not for progestogen only methods) is mandatory before initiating oral contraception. The UK Faculty of Family Planning and Reproductive Health Care concurs with this.[52] In a study of continuation rates of oral contraceptives among teenagers, the only provider–client variable significantly related to inconsistent use was the dispensing of only one packet of pills with continuation dependent upon the teenager returning for additional medical tests.[53]

Concern that oral contraceptives do not protect against sexually transmitted infections has no bearing on their prescription status and, as discussed above, it is by no means clear that counselling in a traditional medical setting increases perfect use. A number of off-prescription options have been suggested which involve assessing a woman's knowledge of the pill before providing it.[50] Alternatively, off-prescription oral contraceptives could be available only to established users whose medical eligibility had been confirmed by a recognised provider, allowing women to obtain supplies free of charge from any UK pharmacist every 6 months for 3 years (the time interval for cervical screening in the UK).

Even if oral contraceptives were not made available off-prescription, a number of simple changes in prescribing could greatly enhance availability and facilitate consistent use. Making small amounts of pills (say ten tablets) available from pharmacies at minimal cost to tide women over between running out of supplies and arranging to attend a health service could increase adherence. So, too, could the practice of giving women supplies sufficient to last 1 year before returning for a review appointment. The UK SPR recommends only annual follow-up for women using oral contraception allowing a supply sufficient for 1 year to be given.[52] While a percentage of women will change their method, stop using contraception or lose their supplies before the year is up, the cost to the NHS of a consultation is greater than that of the pills and the convenience to the user is significant. A quick assessment of pregnancy intention and satisfaction with the method at annual follow up would, in any case, identify many of the women likely to discontinue the method early.

It has been argued that increased use of emergency contraception could reduce unintended pregnancy rates. To be effective, emergency contraception must be used within 72 hours of intercourse and the sooner it is used the more effective it may be. Most unprotected sex probably occurs at weekends when emergency contraception is less easily available. Making emergency contraception available off-prescription has made it more accessible but in the UK it is expensive (£25 per course). A number of studies undertaken in the UK and elsewhere in the world have all demonstrated increased use – and earlier use – of emergency contraception when it is supplied in advance of need.[54] Women with a supply of emergency contraception at home are two or three times more likely to use it than women who have to make arrangements to visit a health service to obtain it or to buy it off-prescription.

Access even to injectable contraception can be made easier by allowing self-administration to women who wish it. A micronised formulation of Depo-Provera has allowed the development of a subcutaneous injection (with the same efficacy and duration of use as the intramuscular formulation) which can be self-administered.[55] A survey of 176 Edinburgh women using Depo-Provera demonstrated that 67% would like to give the injections themselves, thereby reducing the need to visit a clinic to only once a year.[56] Studies in Brazil demonstrated that women were competent to administer the combined injectable contraceptive themselves.[57]

Can service changes make a difference?

It is not difficult to list simple strategies to improve service provision with the potential to improve patterns of contraceptive use. It is much more difficult to show that these approaches make a difference in practice. While some interventions, but by no means all, have been shown to improve knowledge, uptake and even continuation rates of contraception, there are almost none that demonstrate a lasting difference and none at all which clearly shows an effect on pregnancy rates. Interim endpoints are, of course, much easier to measure than a reduction in unintended pregnancy, which is relatively rare and influenced by so many factors. It is not even easy to define an unintended pregnancy and, even if conception is truly unintended, with time, a pregnancy often becomes 'wanted' so the endpoint can be a 'moveable feast'. Groups at high risk, such as women having a therapeutic abortion, are often reluctant to participate in research. Most women having an abortion simply want to put it behind them and move on. In developed countries, most populations of women of reproductive age are geographically mobile. Years of follow-up are required to capture pregnancies, making randomised controlled trials almost impossible. People prepared to take part in research are often different from the general population and the fact of participation often changes their behaviour.

Some well-designed studies have demonstrated an improvement in continuation rates of contraception when women are given structured counselling about a method and its adverse effects.[40] These studies, however, were mostly carried out in developing country settings where women are often poorly informed about contraception. It is also likely that the routine counselling with which the interventions were compared was sometimes rather minimal. A randomised controlled trial of an intervention designed to increase condom use for prevention of sexually transmitted diseases demonstrated significantly more consistent use in a group of very young African-American girls in the USA followed up for one year.[58]

Although some studies have shown improved knowledge in populations more typical of the UK, the knowledge is often quite sophisticated (such as missed-pill rules) and the testing performed rather soon after the intervention.[38] It may be much harder to demonstrate changes in behaviour in settings where women are generally well informed about contraception and reproductive health. A limited randomised trial of condom promotion in women attending inner-city GP surgeries for cervical smears made no difference to condom use.[59] Counselling women about postpartum contraception is often poorly performed[60] and the provision of written administration has been shown (albeit in a rather poor trial) to enhance self-reported method choice.[37] A cluster randomised trial of specialist contraceptive advice, however, backed up with written information, made no difference to patterns of contraceptive use (either switching or continuation rates) in a cohort of postpartum women in both developed and developing countries.[61] Unintended pregnancy rates were lowest in the South African centre where use of a long-acting method of contraception (depot medroxyprogesterone acetate, DMPA) predominated. In a similar randomised controlled trial in which women undergoing therapeutic abortion in a UK hospital were randomised to receive routine contraceptive counselling or specialist advice and enhanced provision, the findings were equally disappointing. While contraceptive uptake at the time of discharge from hospital was highly significantly increased by the intervention and more women chose long-acting methods of contraception, by 16 weeks after the abortion, there were no differences between the two groups of women.[48] A case-note review (with all its limitations) showed no effect of the intervention on rates of repeat abortion two years later.

A questionnaire study of US women undergoing abortion suggested that increased use of emergency contraception prevented up to 51 000 pregnancies in 2001.[62] In contrast, researchers from Sweden, a country with extremely reliable figures for unintended pregnancy rates (in contrast to the USA), have reported that easier access and increased use of emergency contraception appears to have made no difference to abortion rates.[63] Emergency contraception use among women having abortions in the UK has increased significantly in the UK from around 1% in the 1980s[64] to 6% in the mid-1990s[65] and 11–12% in 2002–03[35,48] and yet abortion rates have continued to rise. While all of the trials that have looked at advanced provision of emergency contraception have demonstrated increased use, four studies, three of them randomised controlled trials[66–68] and the other a large community intervention study,[54] have failed to shown any effect on pregnancy or abortion rates. All four showed that many women failed to use emergency contraception even although they had a supply. Most of the authors attributed this observation to a failure to recognise or acknowledge a risk of pregnancy.

Surprisingly, even interventions which intuitively seem promising and easy to measure turn out not to make a difference. A randomised trial designed to test an intensive reminder system among 250 women using Depo-Provera in the USA did not improve compliance.[69] Women receiving reminders were no more likely to return to the clinic on time than women given an appointment at the time of the first injection. A randomised trial of self-administration of DMPA versus clinic administration might determine whether it is the need to make arrangements (including travel and possibly taking time off work) to attend a clinic that leads to mistimed injections.

A Cochrane review of strategies to improve compliance and acceptability of hormonal methods of contraception[70] is continuing but as most of the published studies have many weaknesses,[41] the conclusions are unlikely to be helpful in designing service change.

A few studies have been set up to attempt to understand what factors determine effective use of contraception. In a study of diaphragm users, reservations about the method used, the partner's support of the method chosen and beliefs about the couple's own fertility were important determinants of adherence.[71] In a study of compliance with the oral contraceptive pill, women who did not consider it especially important to avoid pregnancy missed more pills.[72] A study of young inner-city African-American women followed for 2 years showed that only when a young woman unequivocally wants to avoid childbearing or is unequivocally positive towards contraception does her attitude have a significant effect on her behaviour.[73] In a multicentre study of the ovulation method of family planning, most of the pregnancies arose because of rule breaking. Couple who wanted no more children had fewer pregnancies that those who were using the method to 'space' their families.[74] Although it is widely held, certainly in the UK, that unintended pregnancy is related to lack of a strong desire to avoid pregnancy, for example because of lower career aspirations, it appears difficult to prove at the level of the individual.

Conclusion

In conclusion, many changes could be made to contraceptive services which, common sense dictates, should make a difference to patterns of contraceptive use. Demonstrating that the changes make a difference is not easy. Demonstrating that they result in a reduction in rates of unintended pregnancy presents an enormous challenge.

References

1.   Dawe F, Rainford L. *Contraception and Sexual Health 2003. A report on research using the ONS Omnibus Survey produced by the Office for National Statistics on behalf of the Department of Health, London*. London: Office for National Statistics; 2004.
2.   Trussell J. The essentials of contraception: efficacy, safety, and personal considerations. In: Hatcher RA, Trussell J, Stewart F, Cates W, Stewart GK, Kowal D, *et al.*, editors. *Contraceptive Technology*. 18th

ed. New York: Ardent Media; 2004.

3. Mosher WD, Pratt WF. AIDS-related behaviour among women 15–44 years of age: United States, 1988 and 1990. *Adv Data* 1993;239:1–15.

4. Rosenberg MJ, Waugh MS. Causes and consequences of oral contraceptive noncompliance. *Am J Obstet Gynecol* 1999;180:S276–9.

5. Rosenberg MJ, Waugh MS. Oral contraceptive discontinuation: a prospective evaluation of frequency and reasons. *Am J Obstet Gynecol* 1998;179:577–82.

6. Pratt WF, Bachrach CC. What do women use when they stop using the pill? *Fam Plann Perspect* 1987;19:257–66.

7. Duncan G, Harper C, Ashwell E, Mant D, Buchan H, Jones L. Termination of pregnancy: lessons for prevention. *Br J Fam Plann* 1990;15:112–17.

8. Mahmood TA, Lim BH, Lees DA. The characteristics of and the contraceptive practice among women seeking therapeutic termination of pregnancy in the Scottish Highlands. *Health Bull* 1998;46:330–6.

9. Free C, Dawe A, Macey S, Mawer C. Evaluating and developing contraceptive services: the results of an audit of the North Lambeth Primary Care commissioning Group. *J Fam Plann Reprod Health Care* 2001;27:22–8.

10. Clements S, Stone N, Diamond I Ingham R. Modelling the spatial distribution of teenage conception rates within Wessex. *J Fam Plann Reprod Health Care* 1998;24:61–71.

11. Santelli J, Kouzis A, Newcomer S. School-based health centres and adolescent use of primary care and hospital care. *J Adolesc Health* 1996;19:267–75.

12. Mackie CM, Elliot L, Bigrigg A, McAllister KF. Public and private collaboration in establishing a young person's sexual health clinic in a commercial setting. *J Fam Plann Reprod Health Care* 2002;28:201–3.

13. Campbell P. The role of nurses in sexual and reproductive health. *J Fam Plann Reprod Health Care* 2004;30:169–70.

14. Miles K, Penny N, Mercey D, Power R. Sexual health clinics for women led by specialist nurses or senior house officers in a central London GUM service: a randomised controlled trail. *Sex Transm Infect* 2002;78:93–7.

15. Campbell P. Nurse prescribing for contraceptive care and sexual health. *J Fam Plann Reprod Health Care* 2004;30:255–6.

16. Miles K, Penny N, Power R, Mercey D. Comparing doctor- and nurse-led care in a sexual health clinic: patient satisfaction questionnaire. *J Adv Nurs* 2003;42:64–72.

17. Masters L, Nicholas H, Bunting P, Welch J. Family planning in genitourinary medicine: an opportunistic service? *Genitourin Med* 1995;71:103–5.

18. Teenage Pregnancy Unit, Department of Health. *Best Practice Guidance on the Provision of Effective Contraception and Advice Services for Young People*. London: DH; 2002. p. 1–5 [www.info.doh.gov.uk/tpu/tpu.nsf].

19. Todd CS, Plantigna LC, Lichenstein R. Primary care services for an emergency department population: a novel location for contraception. *Contraception* 2005;71:40–4.

20. Bacon L, Savage I, Cook S, Taylor B. Training and supporting pharmacists to supply progestogen-only emergency contraception. *J Fam Plann Reprod Health Care* 2003;29:17–22.

21. Cromer BA, McCarthy M. Family planning services in adolescent pregnancy prevention: The views of key informants in four countries. *Fam Plann Perspect* 1999;31:287–93.

22. Lewin J, King M. Sexual medicine: towards an integrated discipline. *BMJ* 1997;314:1432.

23. Fairhurst K, Wyke S, Seaman P, Ziebland S, Glasier A. "Not that sort of practice". The views of primary care practitioners in a study of advanced provision of emergency contraception. *Fam Pract* 2005;22:280–6.

24. Fairhurst K, Zielband S, Wyke S, Seamann P, Glasier A. Emergency contraception: why can't you give it away? Qualitative findings from an evaluation of advance provision of emergency contraception. *Contraception* 2004;70:25–9.

25. Rosenberg MJ, Waugh MS, Burnhill MS. Compliance, counseling and satisfaction with oral contraceptives: a prospective evaluation. *Fam Plann Perspect* 1998;30:89–92,104.

26. Hippisley-Cox J, Allen J, Pringle M, Ebdon D, McPhearson M, Churchill D, *et al.* Association between teenage pregnancy rates and the age and sex of general practitioners: cross sectional survey in Trent. *BMJ* 2000;320:842–5.

27. Frank E, Harvey LK. Prevention advice rates of women and men physicians. *Arch Fam Med* 1996;5:215–19.

28. The Alan Guttmacher Institute. Can more progress be made? Teenage sexual and reproductive behavior in developed countries New York: Alan Guttmacher Institute; 2001 [www.guttmacher.org/pubs/fb_teens.html].

29. Baraitser P, Fettiplace R, Dolan F, Massil H, Cowley S. Quality, mainstream service with proactive and targeted outreach: a model of contraceptive service provision for young people. *J Fam Plann Reprod Health Care* 2002;28:90–4.

30. Audet MC, Moreau M, Koltun WD, Waldbaum AS, Shangold G, Fisher AC, *et al*. Evaluation of contraceptive efficacy and cycle control of a transdermal contraceptive patch vs an oral contraceptive. A randomized controlled trial. *JAMA* 2001;285:2347–54.

31. McGuire A, Hughes D. *The Economics of Family Planning Services. A report prepared for the Contraceptive Alliance.* London: Family Planning Association; 1995.

32. Stevens-Simon C, Kelly L, Kulick R. A village would be nice but … It takes along-acting contraceptive to prevent repeat adolescent pregnancies. *Am J Prev Med* 2001;21:60–5.

33. Darney PD, Callegari LS, Swift A, Atkinson ES, Robert AM. Condom practices of urban teens using Norplant contraceptive implants, oral contraceptives and condoms for contraception. *Am J Obstet Gynecol* 1998;180:929–37.

34. Kumar U, Baraitser P, Morton S, Massil H. Peri-abortion contraception: a qualitative study of users' experiences. *J Fam Plann Reprod Health Care* 2004;30:55–7.

35. Garg M, Singh M, Mansour D. Peri-aborion contraceptive care: can we reduce the incidence of repeat abortions? *J Fam Plann Reprod Health Care* 2001;27:77–80.

36. Kane R, MacDowall W, Wellings K. Providing information for young people in sexual health clinics: getting it right. *J Fam Plann Reprod Health Care* 2003;141–5.

37. Johnson JK, Edelman A, Jensen J. Patient satisfaction and the impact of written material about postpartum contraceptive decisions. *Am J Obstet Gynecol* 2003;188:1202–4.

38. Little P, Griffin S, Kelly J, Dickson N, Sadler C. Effect of educational leaflets and questions on knowledge of contraception in women taking the combined contraceptive pill: randomised controlled trial. *BMJ* 1998;316:1948–52.

39. Danielson R, Marcy S, Plinkett A, Wiest W, Greenlick MR. Reproductive health counselling for young men: what does it do ? *Fam Plann Perspect* 1990;22:115–21.

40. Hubacher D, Goco N, Gonzalez B, Taylor D. Factors affecting continuation rates of DMPA. *Contraception* 2000;60:345–51.

41. Moos M-K, Bartholomew NE, Lohr KN. Counseling in the clinical setting to prevent unintended pregnancy: an evidence based research agenda. *Contraception* 2003;67:115–32.

42. Trussell J, Koenig J, Vaughan B, Stewart F. Evaluation of a media campaign to increase knowledge about emergency contraception. *Contraception* 2001;63:81–7.

43. Keller SN, Brown JD. Media interventions to promote responsible sexual behaviour. *J Sex Res* 2002;39:67–72.

44. Healthy Respect [www.healthy-respect.com].

45. Grilli R, Ramsay C, Minozzi S. Mass media interventions: effects on health services utilisation. *Cochrane Database Syst Rev* 2002;(1):CD000389.

46. Wellings K. Teenage sexual and reproductive behaviour in developed countries. Country report for Great Britain. Occasional Report No. 6, November 2001. [www.guttmacher.org/pubs/covers/euroteen_or.html].

47. Sex Education Forum. Supporting the needs of boys and young men in sex and relationships education. Forum Fact Sheet 11. London: National Children's Bureau; 1997 [www.ncb.org.uk/sef/res_detail.asp?id=151].

48. Schunmann C, Glasier A. Contraception after abortion. A report for Healthy Respect (in preparation).

49. Cohen JP, Paqette C, Cairns CP. Switching prescription drugs to over the counter. *BMJ* 2005;330:39–41.

50. Trussell J, Stewart F, Potts M, Guest F, Ellertson C. Should oral contraceptives be available without prescription? *Am J Public Health* 1993;83:1094–99.

51. Reproductive Health and Research, World Health Organization. *Medical Eligibilty Criteria for Contraceptive Use.* 3rd ed. Geneva: WHO; 2004 [www.who.int/reproductive-health/publications/MEC_3/index.htm].

52. Faculty of Family Planning and Reproductive Health Care. *UK Selected Practice Recommendations for Contraceptive Use.* London: FFPRHC; 2002.

53. Balassone ML. Risk of contraceptive discontinuation among adolesecents. *J Adolesc Health Care* 1989;10:527–33.

54. Glasier A, Fairhurst K, Wyke S, Ziebland S, Seaman P, Walker J, *et al*. Advanced provision of emergency contraception has not reduced abortion rates. *Contraception* 2004;69:361–6.

55. Jain J, Dutton C, Nicosia A, Wajszczuk C, Bode FR, Mishell DR. Pharmacokinetics, ovulation suppression and return to ovulation following a lower dose subcutaneous formulation of Depo Provera®. *Contraception* 2004;70:11–18.

56. Lakha F, Henderson C, Glasier A. The acceptability of self-administering Depo-Provera. *Contraception*. 2005; 72:14–18.

57. Bahamondes L, Marchi NM, Nakagava HM, de Melo ML, Cristofoletti Mde L, Pellini E, *et al.* Self-administration with UniJect of the once-a-month injectable contraceptive Cyclofem. *Contraception* 1997;56:301–4.

58. DiClemente RJ, Wingood GM, Harrington KF, Lang DL, Davies SL, Hook EW III, *et al.* Efficacy of an HIV prevention intervention for African American adolescent girls: a randomized controlled trial. *JAMA* 2004;292:171–9.

59. Oakeshott P, Kerry S, Hay S, Hay P. Condom promotion in women attending inner city general practices for cervical smears: a randomised controlled trial. *Fam Pract* 2000;17:56–9.

60. Glasier AF, Logan J, McGlew TJ. Who gives advice about post partum contraception? *Contraception* 1996;53:217–20.

61. Smith KB, van der Spuy ZM, Cheng L, Elton R, Glasier A. Is postpartum contraceptive advice given antenatally of value? *Contraception* 2002;237–243.

62. Jones RK, Darroch JE, Henshaw SK. Contraceptive use among US women having abortions in 2000–2001. *Perspect Sex Reprod Health* 2002;34:294–303.

63. Tyden T, Aneblom G, von Essen L, Haggstron-Nordin E, Larsson M, Odlind V. No reduced number of abortions despite easily available emergency contraceptive pills. Studies of women's knowledge, attitudes and experience of the method. *Lakartidningen* 2002;99:4730–2.

64. Johnston TA, Howie PW. Potential use of postcoital contraception to prevent unwanted pregnancy. *BMJ* 1985;290:1040–1.

65. Gordon AF, Owen P. Emergency contraception: change in knowledge of women attending for termination of pregnancy from 1984–1996. *Br J Fam Plann* 1999;24:121–2.

66. Lo SST, Fan SYS, Ho PC, Glasier AF. Effect of advanced provision of emergency contraception on women's contraceptive behaviour: a randomized controlled trial. *Hum Reprod* 2004;19:2404–10.

67. Raine TR, Harper CC, Rocca CH, Fischer R, Padian N, Klausner JD, *et al.* Direct access to emergency contraception through pharmacies and effect on unintended pregnancies and STIs. A randomized controlled trial. *JAMA* 2005;293:54–62.

68. Hu X, Cheng L, Hua X, Glasier A. Advanced provision of emergency contraception to postnatal women in China makes no difference to abortion rates. A randomised controlled trial. *Contraception* 2005;72:111–16.

69. Keder LM, Rulin MC, Gruss J. Compliance with depot medroxyprogesterone acetate: a randomized controlled trial of intensive reminders. *Am J Obstet Gynecol* 1995;169:583–5.

70. Grigorieva V, Gallo MF, Grimes DA. Strategies to improve compliance and acceptability of hormonal methods of contraception. Protocol. *Cochrane Database Syst Rev* 2005:1. doi: 0.1002/14651858.CD004317 [www.mrw.interscience.wiley.com/cochrane/clsysrev/articles/CD004317/frame.html].

71. Jaccard J, Helbig DW, Wan CK, Gutman MA, Kritz-Silverstein DC. Individual differences in attitude-behaviout consistency: the prediction of contraceptive behaviour. *J Appl Soc Psychol* 1990;20:575–617.

72. Oakley D, Potter L, de Leon-Wong, Visness C. Oral contraceptive use and protective behaviour after missed pills. *Fam Plann Perspect* 1997;29:277–9, 287.

73. Zabin LS, Astone NM, Emerson MR,. Do adolescents want babies? The relationship between attitudes and behaviour. *J Res Adolesc* 1993;3:67–86.

74. World Health Organization, Task Force on Methods for the Determination of the Fertile Period, Special Programme of Research, Development and Research Training in Human Reproduction. A prospective multicentre trial of the ovulation method of natural family planning. II. The effectiveness phase. *Fertil Steril* 1981;36:591–8.

Chapter 21
Improving sexual health education

Judith M Stephenson

Introduction

Globally, there is a continuing, urgent need to improve sexual health education for young people by developing demonstrably effective interventions to combat the spread of HIV/AIDS, unintended teenage pregnancy and their consequences. However, the challenges faced in developing countries, where effective behavioural interventions are woefully lacking, are formidable and beyond the scope of this chapter.[1] Much of the research relating to the effectiveness of sexual health education comes from the USA, where teenage pregnancy rates are substantially higher than in the UK.[2] While recognising the importance of that research, this chapter deals principally with the UK context for two reasons: considerable recent effort has been applied to improving sexual health education through two government-led national strategies;[3] and two of the most rigorous trials to evaluate the effects of different approaches to school based sex education have been conducted in the UK.[4,5]

In this chapter, the purpose of sexual health education is interpreted in a public health sense; that is, it goes beyond transfer of knowledge about sexual health and encompasses behavioural change to prevent the adverse consequences of sexual activity, including sexually transmitted infections and unwanted pregnancy. This reflects ample evidence that improving knowledge about sexual health does not necessarily lead to changes in related behaviours and that changing sexual lifestyles and behaviours is a much more complex and challenging task than merely improving knowledge.[6] While the interpretation of sexual health in this chapter emphasises the prevention of adverse outcomes of sexual behaviour, it does not ignore or undermine the importance of 'sex positive' approaches to sexual health education that aim specifically to improve the quality of sexual relationships.

Sexual health education may take place through awareness-raising campaigns at national level and access to information in sexual health services at local level, as well as in the school setting. The chapter begins by describing the UK context and relevant parts of the national strategies and then focuses on sex and relationships education in schools, including evidence for the effectiveness of different approaches with particular reference to two continuing trials, one in Scotland (SHARE) and one in England (RIPPLE). It ends by summarising what we have learnt about improving sexual health education and possible directions for future investment.

The UK policy context

The sexual health of people in the UK has caused increasing concern for many years. It is now more than a decade since sexual health was made one of five priority areas in the Health of the Nation (1992),[7] the first government initiative to set specific targets for reduction in sexually transmitted infection (gonorrhoea) and teenage conceptions (under 16 years). Despite this, rates of sexually transmitted infections and HIV have risen sharply over the last few years[8] and, in 2003, the Government Health Select Committee declared that England was currently witnessing a rapid decline in its sexual health.[9]

There has been a modest decline in under 18 pregnancy rates in the last few years[10] but comparison of UK figures with other Western European countries remains unfavourable and the association between unintended teenage pregnancy and poor health, economic and social outcomes persists for both mother and child.[11] Analysis of the first and second national surveys of sexual attitudes and lifestyles (Natsal 1990 and Natsal 2000), conducted ten years apart in 1990 and 2000 respectively, confirms that early age of first intercourse is significantly associated with pregnancy under 18 years, and that the proportion of women reporting first intercourse before 16 years rose up to, but not after, the mid-1990s.[6] These findings are described in more detail in Chapter 3.

Against this backdrop of rising infection rates and high teenage pregnancy and abortion rates, two further government initiatives were launched: the Teenage Pregnancy Strategy in 2000 and the National Strategy for Sexual Health and HIV in 2001. Both strategies emphasise the importance of improving sexual health education within and outside schools so that people can make informed decisions about preventing sexually transmitted infections and unwanted pregnancy, and both strategies have run sustained national media campaigns to raise awareness of sexual health issues and reduce sexual risk behaviours.

Teenage Pregnancy Strategy for England

With its dual aims of halving conceptions in the under-18 years age group by 2010 and supporting teenage parents, the Teenage Pregnancy Strategy is a multifaceted strategy with four major components:

- a national media awareness campaign via independent radio and teenage magazines
- joined up action to ensure that action is coordinated nationally and locally across all relevant statutory and voluntary agencies
- better prevention through improving sex and relationships education and improving access to contraception and sexual health services
- support for teenage parents to increase the proportion returning to education, training or employment (see Chapter 18).

The Teenage Pregnancy Strategy takes a multifaceted approach to sex and relationships education. The media campaign includes targeted materials in magazines for boys and girls and local independent radio, with key messages about resisting peer pressure to engage in early sexual activity, the use of contraception for those who are sexually active and the availability of confidential advice on contraception and sex and relationship issues. The campaign is backed up by a dedicated helpline – Sexwise – to provide information to young people and details of local services and a supporting website (www.ruthinking.co.uk). The thinking behind the campaign is similar to that for the Sex Lottery described below.

The strategy also addresses the need to help and encourage parents to discuss sex and relationships issues with their children. Several studies, including Natsal 1990 and 2000,[12] show that parents and school are preferred sources of information on sexual matters for both young men and young women. Yet parents often feel poorly equipped to discuss sexual matters with their children and the proportion of young people who would like to have received most of their information from parents is considerably higher than the proportion who actually did.[12] The teenage pregnancy strategy aims to encourage and support parents to discuss sex and relationships issues with their children through the 'Time to Talk' initiative, promoted in a range of parent-oriented media, supported by the Parentline Plus helpline and website. The fpa also runs a programme to improve parent–child communication called 'Speakeasy'.

A further plank of the strategy in relation to sex education focuses on efforts to improve sex and relationships education in schools, including the provision of nonstatutory guidance that highlights the importance of targeting boys as well as girls and a certification programme for specialist teachers of personal, social and health education and for community nurses working with vulnerable groups such as children in care.

There is some evidence that sex and relationships education is more effective when it involves specific links with local sexual health services;[13] for example, organising school group visits to local clinics to improve accessibility and boost confidence or providing clinics on school premises to promote access to information, advice and methods. The Teenage Pregnancy Strategy aims to improve access to contraception and sexual health services for both boys and girls at a range of community settings, including school-based services at the discretion of individual governing bodies, in consultation with parents. Where school clinics have been set up with appropriate consultation and support, they appear to be well received, especially in rural areas. The Teenage Pregnancy Unit has also worked with the Royal College of General Practitioners on a joint initiative called 'Getting it Right For Teenagers in Your Practice', which is aimed at improving young people's uptake of advice from general practice on various health issues including teenage pregnancy and sexual health.

Evaluation of the Teenage Pregnancy Strategy

An evaluation of the Teenage Pregnancy Strategy was conducted by an independent research team from the London School of Hygiene and Tropical Medicine, University College London and the British Market Research Bureau[14] with the aim of assessing the extent to which the aims of the strategy were achieved and identifying factors that enhanced or hindered its implementation (see Chapter 18). Detailed reports of the evaluation team's findings are available from the Teenage Pregnancy Unit's website (www.dfes.gov.uk/teenage pregnancy) and are summarised briefly here.

The evaluation monitored treatment of sex and relationships education in the national and regional press. Stories about sex education attracted considerable media interest, with peak reporting about school clinics and the role of parents in educating their children. The research also showed a positive shift in the tone of newspaper articles, particularly in mid-ground tabloids, such as the *Daily Mail*, in which 52% of articles were negative in the first year of the strategy, compared with 39% in the second year. Awareness of the media campaign was seen to be high among young people.

After four years of campaigning, 76% of 13–17 year olds recognised the campaign materials. Awareness of chlamydia increased from 32% in 2001 to 64% in 2004.

Findings in relation to school sex and relationships education, from the tracking survey used in the evaluation, support its importance as a source of learning about sex for young people, including those from deprived areas. Young people are increasingly using school-based services, help lines and websites to gain contraceptive advice. There was, however, little observable change in behaviour in the first four years of the strategy. The proportion of young people having sexual intercourse before the age of 16 years remained relatively stable over the 4 years 2000–04, at just under 30% of young people aged 16–21 years. Furthermore, despite the high proportion of young people (84% of women and 83% of men) who used contraception at first sexual intercourse, the proportions having protected sex in the last 4 weeks decreased over time (from 88% in the first year to 78% in the fourth year for women, $P = 0.003$, and from 86% to 81% for men, $P = 0.15$).[14]

National Strategy for Sexual Health and HIV: the Sex Lottery campaign

Key recommendations in the National Strategy for Sexual Health and HIV have also led to a national campaign aimed at raising awareness of sexually transmitted infection and motivating safer sex. The aim of the Sex Lottery campaign has been to reduce rates of sexually transmitted infection by informing the public of the increased risk in the short term, with the longer-term aim of changing behaviour. Research shows that campaigns aimed at changing sexual behaviour need to give consistent, simple messages over the long term. Behaviour change is most likely to be achieved with communications that have a high degree of personal relevance, which reflect behaviour accurately and realistically and which state the message clearly and authoritatively. They are also more likely to be more effective if they are empowering rather than directive, if they are sex positive and gender-specific and if they employ humour. Further desirable feature include the offer of a call to action in the form of telephone help lines or websites, clear branding, a consistent strapline and a constant presence. These findings were all incorporated into the Sex Lottery. Results of a tracking survey to evaluate the impact of the campaign are awaited.

School-based sex and relationships education

School-based sex and relationships education offers a potentially efficient means of reaching the vast majority of young people in the UK. As noted above, it is a preferred source of sex education for many young people and has assumed increasing prominence, particularly for men. Natsal 1990 and 2000 have shown that the proportion of men reporting school as their main source of sex education has doubled in the last two decades.[12] In some countries, the importance of school sex education is acknowledged through legislation. The combination of guidance and legislation surrounding sex and relationships education in schools in England[15] can be summarised, at the risk of oversimplification, as follows. Under the 1996 Education Act, the sex and relationships education elements in the National Curriculum Science Order are mandatory for all pupils of primary and secondary school age. This tends to cover the more biological aspects of reproduction and sexual health and may include information about sexually transmitted infections and HIV/AIDS, which all secondary schools are required to provide. All schools must have an up-to-date policy that describes the content and organisation of sex and relationships education provided outside the National Curriculum Science Order. The Office for Standards in Education (Ofsted) is statutorily required to evaluate and report on the spiritual, moral, social and cultural development of pupils at any schools it inspects and this includes the school's sex and relationships education policy. Sex and relationships education guidance builds on legal requirements under the Learning and Skills Act 2000 and recommends that sex and relationships education is planned and delivered as part of personal, social and health education and citizenship but parents have the right to withdraw their children from this part of the curriculum. Since research has consistently shown that pupils think that there is too much emphasis on the biological aspects of sex and reproduction, at the expense of the more emotional and social aspects of sexual relationships, considerable pressure has been brought to bear on the Government to make sex and relationships education within personal, social and health education a statutory requirement.

How is school sex education perceived?

As noted above, there has been a positive shift in media reporting of the teenage pregnancy strategy and its efforts to improve sex education. Until quite recently, debate about the benefits, harms, or ineffectiveness of sex education in relation to young people's sexual health persisted in the absence of reliable evidence to support one or other view. Many health professional and other groups have argued for the benefits of sex education, particularly where it is aimed at improving skills as well as knowledge, thereby enabling young people to make informed choices about sexual relationships and to protect their sexual health. Others, from a more sociological viewpoint, have argued that sex education is unable to dominate more socially determined influences on sexual behaviour, risk-taking and early parenthood. Still others have claimed that explicit sex education, such as practical instruction in the use of contraception, causes harm by hastening the onset of sexual activity that would not otherwise have occurred.

Evidence for the effectiveness of school sex education

Indirect evidence in support of school sex education came from retrospective surveys in which people who obtained most of their information about sexual matters from school lessons started having sex at an older age than those citing a different source.[16] Evidence from intervention trials, conducted mainly in the USA, on the effectiveness of sex education programmes varies according to study methodology which has frequently been found wanting. One of the first broad-ranging reviews of sexual health promotion interventions for young people, conducted in the mid-1990s,[17] found that only 12 (18%) of 65 studies evaluating the outcome of interventions were considered methodologically sound and only two of the sound evaluations (both from North America) showed an impact on self-reported sexual behaviour. The review, commissioned by the Medical Research Council (MRC) of the UK, recommended that evaluation of sexual health interventions should incorporate experimental designs (randomisation), adequate sample sizes and long-term follow-up of participants. Accordingly, in a climate of concern and uncertainty about the effectiveness of behavioural interventions, the MRC funded two cluster, randomised trials of sex education in schools that would provide complementary evidence on different approaches to reducing teenage abortion. SHARE (Sexual Health and Relationships: Safe Happy and Responsible) is comparing the effects of a theory-based, teacher-delivered sex and relationships education programme with convent-ional teacher-led SRE, while RIPPLE (Randomised Intervention trial of PuPil Led sex Education in schools in England) is comparing peer-led sex and relationships education with conventional teacher-led education. The main aspects of these trials are summarised below; detailed descriptions of the interventions themselves and their effects on sexual health outcomes are available elsewhere.[18,19]

SHARE

The SHARE intervention was informed by psychosocial and sociological theory, primarily an extended theory of planned behaviour,[20] which emphasises personal susceptibility, perceived benefits of behaviour, social approval, perceived self-efficacy, intention formation and context-specific planning. The programme combined active learning (for example working in small groups) and games, information leaflets on sexual health and development of skills, mainly through the use of interactive video but also through roleplay. It incorporates the ten characteristics that were identified from research conducted mainly in the USA as necessary for effective sex education programmes.[2] The intervention consisted of a 5-day teacher training programme plus a 20-session pack: ten sessions to be delivered in the third year of secondary school (at age 13–14 years) and ten in the fourth year (age 14–15 years). The programme was intended to reduce unsafe sexual behaviours, reduce unwanted pregnancies and improve the quality of sexual relationships. The rationale for a teacher-delivered programme was primarily based on resources: this was the only means of implementing a substantial programme, that is, 20 sessions over a period of 2 years. The programme was developed and piloted in Scotland over 2 years, in consultation with teachers, sex education specialists and health promotion departments

RIPPLE

The peer-led sex and relationships education programme was shorter than the SHARE programme. Unlike SHARE, the RIPPLE programme was not designed explicitly around any particular theoretical framework but was based on a similar peer education programme that had already been used in a number of schools in England. RIPPLE consisted of three sessions, each lasting around 1 hour, and used participatory learning methods and activities focusing on relationships, sexually transmitted infections and contraception. The programme was designed by an external team of health promotion practitioners with experience of delivering peer-led sexual health programmes in schools The programme was piloted to ensure that it was acceptable to teachers and pupils and could be implemented in a standardised way across different types of schools.[21] Peer educators were recruited from Year 12 (aged 16–17 years) in the schools and trained to prepare classroom sessions aimed at improving the younger pupils' skills in sexual communication and condom use, and their knowledge about pregnancy, sexually transmitted infections, contraception and local sexual health services. Continuing support was provided by teachers, who organised suitable times for teams of peer educators to deliver three sessions of sex and relationships education to Year 9 pupils (aged 13–14 years). Teachers were not present in the classroom when the sessions were delivered. These sessions replaced the usual teacher-led sex and relationships education delivered during personal, social and health education in intervention schools. The control schools continued with their usual teacher-led sex and relationships education.

Experimental evaluation of SHARE and RIPPLE

The two trials were designed semi-independently but arrived at a similar trial design and methodology to evaluate the effects of the different interventions: Twenty-five state schools in Tayside and Lothian regions in Scotland were randomly allocated to deliver the SHARE programme or to continue with their existing sex education; 27 schools in central and southern England were randomly allocated to deliver the RIPPLE programme or to continue with their existing sex education. Over 7000 pupils participated in the SHARE trial and over 9000 in the RIPPLE trial. Both trials were statistically powered to detect a 33% reduction in the primary endpoint; that is, the cumulative abortion rate by age 20 years. In both trials (which are still continuing) the primary endpoint is being ascertained through anonymised linkage of all girls entering the trial to statutory abortion data in England and Scotland – thereby minimising loss to follow-up for this outcome – as well as through self-reported abortion. Live birth rates are also being estimated via anonymised data linkage to help interpret differences in abortion rates. In both trials, self-completion questionnaires were filled out in school classrooms pre- and post-intervention when pupils were aged 13–14 years and 15–16 years, respectively. Both trials carried out extensive process evaluation, through observation of sex and relationships education sessions, focus discussion groups with pupils (and peer educators in RIPPLE) and interviews with school staff.

Interim findings from the SHARE trial[5] showed that, compared with conventional school sex education, SHARE was more highly regarded by pupils and teachers, it increased practical sexual health knowledge and slightly improved the quality of sexual relationships, mainly through reducing regret in relation to first sexual intercourse with most recent partner. Overall, 41% of all girls and 31% of all boys reported having had sexual intercourse at follow-up (average age 16 years and 1 month), of whom over 70% of girls and 78% of boys used a condom at first sex. However, among those reporting first sex after receiving sex and relationships education there was no significant difference in the prevalence of reported sexual intercourse, condom or contraceptive use between those allocated to the SHARE programme and those in the control group: 5.2% of all boys in the intervention group and 5.7% in the control group reported first intercourse without a condom at follow-up ($P = 0.63$); corresponding figures for the girls were 9.7% and 9.1% ($P = 0.66$). Lack of an effect on sexual behaviour could not be linked to differences between schools in the quality of delivery of the intervention. The authors concluded that the impact of a 20-period schools sex education programme was probably relatively unimportant compared with long-term and pervasive influences from family, local culture and the mass media. Due largely to its popularity with pupils and teachers, the SHARE programme is increasingly being implemented in schools across Scotland.

Interim findings from the RIPPLE trial,[18] when recipients of the intervention were aged 16 years, showed that, compared with more traditional sex education, this type of peer-led sex and relationships education was associated with greater satisfaction among pupils and improved knowledge about prevention of sexually transmitted diseases. However, no significant reduction in unprotected first sexual intercourse by age 16 years was reported in 8.6% of all girls in the intervention group and 8.3% in the control group; and by 6.2% and 4.7% of boys, respectively. There was no significant reduction in regretted first sex for either gender. However, significantly fewer girls in the peer-led arm of the trial reported having had sexual intercourse (34.7% versus 40.8% in the control group, $P = 0.0008$) and there were somewhat fewer reported unintended pregnancies (2.3% versus 3.3%, $P = 0.07$). Further follow-up will determine whether the reported difference in teenage pregnancy becomes statistically significant over time and whether it is corroborated by analysis of statutory abortion data. Overall, reported use of contraception at first sexual intercourse was high (reported by 82% of girls and 84% of boys). Although both girls and boys were significantly more satisfied with peer-led than teacher-led sex education, 57% of girls and 32% of boys wanted at least some of their sex education in single-sex groups. The final results from these two trials are awaited. To summarise the interim findings, both trials have shown that pupils are more satisfied with the new sex and relationships education programmes than the conventional ones (which may not surprise, given the level of investment in the new programmes), that around four of five young people use contraception the first time they have sex and that around one-third of girls and up to one-fifth of boys expressed regret about the first occasion they had sex. Differences in sexual behaviour between the experimental and control groups were not apparent in SHARE and were small in RIPPLE.

Features that distinguished good sex and relationships education, according to pupils in RIPPLE,[22] are: use of participative/active methods; practising key skills; being provided with key information; lessons that include fun and humour, feeling positive about the sex educator; learning something new and feeling satisfied with the coverage of key topics. These features could be found in both types of sex and relationships education but were more common in peer-led than teacher-led sex and relationships education. The personal characteristics of sex educators (whether teachers or peers) and how they interacted with pupils were crucial. Pupils felt that peer educators had greater expertise and respect for pupils than teachers. They were described as more confident, empathetic, caring and trustworthy and less moralistic and patronising. Pupils also felt that peer educators provided more relevant, detailed information and held similar sexual values. Weaknesses of peer educators included shyness and embarrassments and difficulties with managing the disruptive behaviour of some pupils. Pupils also identified skill-based activities as important. These included practising putting a condom on a penis-like object and activities that involved moving around, working in small groups and discussion, all of which were more common in the peer-led programme.[23] Quantitative analysis of RIPPLE data suggests that the modest effect of peer-led sex and relationships education on sexual behaviour may have been 'mediated' by active teaching methods and practising key skills.

Other evidence

Since the RIPPLE and SHARE trials began, further systematic reviews in this area have been published.[24-27] The first compared the results of randomised trials with observational studies of interventions to prevent adolescent pregnancy. Thirteen trials and 17 observational studies were identified. Based on four comparable outcomes (sexual intercourse, contraceptive use, responsible sexual behaviour and pregnancy), the review found that the observational studies yielded systematically greater estimates of intervention effects than randomised trials. Since it is unlikely that the interventions in the observational studies were inherently more effective than those studied in randomised trials, the findings may indicate that adolescents assigned to the intervention in the observational studies were destined to have better outcomes than control adolescents irrespective of the intervention. The review concluded that, wherever possible, recommendations and public policy should be based on randomised trials.

A second systematic review pooled findings from 26 randomised trials of interventions aimed at reducing unintended pregnancies among adolescents.[25] Some of these trials were school-based and included peer-led education, although none was aimed at improving the quality of sexual relationships. The strategies evaluated did not delay the start of sexual intercourse or improve use of contraception and neither did they reduce pregnancies in young women. Meta-analysis of five abstinence programmes showed at best no effect and, at worst, an increase in pregnancy in the partners of male participants.[25] One of the conclusions of this review is that sex education programmes may need to start much earlier than they currently do. In a more recent meta-analysis,[26] small improvements were reported in sexual risk reduction skills and behaviours in adolescents after intervention, although average follow-up was only 14 weeks and 23% of studies did not randomise participants to intervention or comparison groups, which might weaken their findings. Finally, a review of reviews concluded that there is now sufficient review-level evidence that school-based sex education can be effective in reducing sexual risk behaviour and is not, as critics have suggested, associated with increased sexual activity.[13]

Conclusions

Indicators of the sexual health of young people in the UK present a mixed picture. Rates of sexually transmitted infections including HIV are clearly rising and England continues to have the highest teenage pregnancy rate in Western Europe. However, the decline in age at first sexual intercourse has stabilised, condom use at first intercourse is high and the conception rate in under 18s has fallen.

Improving sexual health through reducing sexual risk behaviour is no easy task. Rigorous evaluation of specific sexual health intervention programmes shows at best only modest effects on sexual behaviour. Furthermore, these trials have been crucial in showing that the benefits of promising interventions should not be assumed or overestimated, as even well-designed, carefully executed interventions may have the capacity to do more harm than good.[28] Evaluation of process in such trials helps to understand the nature of sex education programmes that appeal to pupils and that may have more chance of success. One of the many challenges in providing good sex education is to cater simultaneously for the needs of young people at different stages of sexual maturity. Delaying sexual activity is an important objective for reducing the risk of unwanted pregnancy and sexually transmitted infections but sex education must not ignore the needs of the minority who are already sexually active and who are at greatest risk.

Broader approaches to improving sexual health education outside the classroom are being taken through national awareness-raising campaigns and through improving access to sexual health services. Future efforts should build on the desire of young people and their parents for more parental involvement in their sex education. Evaluation of interventions to improve parent–child communication should include randomised trials of families that do and do not participate in well-designed and piloted interventions. Other research methods should be developed to evaluate the usefulness of school clinics in improving young people's sexual health. The experience of other countries, such as the Netherlands, where teenage pregnancy rates have fallen steadily since the 1960s reminds us that behaviour change over the long term is an achievable goal.

References

1. Stephenson JM, Obasi A. HIV risk-reduction in adolescents. *Lancet* 2004;363:1177–8.
2. Kirby D, Short L, Collins J, Rugg D, Kolbe L, Howard M *et al.* School-based programs to reduce sexual behaviors: a review of effectiveness. *Public Health Rep* 1994;109:339–60.

3. Department of Health. *Better Prevention, Better Services, Better Sexual Health. The National Strategy for Sexual Health and HIV.* London: DH; 2001.

4. Stephenson JM, Oakley A, Johnson AM, Forrest S, Strange V, Charleston S, *et al.* A school-based randomised controlled trial of peer-led sex education in England. *Control Clin Trials* 2003;24:643–57.

5. Wight D, Raab GM, Henderson M, Abraham C, Buston K, Hart G, *et al.* Limits of teacher delivered sex education: interim behavioural outcomes from randomised trial. *BMJ* 2002;324:1430–3.

6. Wellings K, Nanchahal K, Macdowall W, McManus S, Erens B, Mercer CH, *et al.* Sexual behaviour in Britain: early heterosexual experience. *Lancet* 2001;358:1843–50.

7. Department of Health. *The Health of the Nation. A Strategy for Health in England.* London: HMSO; 1992.

8. UK Collaborative Group for HIV and STI Surveillance. *HIV and other Sexually Transmitted Infections in the UK in 2003. 2nd Annual Surveillance Report.* London: Health Protection Agency Centre for Infections; 2004.

9. House of Commons Health Committee. Sexual Health. *Third Report of Session 2002–03.* HC 69-I. Session 2002-03 69-II. London: The Stationery Office; 2003.

10. Teenage Pregnancy Strategy Evaluation Team. Implementation of the Teenage Pregnancy Strategy: Implementation Report. TP(IAG)97. London: Teenage Pregnancy Unit; 2004.

11. Botting B, Rosato M, Wood R. Teenage mothers and the health of their children. *Popul Trends* 1998;93:19–28.

12. Macdowall W, Wellings K, Mercer CH, Nanchahal K, Johnson AM, Copas AJ, *et al.* Results from the 2000 National Survey of Sexual Attitudes and Lifestyles ('Natsal 2000'). *Health Education and Behaviour* 2005. In press.

13. Health Development Agency. *Teenage Pregnancy: An update on key characteristics of effective interventions.* London: Health Development Agency; 2001.

14. Teenage Pregnancy Strategy Evaluation Team. *Final Report Synthesis.* London: Teenage Pregnancy Unit; 2004.

15. Sex Education Forum, National Association of governors and Managers, National Children's Bureau. *Sex and Relationships Education: Support for School Governors.* PHSE and Citizenship Spotlight Series. London: National Children's Bureau; 2005 [www.ncb.org.uk/resources/sef_schoolgov.pdf].

16. Wellings K, Field J, Wadsworth J, Johnson AM, Anderson RM, Bradshaw SA. Sexual lifestyles under scrutiny. *Nature* 1990;348:276–8.

17. Oakley A, Fullerton D, Holland J, Arnold S, France-Dawson M, Kelley P, *et al. Review of the Effectiveness of Sexual Health Promotion Interventions for Young People.* London: EPI-Centre; 1999.

18. Stephenson JM, Strange V, Forrest S, Oakley A, Allen E, Babiker A *et al.* Pupil-led Sex Education in England (RIPPLE study): cluster-randomised intervention trial. *Lancet* 2004;364:338–46.

19. Wight D, Dixon H. SHARE: The rationale, principles and content of a research-based teacher-led sex education programme. *Education and Health* 2004;22:3–7.

20. Ajzen I. The theory of planned behavior. *Organizational Behavior and Human Decision Processes* 1991;50:179–211.

21. Stephenson JM, Oakley A, Charleston S, Brodala A, Fenton K, Petruckevitch A, *et al.* Behavioural intervention trails for HIV. STD prevention in schools: are they feasible? *Sex Transm Infect* 1998;74:405–8.

22. Oakley A, Strange V, Stephenson J, Forrest S, Monteiro H, The RIPPLE Study Team. Evaluating processes: a case study of a randomized controlled trial of sex education. *Evaluation* 2005. In press.

23. Forrest S, Strange V, Oakley A, The RIPPLE Study Team. A comparision of students' evaluations of a peer-delivered sex education programme and teacher led provision. *Sex Education* 2002;2:195–214.

24. Guyatt GH, DiCenso A, Farewell V, Willan A, Griffith L. Randomised trials versus observational studies in adolescent pregnancy prevention. *J Clin Epidemiol* 2000;53:167–74.

25. DiCenso A, Guyatt G, Willan A, Griffith I. Interventions to reduce unintended pregnancies among adolescents; systematic review of randomised controlled trials. *BMJ* 2002;324:1426–30.

26. Johnson BT, Carey MP, Marsh KL, Levin KD, Scott-Sheldon LAJ. Interventions to reduce sexual risk for the human immunodeficiency virus in adolescents, 1985–2000. *Arch Pediatr Adolesc Med* 2003;157:381–8.

27. NHS Centre for Reviews and Dissemination. Prevention and reducing the adverse effects of unintended teenage pregnancies. *Effective Health Care Bull* 1997;1:1–12.

28. Stephenson JM, Imrie J. Why do we need randomised controlled trials to assess behavioural interventions? *BMJ* 2001;316:611–13.

SECTION 3
CONSENSUS VIEWS

Chapter 22

Consensus views arising from the 49th RCOG Study Group

Introduction

The focus of this meeting was on contraception and contraceptive use in developed countries, particularly in the UK. Other issues relating to fertility control, such as abortion, were addressed tangentially. Only passing reference was made to other parts of the world, including resource-poor countries. This summary of consensus views records briefly the key points made during the course of the meeting, followed by their implications for action. It reflects the views of the members of the Study Group and is not a comprehensive review.

Demographic and lifestyle trends

Population is still a vitally important policy area in both developed and developing countries. Patterns of and trends in fertility are now as important a focus in public health terms as absolute fertility rates have been to date.

The so-called 'second demographic transition', characterised by declining age at first intercourse (to an average age of 16 years for today's teenagers) and increasing age at first childbirth (average age 27 years for women and 29 years for men), creates an extended interval during which people are at risk of unintended pregnancy and sexually transmitted infection. Increasing proportions of women are delaying childbearing until their fourth decade.

The trend towards later marriage and the greater prevalence of cohabitation, delayed pregnancy and smaller families has major implications for contraceptive use and the demand for abortion.

Condom use at first intercourse has increased dramatically over the past two decades. Comparative studies, however, show the prevalence of intercourse before age 16 years in England to be the second highest, and recent condom use among young people to be the fifth lowest, in Europe.

Abortion rates in the UK are comparable to those in other Western European countries in which contraceptive prevalence is high. Abortion ratios (the proportion of all pregnancies which are terminated) have been increasing, especially among teenage women. However, the figures for the UK remain considerably lower than those in other European countries.

Teenage conception rates in the UK have remained relatively stable over recent decades unlike those in some Western European countries, where rates have fallen. Rates in the UK remain amongst the highest in developed countries.

Implications for action

Health policy/education

1. Sexual health strategies need to continue to take account of our persistently unfavourable situation with regard to teenage pregnancy in comparison with other European countries.
2. Contraception and abortion elements of the National Sexual Health Strategies need to be prioritised by UK Government, the Department of Health and Commissioners, by establishing a National Service Framework or its equivalent.

Contraceptive use

Given the increasing interval between the onset of sexual activity and the start of childbearing, considerable achievements have been made in helping people to regulate their fertility.

Men and women take into account a number of criteria when choosing a contraceptive method (from a list which might include effectiveness, safety, positive and negative side effects and acceptability of use) according to their health and situation in life. Couples in the UK who have completed their families still tend to choose sterilisation, despite the availability of long-acting methods that are easy to use and reversible in the event of wishing to resume childbearing with a new partner.

Most women need to use contraception for over 30 years. During the perimenopause, declining fertility, an increasing tendency towards menstrual irregularity and increasing background risks of both cardiovascular disease and breast cancer influence contraceptive choice and eligibility.

Contraceptive continuation rates, in common with other health behaviours, increase with age and experience. With reversible methods, continuation rates have been shown to be highest with long-acting methods of contraception. Evidence from the USA suggests that increasing the uptake of injections and implants has contributed to a reduction in teenage pregnancy. The causes of discontinuation are not well understood but side effects, perceived or real, play a major part. Evidence is emerging of a beneficial effect on continuation rates of high quality information and advice.

Failure to use contraception at all, or to use it effectively and consistently, is often used as an indicator of unplanned pregnancy. Research has shown pregnancy intentions to be complex and so a simple measurement strategy is likely to provide poor estimates of the prevalence of unplanned pregnancy. Moreover, the value attached to the outcome of pregnancy varies with life stage and situation. Although a new evidence-based measure of unintended pregnancy has been developed, taking account of these factors, it has not yet been used to estimate prevalence. Furthermore, there is almost no detailed research on how women experience pregnancy, make decisions on outcomes and seek and use abortion services.

In the context of the need for prevention of sexually transmitted infections, there is an increasing necessity to ensure that protection against both pregnancy and infection are practised in tandem.

Implications for action

Policy

1. The RCOG guidelines on offering the full range of contraceptive methods to women after abortion should be reaffirmed.
2. Efforts should be made to educate the public about the safety and convenience of modern, long-term, reversible methods of contraception as an alternative to sterilisation.

Clinical practice

1. Given their relatively high continuation rates, long-acting non-user-dependent methods of contraception should be promoted among women likely to benefit most from their use.
2. Counselling for male and female sterilisation should be provided in services that can offer all contraceptive methods on site.
3. Contraceptive method counselling should include sexually transmitted infection prevention messages and discussion of the effective use of condoms for all women not in an exclusive sexual relationship.
4. There is a need for the development and use of a simple tool, for use in clinical practice, which will identify women at high risk of unintended pregnancy.
5. The newly available, validated British measure of unintended pregnancy should be used in research and in clinical practice to provide data that will inform the development and effective targeting of contraceptive services.

Research

1. More research is urgently needed in the UK to understand patterns of contraceptive use, the reasons for these patterns and the effectiveness of interventions designed to enhance use.
2. Further research is needed on premature discontinuation, with particular attention to the meaning for men and women of side effects of specific methods and how this interacts with ambivalence towards use of the method.
3. Research is needed to generate an understanding of why women seek abortion and their experience of doing so (including at later gestational stages).
4. Research is needed to examine and increase understanding of the interface between combined hormonal contraception and hormone replacement therapy relating to providing ongoing contraception, cycle control and relief of menopausal symptoms in older women.
5. Research should be undertaken into the biochemistry of the perimenopause to identify factors which might predict with greater precision the likelihood of further ovulation and hence the need for use of ongoing contraception.

Contraceptive methods risks, benefits and new developments

A variety of different methods of contraception are available. All are generally extremely safe compared with the risks associated with pregnancy and childbirth. Not all methods are suitable for everyone. Combined hormonal methods, in particular, are contraindicated for women with certain medical conditions.

Summaries of product characteristics and patient information leaflets produced by the manufacturers of contraceptives are often at odds with evidence and with national guidance and can cause confusion.

While there is evidence for an increased relative risk of breast and cervical cancer and cardiovascular disease in association with hormonal contraception, particularly the combined pill, the absolute risk is very small.

Since most cardiovascular events among oral contraceptive users occur in women with well-recognised risk factors (including smoking, hypertension and adverse lipid profiles), the most important preventive strategy in reducing cardiovascular risk among women of reproductive age is to reduce these risk factors.

Concern persists about the effect hormonal contraception may have on the risk of sexually transmitted infections and HIV infection acquisition and transmission.

The noncontraceptive health benefits of different methods (such as the reduction in menstrual dysfunction and ovarian, colorectal and endometrial cancer associated with the combined pill) have potentially enormous consequences for public health. These benefits may also increase uptake and continuation rates.

The prospect of new systemic methods of contraception, which depart from the theme of steroid hormones, remains distant. While antiprogestogens have been shown to have a wide range of contraceptive effects, their development has been hampered by their association with abortion.

Important advances have been made in the last decade in the development of hormonal methods for men.

Implications for action

Policy

1. Discussion on the content of summaries of product characteristics and patient information leaflets should involve the Medicines and Healthcare products Regulatory Agency, European regulatory authorities and consumer representatives and should reflect national guidance.

Clinical practice

1. Users of combined oral contraceptives should be told that they may have an increased relative risk of having breast and cervical cancer (particularly after prolonged periods of use) diagnosed while using hormonal methods of contraception.
2. When discussing the harmful effects of hormonal contraception, however, absolute as well as relative risks should be discussed and any beneficial effects highlighted.
3. Women should be informed of the risk factors associated with specific adverse health outcomes (such as smoking) and encouraged to reduce them.
4. Evidence-based guidelines, such as the World Health Organization's Medical Eligibility Criteria, the UK Faculty of Family Planning and Reproductive Health Care (FFPRHC) Guidance and the American College of Obstetricians and Gynecologists Practice Bulletin, should include recommendations based on different levels and combinations of risk factors.
5. Women with conditions that may be exacerbated by oestrogen should use progestogen-only rather than combined methods.

Research

1. Additional high-quality prospective studies are needed to evaluate the effect of intrauterine contraception, oral and injectable contraceptives and newer hormonal methods on the risk of acquisition of sexually transmitted infections.
2. Continued research is needed regarding the combined effects of hormonal contraception and cardiovascular risk factors, especially for newer combined formulations and for progestogen-only formulations.
3. The development of new methods should take account of the need for contraceptives which have added health benefits, such as the prevention of breast or prostate cancer. Ideally, future developments in contraception should offer protection against both pregnancy and sexually transmitted infections.
4. The development of hormonal methods for men should continue as a priority.

Provision of contraceptive education

Broad-spectrum dedicated campaigns, using the mass media, have been shown to be of value in raising awareness of the need for safer sex and contraception. By contrast, routine coverage in the print and broadcast media has contributed greatly to successive sensationalised 'pill scares', which have hindered progress in terms of preventing unplanned pregnancy.

Research has shown benefits of personal and sex education in schools in terms of increased likelihood of contraceptive use at first intercourse.

Implications for action

Policy

1. Sex and relationships education should be made a statutory component of personal, social and health education and citizenship within schools and efforts should continue to be made to incorporate it into teacher training.
2. Sex and relationship education needs to take account of the wider social context in which it takes place.

Clinical practice

1. Efforts should be made to use the media to educate contraceptive users and to influence the ways in which contraceptive issues are presented in the press.
2. Thought needs to be given to ways of presenting risk in a way that is easily understood by both professionals and the public, particularly with regard to relative and absolute risk.
3. Efforts should be made to increase awareness and knowledge of long-acting methods of contraception among both healthcare professionals and the public.

Research

1. Future research should focus on those at highest risk, with the aim of developing and evaluating interventions, including specifically parental involvement, to improve sexual health education.

2. Methods of developing and evaluating promising interventions in schools should be explored.
3. Research is needed on how healthcare professionals communicate risk and harm and on how this may influence uptake, adherence and continuation of contraceptives.

Provision of contraceptive services

Despite the many potential interventions for improving service delivery, there are few good data demonstrating that they improve contraceptive uptake, compliance or continuation rates, and none showing an effect on rates of unintended pregnancy. There is disappointingly little evidence, as yet, of any impact of protocols and guidelines on effectiveness of service provision. There is, however, evidence that contraceptive access is improved by provision of services in a range of settings, including nonclinical venues. There is also evidence from other countries, most notably the Netherlands, that the dismantling of services is quickly followed by a deterioration of sexual and reproductive health status.

Research shows confidentiality to be paramount in young people's decision to choose and use a service.

Implications for action

Policy

1. Consideration should be given to the more frequent and widespread use of independent and supplementary prescribing and Patient Group Directions so as to improve access to contraceptive and sexual health services.
2. Given the strength of the evidence of young people's need to access confidential services, members of the Study Group oppose any changes that would jeopardise this.

Clinical practice ˙

1. Access to all forms of fertility control should be increased by optimising opening hours and broadening the range of outlets, including those in innovative settings such as schools.
2. Training should address clinical skills and knowledge, attitudes, values and communication in contraception and sexual health.
3. Sexual health training in relevant healthcare subjects needs to start in the undergraduate years and continue throughout postgraduate careers.
3. All professionals providing contraceptive services should be appropriately trained.
4. Every health policy maker, head of service and clinical team should routinely have a system in place to draw attention to recently published guidelines, standards, consensus statements (such as these Study Group proceedings) and policy documents relevant to their area of practice.
5. Policy makers, heads of services and clinical teams should compare their own practice with the recommendations in these identified documents. If necessary, local audits should be undertaken to assess the extent to which practice measures up to recommendations.

6. For each aspect of practice for which a need for change is identified, a three-point action plan for change should be adopted:
   - What are we going to do?
   - Who is going to make it happen?
   - When will it be done?

Index

abortion
    age and 9–10, 34, 35, 174–5
    contraception and 36–7, 41, 108, 236,
        240
    England and Wales 9–10, 33–4, 174–5,
        261
    fertility rates and 9–10, 40–1
    'late' 33–5, 41–2
    service provision 48
    social acceptability of 40–1
    Study Group findings 261, 263
    Sweden 103, 105–6
    unintended pregnancies 19, 27
    young people 35, 174–5
adverse effects
    cancer see cancer
    cardiovascular see cardiovascular disease
    contraceptive type
        barrier methods 62, 63
        DMPA injections 57, 113–14, 145,
            159
        emergency contraception 67, 68
        implants 58, 114, 160
        IUDs 61, 68, 103, 113
        LNG-IUS 60
        oral contraceptives 55–6, 103, 113,
            137–45, 148–63, 187–8
        sterilisation 63–4, 65
    discontinuation rates 103, 104–5,
        112–14
    in older women 187–8, 189
    osteoporosis 57, 179, 189–90
    risk assessment 136–7
    Study Group findings 263–5
    in the young 179, 180
age
    abortion rates 9–10, 34, 35, 174–5
    cancer risk 138–9, 188
    cardiovascular risk 153, 155, 187–8
    consent 177–8

discontinuation rates 110, 112, 180
fertility rates 7, 8, 10–11, 37
    older women 171, 184–5
    teenagers 17, 172–3, 222
patterns of contraceptive use 93–4,
    100–2, 175–7, 185–6, 189–91
sexual behaviour 13, 14–15, 17, 169–72,
    177, 185, 252
STIs 173–4
stopping contraception 191–2
see also older women; young people
AIDS see HIV
air travel 157
American College of Obstetricians and
    Gynecologists (ACOG) 161–2
androgen replacement 209–11
    plus progestogens 211–13
angiogenesis, inhibitors 202
Asia
    male hormonal contraception 211, 214
    patterns of contraceptive use 92–3
audit 51, 230–1
Avon Brook Advisory Centre 178

barrier methods see individual methods
benefits of hormonal contraception 55, 56,
    57, 58, 59, 264
    cancer risk 55, 145, 188
    menstrual 188, 190–1
    osteoporosis risk 189
birth rates see fertility rates
blood pressure, high 152, 154, 155, 158,
    159
Bone, Margaret 21
bone mineral density
    COCs 189
    progestogen-only methods 57, 179,
        189–90
BRCA genes 141, 142
breast cancer 55, 137–42, 188, 198

breastfeeding
  contraception during 56, 57
  as contraceptive method 65–6

C-reactive protein 157
Cairo Conference on Population and
  Development 4
cancer
  breast 55, 137–42, 188, 198
  cervical 55, 143–5, 188, 204
  protective effects of COCs 55, 145, 188
  Study Group findings 264
caps 60–1, 191
cardiovascular disease (refers to COCs unless
  stated otherwise)
  clinical trials 149–51
  guidelines for COC use 160–2, 264
  morbidity and mortality rates 157–9
  myocardial infarction 152–3, 187
  non-oral combined methods 159, 163
  progestogen-only methods 159–60, 163
  risk factors 160, 163, 264
    age 153, 155, 187–8
    clinical markers 157, 159
    genetic 156
    hypertension 152, 154, 155, 158,
      159
    migraine 154–5
    progestogen type 148, 153, 154,
      156, 157, 158, 180
    smoking 152, 154, 155, 158, 159,
      187
  stroke 55, 153–5, 187
  Study Group findings 264, 265
  VTE 55, 155–7, 160, 180, 187–8
Cartwright, Ann 20–1
cerebrovascular accidents 55, 153–5, 187
cervical cancer 143–5, 188, 204
childcare provision 39–40, 221
childlessness 8, 37–8, 39, 171
Children Act (2004) 219
China 204, 211
Chlamydia trachomatis 105, 123, 129, 130,
  131, 174
choice of method
  availability of services 47–8, 69–70,
    83–5
  improving 85–6, 236–40
  Study Group findings 262–3
  users' perception of 78–83
  see also patterns of contraceptive use
Choosing Health: Making Healthy Choices
  Easier (DoH) 48, 219
COC see combined oral contraception
Cochrane reviews 226–34
coils see intrauterine devices
coitus interruptus 66
Collaborative Group on Hormonal Factors in

Breast Cancer reanalysis 138–9
colorectal cancer 145, 188
combined oral contraception (COC)
  advantages and disadvantages 55, 70
  cancer risk 137–45, 188
  cardiovascular risk see cardiovascular
    disease
  osteoporosis 189
  discontinuation rates 110, 111, 113, 114
  formulations 54, 148
  mode of action 199
  patterns of use 69, 90, 91, 92, 102–3
    older women 93, 185, 187, 191
    younger women 93, 176
  Study Group findings 264
Committee on Safety of Medicines (CSM) 57,
  72
communication see education; information
  provision
community health services 46, 68–70, 175,
  237, 242
competence to give consent
  to intercourse 171–2
  to treatment 177–8
compliance see discontinuation rates
condoms
  female 61, 91
  patterns of use 89, 90, 90–1, 102, 105
    younger people 93, 176
  prophylaxis against STIs 14, 120–1, 131,
    179, 191
confidentiality 179, 266
consent 84, 177–8
consultations 52–4, 84–5, 239
continuation rates see discontinuation rates
Contraceptive Choices for Young People
  (FFPRHC) 177, 180
copper 60, 67
corpus luteum 201
cost of contraceptives 44, 72–3, 95–6,
  239–40
counselling
  during consultations 52–4, 84–5, 239
  see also information provision
cyclo-oxygenase-2 inhibitors 201
cyproterone acetate 156, 212

demography
  abortion rates 9–10, 33–4, 40–1
  fertility rates 6–11, 37–8, 184–5, 222
  rationale for birth control 3
  'second demographic transition' 37–41,
    261
  Study Group findings 261–2
  see also patterns of contraceptive use
Department for Education and Skills (DfES)
  218–19, 220
Depo-Provera see DMPA

depot medroxyprogesterone acetate *see* DMPA
desogestrel
    in men 212–13
    in women 54, 148, 153, 156
DFFP (Diploma in the Faculty of Family Planning) 70, 71, 181
diabetes 56
diaphragms 60–1, 191
discontinuation rates
    adverse effects and 103, 104–5, 112–14
    desire for pregnancy (or lack thereof) 108, 114–15, 245
    by duration of use 111–12
    family influences 115, 116
    provider attitudes 239
    reduction of 115–17, 240–1, 242–5
    research into 108–9, 245
    Study Group findings 262, 263
    by type of contraceptive 109–11
    by user characteristics 112, 180
DMPA (depot medroxyprogesterone acetate) injections 56–7
    adverse effects 57, 113–14, 145, 159
    discontinuation 110, 113–14, 245
    in men 212
    in older women 189–90
    self-administered 243
    STI risk 120, 123, 124–8, 129, 130, 131–2
    in the young 57, 177, 179
drospirenone 152
drug development *see* research
Dunnell, Karen 21
dysmenorrhoea 55, 57

economic issues
    cost of contraceptives 44, 72–3, 95–6, 239–40
    funding of services 49–52, 75
    professional remuneration 50, 231–2
education
    of healthcare professionals
        changing practice 227–31, 232–3
        training 70–1, 74, 181, 266
    of users
        choice of method 79, 80–1, 84–6, 240–1
        compliance rates 116, 240–1, 244
        information leaflets 116, 241, 264
        STI risks 131–2
        Study Group findings 264, 265–6
    of women (educational status) 10–11
    of young people (sex education) 219–20, 249–57, 265–6
    see also information provision
efficacy *see* failure rates
emergency contraception

attitudes towards 83, 238–9
    changing professional practice 232–3
    patterns of use 94–5, 105, 244–5
    service provision 49, 66–7, 237, 238, 243
    types of 66–8, 190, 204
employment status of women 38–9
endometrial cancer 145, 188, 202
England
    abortion rates 9–10, 33–4, 174–5, 261
    fertility rates 6–11, 37–8
    Teenage Pregnancy Strategy 48–9, 217–24, 250–2
epidemiology *see* patterns of contraceptive use
ethical issues
    conscientious objections by the GP 49
    emergency contraception 204
ethnic differences, male hormonal contraception 211, 213, 214
etonogestrel implants
    in men 213
    in women 190
Europe
    abortion rates 175
    discontinuation rates 113
    patterns of contraceptive use 89, 90, 91–2, 95–6, 119–20
    teenage pregnancies 173, 223–4
    see also individual countries
Every Child Matters (DfES) 219
evidence-based medicine 226

factor V Leiden 156
Faculty of Family Planning and Reproductive Health Care (FFPRHC)
    diploma (DFFP) 70, 71, 181
    guidelines 74
        COC use and cardiovascular risk 161–2
        young people 177, 180
    service provision role 52, 71
failure rates 36, 110–11, 112, 236
    by contraceptive type 53
    male hormonal contraception 210, 211
    POPs 189, 198
Family Planning Association (fpa) 45
family planning clinics 46, 68–70, 175, 237, 242
family size 7–8
fertilisation 202–3
fertility awareness 65–6, 90, 91, 102
fertility rates
    abortion and 9–10, 40–1
    employment of women 39
    marriage and 39, 40, 171
    maternal age 7, 8, 10–11, 37
        older women 171, 184–5

teenagers 17, 172–3, 222
Sweden 103
UK 37–8
England and Wales 6–11
worldwide 6
'fertility transition' 36
FFPRHC see Faculty of Family Planning and Reproductive Health Care
follicle-stimulating hormone (FSH)
in men 209
in women 191–2
folliculogenesis 200–1
France 89, 90, 91
Fraser competence 177–8
funding of services 49–52, 75
future trends see research

General Household Survey (UK) 10, 88, 91, 176
General Medical Service (GMS) contracts 49–51, 52
general practitioners (GPs)
consultations 52–4, 84–5, 239
as providers of contraceptive services 46, 48, 49–52, 68–70, 175, 240
remuneration 50, 231–2
training 70–1, 74, 181, 266
genetic factors
BRCA genes 141, 142
factor V Leiden 156
genitourinary medicine clinics 46
Germany 89, 90, 92
gestodene 148, 153, 156
Gillick competence see Fraser competence
GMS (General Medical Service) contracts 49–51, 52
gonadotrophin-releasing hormone (GnRH)
agonists/antagonists
in men 213–14
in women 198, 200
gonadotrophins
in men 209
in women 191–2, 201
gonorrhoea 123, 125, 129, 130, 174
GPs see general practitioners
guidelines
cardiovascular risk and COC use 160–2, 264
compliance with 227–9, 266
contraception in the young 177, 179, 180
DMPA injections 57
FFPRHC 74, 161–2, 177, 180
prescribing practice 71–2, 74, 242
WHOMEC 74, 161–2, 179, 242

haemorrhagic stroke 155, 187
hCG (human chorionic gonadotrophin) 201

Healthy Schools Programme 220
heart attacks 152–3, 187
hereditary factors
BRCA genes 141, 142
factor V Leiden 156
herpes simplex virus (HSV) 128, 129–30, 174
history of contraceptive use 3–4, 45–6
HIV 13, 131
strategy documents 47, 221–2, 252
hormonal contraception see individual methods
hormone replacement therapy (HRT) 140, 190–1, 192
HPV (human papillomavirus) 126–7, 129, 143, 144, 204
HSV (herpes simplex virus) 128, 129–30, 174
human chorionic gonadotrophin (hCG) 201
human papillomavirus (HPV) 126–7, 129, 143, 144, 204
hypertension 152, 154, 155, 158, 159
hypothalamus 200

immobilisation, risk of VTE 156–7
Implanon® 58, 213
implantation, failure of 201–2
implants
adverse effects 58, 114, 160
discontinuation rates 109–10, 114
for men 210, 211, 212, 213
patterns of use 89, 91
Study Group findings 262, 263
types of 58, 190
information provision
by healthcare professionals 53–4, 79, 80, 84–6, 240–1, 244
by the media
effect on user habits 80–1, 104–5, 114, 231
sexual health campaigns 219, 222, 241, 251–2, 265
by parents 219, 251
by schools 220, 251, 252–7
contraceptives and STI risk 131–2
leaflets 116, 241, 264
misinformation, examples of 82–3
see also education
injections
combined 159
DMPA see DMPA
for men 209–10, 210–11, 212, 213
norethisterone 56, 213
patterns of use 89, 91
Study Group findings 262, 263
'interactional competence' 171–2
International Conference on Population and Development (ICPD) (Cairo, 1994) 4

ternet 74, 241
rauterine devices (IUD) 59–60
   adverse effects 61, 68, 103, 113
   discontinuation rates 111, 113
   emergency contraception 67–8
   for older women 190, 192
   patterns of use 89, 91, 92–3, 102
   service provision 50–1, 52
   STI risk 123, 124–8, 129
   terminology 83
intrauterine systems (LNG-IUS) 59
   discontinuation rates 111, 113
   for older women 190–1
   patterns of use 89, 91
ischaemic stroke 55, 153–4, 187
Italy 89, 90, 95
IUD *see* intrauterine devices
IUS *see* intrauterine systems (LNG-IUS)

Journal of Family Planning and Reproductive Health Care 74

lactational amenorrhoea 65–6
leukaemia inhibitory factor (LIF) 202
levonorgestrel
   in COCs 148
   emergency contraception 190
   LNG-IUS *see* intrauterine systems
   in men 212
   Norplant® 58, 114, 160
lipoproteins 157, 159, 213
LNG-IUS *see* intrauterine systems
luteinising hormone (LH)
   in men 209
   in women 201

male contraception
   condoms
      patterns of use 89, 90, 90–1, 93, 102, 105, 176
      prophylaxis against STIs 14, 120–1, 131, 179, 191
   future trends 202–3, 208–14
   service provision 241–2
   sterilisation 63–5
Malthus, Thomas 3
marriage
   discontinuation rates 112, 115
   fertility rates 39, 40, 171
media
   effect on user habits 80–1, 104–5, 114, 231
   sexual health campaigns 219, 222, 241, 251–2, 265
Medicines and Healthcare Products Regulatory Agency (MHRA) 71
medroxyprogesterone acetate *see* DMPA
men *see* male contraception

menopause 190–1, 191–2, 263
menstruation
   disorders
      effect of contraceptive type 55, 57, 59
      in older women 188, 189, 190–1
   and new contraceptive methods 199
   premenstrual symptoms 191
7α-methyl-19-nortestosterone (MENT) 211
mifepristone 201–2, 204
migraine 154–5
Millennium Cohort Survey (UK) 22
Mirena® *see* intrauterine systems (LNG-IUS)
miscarriage 184–5
misinformation, examples of 82–3
myocardial infarction 152–3, 187

National Institute for Clinical Excellence (NICE) 72, 226
National Service Framework for Children, Young People and Maternity Services (DoH) 219
National Strategy for Sexual Health and HIV 2001 (UK) 47, 221–2, 252
National Survey of Family Growth (NSFG) (USA) 22–4, 110–11
National Survey of Sexual Attitudes and Lifestyles (NATSAL) (UK) 12, 169, 170, 171
natural family planning 65–6, 90, 91, 102
Neisseria gonorrhoeae 123, 125, 129, 130, 174
Netherlands
   patterns of contraceptive use 89, 95
   sexual behaviour in the young 171–2
NICE (National Institute for Clinical Excellence) 72, 226
noncompliance *see* discontinuation rates
nonoxinol-9 61, 203
norethisterone
   in men 213
   in women 56, 148
norgestimate 148
Norplant® 58, 114, 160
Northern Ireland 91, 93
NSFG (National Survey of Family Growth) (USA) 22–4, 110–11
nurses 70, 238

obesity 56, 156
oestrogen
   in COCs 148
   replacement 190–1, 200
Office for National Statistics Omnibus Survey (UK) 88, 89, 91, 236, 237
older women
   cardiovascular risk 153, 155, 187–8
   fertility rates 171, 184–5

menopause 190–1, 191–2, 263
osteoporosis risk 189, 189–90
patterns of contraceptive use 93, 185–6,
    189–91
sexual behaviour 185
Omnibus Survey (UK) 88, 89, 91, 236, 237
on-line resources 74, 241
opinion leaders 230
oral contraception
    adverse effects 55–6, 103, 113
        cancer 137–45, 188
        cardiovascular disease 148–63,
            187–8
    combined *see* combined oral
        contraception
    discontinuation rates 110, 111, 113, 114
    myths concerning 82
    off-prescription use 242–3
    once-a-month pills 201, 202
    patterns of use 69, 89, 90, 92, 93, 102–5
    progestogen-only 54–6, 141, 160, 189,
        192, 202
    STI risk and 123–30, 131
osteoporosis
    COCs 189
    progestogen-only methods 57, 179,
        189–90
outreach visits (to professionals) 230
ovarian cancer 142, 145, 188
ovarian function, as a target for contraception
199, 200–1

papillomavirus (HPV) 126–7, 129, 143, 144,
    204
parents
    effect on discontinuation rates 115
    policies towards 39–40, 221
    as providers of information 219, 251
partners, effect on discontinuation rates 115,
    116
patches
    combined 54, 55, 159
    for men (testosterone) 211
patient group directions 95, 266
patterns of contraceptive use
    age-related 93–4, 100–2, 175–7, 185–6,
        189–91
    availability of services 48, 69–70
    by contraceptive type 89, 90–3, 100–3,
        236
    cost implications 95–6
    emergency contraception 94–5, 105,
        244–5
    by geographical area
        Europe 89, 90, 91–2, 95–6, 119–20
        Sweden 98–106
        UK 69, 88–96, 176–7
        USA 120

worldwide 92–3
parity 102
Study Group findings 262–3
unintended pregnancy 53, 89–90, 103,
    105–6, 236
see also provision of services
pelvic inflammatory disease (PID) 55, 60, 61,
    131
personal medical service (PMS) contracts
    51–2
pharmaceutical development *see* research
pharmacies, emergency contraception 66,
    237, 238
pills *see* oral contraception
POP (progestogen-only pills) 54–6, 141, 160,
    189, 192, 202
population control 3
poverty, failure rates 112
pregnancy
    rates *see* fertility rates
    targets for new contraceptives 199
    unintended
        abortion and 19, 27
        contraceptive method used 53,
            89–90, 103, 105–6, 236
        estimation of rates of 20–7, 31–2,
            262
        policy implications 19, 27–8
        Study Group findings 262, 263
        see also teenage pregnancy
prescribing practice
    guidelines 71–2, 74, 242
    how to change 226–34
    off-prescription use 95, 242–3, 266
    Study Group findings 266
    trends 69–70
primary health care *see* general practitioners
primigravidae, age of 8, 14, 37
prodigy guidance 74
professional practice, changing 226–7,
    233–4
    audit 230–1
    education 227–30, 231
    payments to doctors 231–2
    prescribing practice 232–3
progestogens
    in COCs 148, 152
        cardiovascular risk 148, 153, 154,
            156, 157, 158, 180
    progestogen-only methods
        cancer risk 141–2, 145
        cardiovascular risk 159–60, 163
        emergency contraception 66–7, 190,
            204
        implants *see* implants
        injections *see* DMPA injections
        LNG-IUS *see* intrauterine systems
        for older women 189–90, 192

osteoporosis risk 57, 179, 189–90
pills (POP) 54–6, 141, 160, 189,
    192, 202
targets for new contraceptives 201, 264
    male contraception 211–13
    mifepristone 201–2, 204
provision of information *see* information
provision
provision of services
    abortion 48
    choice of method 48, 69–70, 83–5
    cost effectiveness 44, 72–3, 239–40
    emergency contraception 49, 66–7, 237,
        238, 243
    history of 4, 45–6
    improving 236–45, 266–7
    to men 241–2
    outlet characteristics 46–52, 175, 220–1,
        237–8, 239, 240, 266
    Study Group findings 266–7
    to young people 175, 180, 220–1, 224,
        237
public health initiatives
    *Choosing Health: Making Healthy
        Choices Easier* (2004) 48, 219
    National Service Framework 219
    National Strategy for Sexual Health and
        HIV (2001) 47, 221–2, 252
    Teenage Pregnancy Strategy for England
        (1999) 48–9, 217–24, 250–2
    see also sex and relationship education

qualifications in family planning 70, 71, 181
Quality and Outcome Framework (QOF)
    reviews 51

recertification 52, 71
research
    female contraception 199–202, 203–5,
        264, 265
    male contraception 202–3, 208–14, 265
    need for 197–9, 208
    Study Group recommendations 263,
        265, 265–6
rhythm method *see* natural family planning
rings, vaginal 54, 55, 89, 159
RIPPLE trial 254–6
risks of contraceptive use *see* adverse effects
Royal College of Obstetricians and
    Gynaecologists
    Study Group findings 261–7
    training 70, 71

schools
    provision of contraceptive services 221,
        251
    sex education 220, 251, 252–7, 265
Scotland

implementation of guidelines 227–9
Scottish Intercollegiate Guidelines
Network (SIGN) 74
    Scottish Medicines Consortium (SMC) 72
    SHARE trial 253–4, 255–6
service provision *see* provision of services
Sex Lottery campaign 252
sex and relationship education 220, 249–57,
    265–6
sexual behaviour
    age and 13, 14–15, 17
        older women 185
        young people 13, 17, 169–72, 177,
            178, 252
    first intercourse 13, 17, 172, 178, 252
    frequency of intercourse 169, 185
    gender convergence 15, 16
    partner numbers 13, 14, 15, 170–1
    policy implications 17
    risk behaviour 13–14, 78
    social attitudes 16–17
    Study Group findings 261–2
    survey methodology 12, 15–16, 121–3
Sexual Health Strategy 2001 (UK) 47, 221–2,
    252
Sexually Transmitted Infection Foundation
    (STIF) Course 181
sexually transmitted infections (STIs)
    contraceptive use and 119–32, 203
        condom prophylaxis 14, 120–1, 131,
            179, 191
    and general practice 175
    research 130–1, 203–4
    sexual behaviour and 13, 17
    Study Group findings 262, 263, 264, 265
    Sweden 105
    young people in the UK 173–4
Sexwise help line 219
SHARE trial 253–4, 255–6
side effects *see* adverse effects
smoking
    cardiovascular risk 152, 154, 155, 158,
        159, 187
    Sweden 103, 106
social policy *see* public health initiatives
social status, failure rates 112
Spain 89, 90, 95
sperm
    spermicides 61, 203
    as targets for new contraceptives 202–3,
        209–14
sterilisation
    female 62–3, 191
    male 63–5
    patterns of use 90, 91–2, 93, 191
STI *see* sexually transmitted infections
STIF Course (Sexually Transmitted Infection
    Foundation) 181

stroke 55, 153–5, 187
Sweden 98–106
syphilis 128, 130

teenage pregnancy
    abortions 35, 175
    Europe 173, 223–4
    maternity services 221
    Study Group findings 262
    Teenage Pregnancy Strategy for England
        48–9, 217–24, 250–2
    UK 17, 172, 222
    USA 177
    see also young people
termination of pregnancy see abortion
testosterone replacement 209–11
    plus progestogens 211–13
thromboembolism 55, 155–7, 160, 180,
    187–8
'Time to Talk' initiative 219, 251
training 70–1, 74, 181, 266
    changing professional behaviour 227–30,
        232–3
transdermal preparations see patches
Treponema pallidum 128, 130
trichomoniasis 126, 129, 130

UK
    fertility rates 6–11, 37–8
    patterns of contraceptive use 69, 88–96,
        176–7
    provision of services see provision of
        services
    public health initiatives see public health
        initiatives
    sexual behaviour in the young 169–72
    STIs in the young 173–4
    teenage pregnancies 17, 172, 222, 262
    unintended pregnancies 20–2, 24–8,
        31–2

    see also England; Northern Ireland;
        Scotland
USA
    discontinuation rates 108–15
    patterns of contraceptive use 120
    unintended pregnancies 22–4, 108, 177
uterus
    as target for new contraceptives 201–2
    see also intrauterine devices and systems

vaginal rings 54, 55, 89, 159
vasectomy 63–5
venous thromboembolism (VTE) 55, 155–7,
    160, 180, 187–8

warts, genital 174
World Fertility Survey 21, 22
World Health Organization (WHO) Medical
    Eligibility Criteria 74, 242
    COCs and cardiovascular risk 161–2
    young people 179

young people
    abortion rates 35, 174–5
    contraceptive use 93, 96, 175–82
        adverse effects 179, 180
        discontinuation rates 110, 112, 115,
            180
        service provision 175, 180, 220–1,
            224, 237
    fertility rates 17, 172–3, 222
    sex education 219–20, 249–57, 265–6
    sexual behaviour 13, 17, 169–72, 177,
        178, 252
    STIs 173–4
    Study Group findings 261, 262, 265–6
    Teenage Pregnancy Strategy for England
        48–9, 217–24, 250–2
    see also teenage pregnancy
    Youth Matters (DfES) 219

Coventry University